W0105740

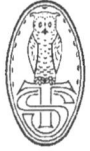
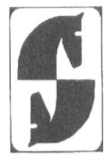

Symposium on
Ambulatory Blood Pressure Monitoring
November 13, 1983
Newport Beach, California

Michael A. Weber · Jan I. M. Drayer (Eds.)

Ambulatory Blood Pressure Monitoring

With Contributions by E. Beahm, S. Blank, K. Bolen, N. O. Borhani, E. L. Bravo, H. R. Brunner, P. M. M. Cashman, R. Catania, E. R. Chard, D. L. Clement, F. Colardyn, B. J. des Combes, L. Cordone, C. Dal Palù, R. B. Devereux, J. I. M. Drayer, S. Dunkle, F. G. Dunn, P. Eggena, B. Falkner, D. J. Fitzgerald, F. M. Fouad, M. Frisk-Holmberg, E. D. Frohlich, B. N. Garrett, R. W. Gifford jr., I. B. Goldstein, M. S. Golub, B. A. Gould, A. H. Gradman, E. Halberg, F. Halberg, J. Halberg, P. Hanson, T. R. Harman, G. A. Harshfield, R. S. Hornung, R. Jacob, A. Jain, A. M. Johnson, R. I. Jones, H. L. Kennedy, I. Kobrin, A. Kumar, H. Kushner, F. LaBaw, J. H. Laragh, C. Lindahl, M. Littner, J. Lowenstein, D. T. Lowenthal, S. Mann, D. McGinty, F. G. McMahon, F. H. Messerli, C. Nemec, A. J. Neusy, M. Nyby, E. T. O'Brien, P. C. O'Brien, W. Oigman, C. L. O'Keefe, K. O'Malley, L. Packet, P. Palatini, A. C. Pessina, T. G. Pickering, M. Porchet, E. B. Raftery, L. Ramsey, R. A. Reeves, R. J. Rose, J. R. Ryan, J. R. Salcedo, M. P. Sambhi, A. Schirger, A. P. Shapiro, D. Shapiro, S. G. Sheps, J. Sowers, G. Sperti, R. E. Spiekerman, J. M. Steele jr., N. Stern, L. Stroud, R. C. Tarazi, S. C. Textor, C. Thananopavarn, A. M. Thompson, W. Thornton, Y. M. Traub, G. O. Van Maele, E. Ventura, H. O. Ventura, B. Waeber, J. Wallace, A. Ward, M. A. Weber

Springer-Verlag Berlin Heidelberg GmbH

Michael, A. Weber, M.D.
Jan I. M. Drayer, M.D.
Hypertension Center
Veterans Administration Medical Center
5901 East Seventh Street
Long Beach, CA 90822

CIP-Kurztitelaufnahme der Deutschen Bibliothek

Ambulatory blood pressure monitoring / [Symposium on Ambulatory Blood Pressure Monitoring, November 13, 1983, Newport Beach, California]. Michael A. Weber; Jan I. M. Drayer (eds.). With contributions by E. Beahm ...
ISBN 978-3-662-05687-5   ISBN 978-3-662-05685-1 (eBook)
DOI 10.1007/978-3-662-05685-1
NE: Weber, Michael A. [Hrsg.]; Beahm, Edward [Mitverf.]; Symposium on Ambulatory Blood Pressure Monitoring (1983, Newport Beach, Calif.).

Editorial Assistance: Juliane K. Weller – Production: Heinz J. Schäfer

Type-Setting

Foreword

The availability of new technologies that enable blood pressure to be measured and recorded continuously or repetitively during prolonged observation periods has created exciting opportunities for studying the physiology of blood pressure regulation and the characteristics of clinical hypertension.

Ambulatory blood pressure monitoring has been based on three types of approach. The first of these has utilized an intra-arterial catheter that allows blood pressure to be measured directly and continuously during a full 24-hour period. The second approach is based on non-invasive techniques, and utilizes devices capable of automatically inflating conventional arm cuffs and recording blood pressures at pre-set intervals throughout the day. The third, and most simple method, has depended upon semiautomated techniques that require the subject to inflate a cuff at convenient intervals during the period of observation. During the last few years, concerted research into these differing techniques has exposed their strengths and shortcomings. Overall, however, there has been a growing perception that these approaches to the measurement of blood pressure might add considerably to the information obtained in the doctor's office by the traditional single or casual reading.

This book summarizes the state of the art in ambulatory blood pressure monitoring. We have divided the subject matter into three main areas: the available technologies for measuring and recording blood pressure; the use of these techniques for better understanding the physiology and characteristics of blood pressure; and the present state of our experience in employing these techniques for diagnosing and assessing therapy in patients with clinical hypertension. We believe that these innovative approaches for documenting normal and abnormal blood pressure patterns have now become critical components of clinical research studies. Moreover, the evaluation of the single patient by long-term monitoring may soon become part of the physician's diagnostic armamentarium.

This book takes its origins from an international symposium on blood pressure monitoring held recently in Newport Beach under the auspices of the Hypertension Center of the Veterans Administration Medical Center, Long Beach, and the University of California, Irvine. We hope that it will provide a broad background to the subject as well as provide practical clinical and technical guidance.

Acknowledgements

We gratefully acknowledge the assistance we received from Ginger Paselk in the planning of the meeting and the handling of the manuscripts. In addition, we are grateful to Deborah Brewer and Eleanor Chard, who were most active in the organization of the meeting. Finally, we would like to thank Bruce Del Mar and Marna Schnabel for their financial contribution to the meeting.

Contents

Section II: Physiology

VIII

Section III: Therapy

Ambulatory blood pressure monitoring: recorders, applications and analyses

Gregory A. Harshfield, Thomas G. Pickering, Seymour Blank, Cherie Lindahl, Lisa Stroud, John H. Laragh

Summary: We have had considerable experience with ambulatory monitoring of blood pressure and heart rate over the past five years. We have used three different systems to monitor over 800 patients: the Del Mar Avionics Ambulatory Pressurometer II and ECG Recorder (P2), the Del Mar Avionics Ambulatory Pressurometer III (P3), and the Instruments for Cardiac Research system (ICR). We have found that all of these systems provide accurate readings on approximately 80% of the patients tested. The ICR unit has the advantage of being smaller, quieter, and cheaper than either the P2 or P3. The current major problem with all of the systems, however, is a breakdown rate of over 30%. We have also developed our own software to evaluate the 24 hour records and have taken a decidedly behavioral approach to analysis. Specifically we code each blood pressure determination for location, position, activity and mood. We have been able to link these pressures to both target organ damages and personality traits. Finally, we have begun to use the technique of ambulatory monitoring in the evaluation of patients with psychiatric disorders.

Introduction

We have been using the technique of ambulatory monitoring of blood pressure and heart rate in the evaluation of essential hypertension for over five years. During this time we have performed 800 recordings as well as developed our own software for data reduction and analysis. This technique has become the central focus of our continually expanding protocol for the evaluation of borderline hypertension. At the present time, along with the 24 hour recordings, this evaluation consists of a treadmill test, a mental stress test, an echocardiogram, self- monitoring of home pressures, personality profiles, radionuclide cineangiography (when appropriate), and blood and urine tests. Furthermore, we have recently begun to expand the use of ambulatory monitoring to the evaluation of psychiatric disorders.

The purpose of the present paper is three-fold. Firstly, to describe the different units we have used and detail our experience with them; secondly, to describe our approach to data reduction and analysis with a description of our rationale for taking this approach; and finally, to describe some of the applications for ambulatory monitoring in the fields of both hypertension and psychiatry.

Description and experience

We now have experience with three commercially available non-invasive automatic ambulatory blood pressure and heart rate monitoring systems. Two of these systems, the Ambulatory Blood Pressurometer II and ECG Recording System (P2) and the Pressuro-

Cardiovascular Center, The New York Hospital-Cornell Medical Center.

meter III (P3) are manufactured by Del Mar Avionics. The third system is a product of Instruments for Cardiac Research (ICR). I will describe our protocol for ambulatory monitoring prior to a description of each of the three systems in detail along with our impressions of accuracy, durability, patient compliance, and company service.

In our protocol, the patient comes to the Hypertension Center on the morning of testing. The unit is attached to the patient and calibration readings are taken simultaneously by the technician with a mercury column and stethoscope and the ambulatory recorder. Five consecutive readings with the two procedures agreeing to within 5 mmHg for both systolic and diastolic pressure must be obtained to be considered an adequate calibration. If this criterion is not met, the recording is abandoned. If the calibration is successful, the patient is fully briefed as to the operation of the recorder. The patient is also asked to record in a diary each awake reading along with their location, position, activity, and mood at the time of the recording. The diary sheet also describes possible sources of artifactual readings and how to correct them, as well as a telephone number where someone can be reached for help at any time. The patient is then instructed to continue a normal day and return the following morning for a second calibration, removal of the unit, and a debriefing of the high points of the diary. The recorder is set to take a reading automatically every 15 min throughout the 24 h period.

The P2 system, the oldest of the 3 systems, consists of the Pressurometer, a Holter tape recorder, an auscultatory cuff and piezo-electric microphone, and an ECG electrode system. The P2 itself contains the pump and microphone connections, an interval timer (which can be set at standby, 7.5, 15, or 30 min cycles), a manual operation switch, a microphone sensitivity switch, a digital display of pressure (which can be turned off), and a test jack which allows concurrent readings with a mercury sphygmomanometer. The ECG system utilizes 5 precordial leads. The entire system weighs approximately 2.32 Kg. The data are stored on a Holter tape which is read by a Heart Rate and Blood Pressure Trend Analyzer (model 671) which plugs into an ECG scanner (model 660) and provides a raw ECG, a trend of both heart rate and blood pressure, and a digital readout of blood pressure at 1X, 60X, or 120X real time.

We have performed validation studies on the P2 and found it to produce satisfactory recordings (1). Based on a total of 450 readings taken simultaneously with a mercury column on patients who met calibration criteria, we found a correlation of $r = 0.99$ for systolic and $r = 0.94$ for diastolic pressure. Two provisos must be made about the accuracy of the recorders, however. Firstly, in about 20% of the patients we are not able to obtain satisfactory calibrations for a variety of reasons including obesity, a weak brachial pulse, or a muscular arm. (We have improved this percentage considerably with a transducer which is not yet commercially available (2).) Secondly, 10–20% of the obtained readings are artifactual and must be edited out of the record. Recordings are rejected if the pulse pressure is not greater than an empirically derived value of $(0.41 \times$ diastolic pressure$) - 17$, for diastolic pressures between 60 and 150 mmHg.

We have performed over 200 recordings with this system. Based on these recordings we have made several observations: (a) the P2 system provides the most information by recording ECG as well as blood pressure which has proven valuable for some of our studies; (b) the P2 system is also the bulkiest and the least comfortable for patients; (c) this system is considerably more expensive than the other available units; (d) we have lost 30% of our recordings due to intermittent failures which remain undiagnosed by Avionics; and (e) we have not found the field service on these units to be satisfactory.

The P3 system is relatively similar to the P2 system except for a few modifications. Firstly, it uses a solid-state memory rather than the Holter tape recorder for data storage, and consists of one rather than two units. Secondly, the P3 does not record ECG but does give heart rate, requiring 3 ECG leads rather than 5. Lastly, the P3 does not require a scanner for data retrieval but can be interfaced with a number of different computers and printers. The rest of the P3 system is identical to the P2 system including the transducer and cuff assembly and algorithm for determination of blood pressure. Therefore the same performance level apply to this unit as did to the P2.

We also have evidence to indicate that these recorders give valid readings outside the laboratory situation. In 99 patients BP was measured at home both by the P3 recorders and (on separate days) by the patient using a sphygmomanometer and stethoscope (3). The correlations between the two sets of readings were 0.69 for systolic and 0.71 for diastolic pressures. The average diastolic pressures taken manually were identical to those taken by the recorder (89 ± 1 mmHg), but the average manual systolic pressure (138 ± 2 mmHg) was significantly higher (p < 0.05) than the average automatic systolic pressure (133 ± 2 mmHg). This difference could be due to the greater mental and physical activity involved when the patient takes his or her own blood pressure.

We have performed over 500 recordings with the P3 and have made a number of observations on this unit as well: (a) Since the P3 is a single unit it is more comfortable for the patient; (b) the P3 is less expensive than the P2 and does not require purchasing an additional scanner to read the tapes; (c) we have found a failure rate in which the majority of the memory was not retrievable in approximately 34% of the recording trials.

The ICR system is the newest system commercially available. The recorder is 5.5 cm high, 21 cm long, and 11.5 cm wide and weighs 1.89 Kg. The system is divided into three parts: (a) a main section containing the display, an on/off button, a manual operation button, and the cuff connections; (b) a removable RAMPAC containing a programmable memory and the battery storage compartment; and (c) a blood pressure cuff with a piezo-electric microphone. Calibration and operation of the ICR unit is generally similar to the P2 and P3 except the ICR unit does not require ECG leads. Prior to calibration the RAMPAC is programmed with various data including patient name and characteristics, cycle time, and display on/off. One major difference in the functioning of the ICR unit is the way in which a blood pressure determination is made. If the unit is not able to get an accurate reading using the piezo-electric microphone it automatically reverts to an oscillometric mode.

We have performed a preliminary validation study of the ICR system on 48 patients who met our calibration criterion. The patients were 43 males and 5 females, whose age ranged from 23 to 71 (mean = 49), and whose blood pressure ranged from 120/66 to 163/114 mmHg. We found correlations between the ICR recorder and a mercury column of r = 0.97 for systolic pressure and r = 0.95 for diastolic pressure (see Fig. 1). There were no significant differences in the level of pressure between the ICR recorder (mean = 138/90) and the mercury column (mean = 140/90).

We have performed approximately 125 recordings with the ICR system and have made a number of observations on this system as well: (a) the ICR unit is smaller, lighter, quieter, and displays error codes rather than artifactual readings making it more patient-compatible than either the P2 or P3; (b) the ICR unit is considerably less expensive than the other units; (c) we have found the company thus far to be quite responsive to service requirements; and (d) at present the ICR unit also seems to have serious breakdown rates.

3

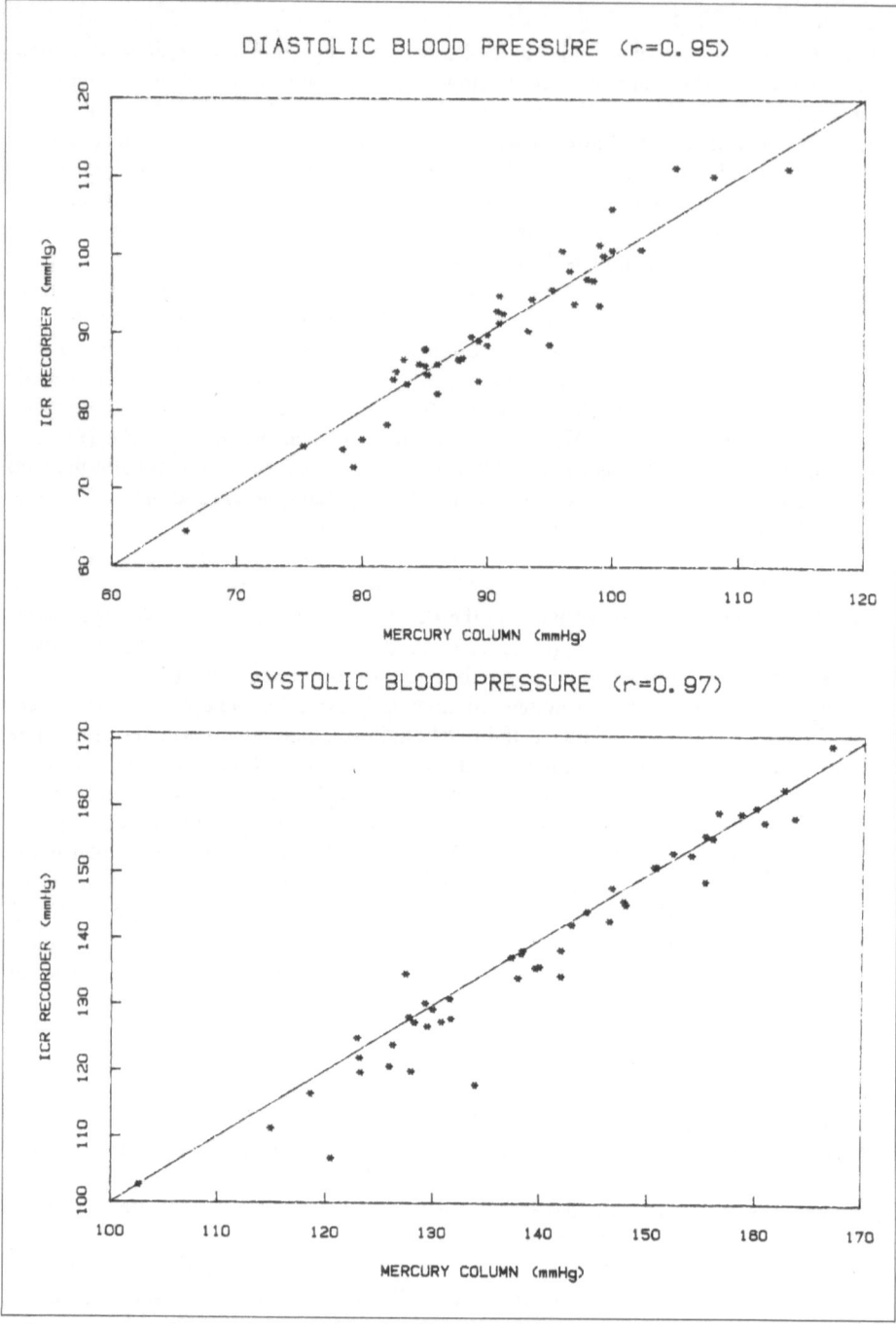

Fig. 1. Correlations between simultaneously determined pressures by mercury column and stethoscope versus ICR recorder for systolic pressure (upper panel) and diastolic pressure (lower panel).

In summary, the ICR unit seems to be superior to the P2 and P3 units in terms of cost, patient compliance and company service. The units do not seem to differ in terms of accuracy and durability, with all 3 units showing acceptable accuracies and poor durability. In fairness to ICR, however, the units we have tested are still in the developmental phase and the durability problem may be corrected.

Data reduction and analysis

We have taken a somewhat different approach to data reduction and analysis than have other groups using ambulatory blood pressure monitoring. Our approach has been decidedly behavioral, examining changes in blood pressure associated with activities. Specifically we code each reading, based on the patient diary, for recording location (physician's office, work, home, miscellaneous, and sleep), position (sitting, standing or reclining) and activity (eating, drinking, walking, smoking, chores, sex, desk work, relaxing, watching TV, talking, business meetings, listening to music, writing, dressing, shopping, talking or transportation), as well as mood (happy, sad, anxious, or angry) and time of day.

The value of this approach can be seen by examining Fig. 2. The top half of this figure is an hourly plot of the blood pressure of a patient in the hospital who remained relatively inactive throughout the 24 hours. This plot shows very little change in pressure throughout the day with only one peak occurring during eating. The bottom half of this figure is a plot of this same patient during a normal day. In this plot he shows several peaks during eating, telephoning, and business meetings.

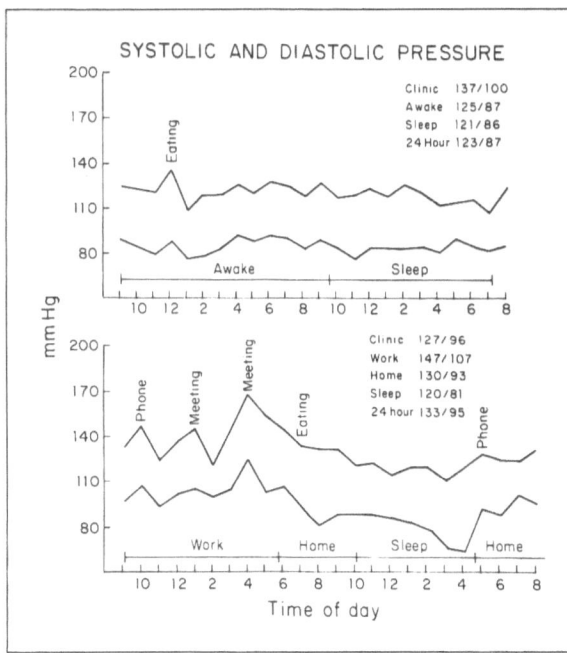

Fig. 2. Two 24 hour recordings in the same patient under different circumstances. Upper panel: while in hospital. Lower panel: during a normal day.

We have already applied this approach in a number of studies with very encouraging results. Thus far we have been able to demonstrate a difference in pressure based on recording location (4) and activity (5) as well as a difference in patterns of pressure between hypertensives and normals (6). Furthermore, we have been able to show promising relationships between pressures obtained on working days and a variety of target organ responses including left ventricular hypertrophy (7), left ventricular dysfunction (8), and premature ventricular contractions. (These studies are reported on in detail in the chapter by Pickering et al.)

Applications

Ambulatory blood pressure monitoring has a variety of applications in the field of hypertension. From a clinical standpoint we feel the technique will be used routinely in the evaluation and diagnosis of essential hypertension as well as in the evaluation of antihypertensive therapy. This will be particularly true for behavioral treatments of hypertension in which ambulatory monitoring can be used to identify situations which are associated with pressor responses for an individual. The behavioral therapy could then be designed to reduce the stress associated with these situations.

The technique of ambulatory blood pressure monitoring, however, need not be restricted to the field of hypertension. We are currently using the P2 system in a study of patients with panic disorder. Using this technique we have been able to demonstrate that panic disorder patients show normal blood pressures and heart rates throughout the day except during panic periods. Furthermore these patients do seem to show significant deviations in blood pressure and heart rate during spontaneous episodes of panic, which are diminished by treatment with imipramine.

In conclusion, the technique of ambulatory blood pressure monitoring has seen great strides in recent years. As more companies get involved in production of the systems the recorders will become smaller, more versatile, more durable, more widely used and cheaper. Furthermore, the techniques will be applied to a variety of other disorders associated with the cardiovascular system, particularly psychiatric disorders. It is particularly important at this time to establish a common method of data reduction and analysis while the technique is still in a developmental phase. Based on a variety of our earlier findings we think a behavioral approach of analyzing blood pressure by activity currently shows the greatest promise.

Acknowledgements

We should like to acknowledge the invaluable assistance of Beth Liebowitz in this work.

References

1. Harshfield GA, Pickering TG, Laragh JH: A validation study of the Del Mar Avionics Ambulatory Blood Pressure System. Ambulatory Electrocardio 1: 7–12 (1979).
2. West JE, Busch-Visniac IJ, Harshfield GA, Pickering TG: Foil electret transducer for blood pressure monitoring. J Acoust Soc Am 74: 680–686 (1983).

3. Marion RM, Sullivan PA, Harshfield GA, Kleinert HD, Pickering TG, Laragh JH: The value of home blood pressure vs. physician office blood pressure. Circulation 68: III–37 (1983).
4. Harshfield GA, Pickering TG, Kleinert HD, Blank S, Laragh JH: Situational variations of blood pressure in ambulatory hypertensive patients. Psychosometric Med 44 (3): 237–245 (1982).
5. Harshfield GA, Pickering TG, Kleinert HD, Denby L, Kleiner B, Kaplan PM, Tucker LW, Laragh JH: The situational reactivity of blood pressure in essential hypertensive patients during normal activities. Psychophysiology 18: 163 (1981) (Abstract).
6. Pickering TG, Harshfield GA, Kleinert HD, Blank S, Laragh, JH: Comparisons of blood pressure during normal daily activities, sleep, and exercise in normal and hypertensive subjects. JAMA 247: 992–996 (1982).
7. Devereux RB, Pickering TG, Harshfield GA, Kleinert HD, Denby L, Clark L, Pregibon D, Jason M, Sachs I, Borer JS, Laragh JH: Left ventricular hypertrophy in patients with hypertension: Importance of blood pressure response to regularly recurring stress. Circulation 68 (3): 470–476 (1983).
8. Jason M, Devereux RB, Borer JS, Pickering T, Fisher J, Harshfield G, Berkowitz A, Laragh J: 24-Hour arterial pressure measurement: Improved prediction of left ventricular dysfunction in essential hypertension. Am J Cardiol 1 (2): 599 (1983).

Address for correspondence:
Gregory A. Harshfield, Ph.D.
Cardiovascular Center
The New York Hospital-Cornell Medical Center
1300 York Avenue
New York, N.Y. 10021

Ambulatory blood pressure – direct and indirect

Brian A. Gould, Robert S. Hornung, Peter M. M. Cashman, Edward B. Raftery

Summary: Ambulatory blood pressures help characterise the behavior of blood pressure away from the hospital environment and may aid in the diagnosis and management of hypertensive patients. These measurements have been obtained either by patient-recorded blood pressures or with automated recorders such as the Remler M2000 and Avionics 1978 Pressurometer. We have evaluated these techniques against indirect pressures measured with the random zero sphygmomanometer and intra-arterial blood pressures recorded with the "Oxford" sytem for ambulatory monitoring. The mean discrepancy for home BP-intra arterial BP was 0/3 mmHg whilst for clinic BP-intra-arterial BP it was -13/1 mmHg. There was a mean error of 3/2 mmHg for Remler-intra-arterial BP and of -2/4 for clinic BP-Remler. There was a mean error of -2/11 mmHg for Avionics -intra-arterial BP and of 3/8 mmHg for clinic BP-Avionics. Morning and evening self-recorded blood pressures (as used by epidemiologists) did not relate well to mean daytime ambulatory pressures. During a clinical trial the observed reductions in blood-pressure, as recorded by intra-arterial and self-recorded pressures, showed good agreement for a group of patients but not for the individual.

A wide scatter of data was found when non-invasive measurements were compared with intra-arterial pressures. All indirect methods over-estimated the diastolic blood pressure. Of the three methods, patient-recorded pressures showed closest agreement with standard indirect measurements, indicating that automated machines provide little advantage over self-recorded pressures.

Introduction

Blood pressure is a continually varying parameter which cannot be characterised by the occasional outpatient (office) indirect recording. Serial measurements throughout the day and night are required. Such measurements may be obtained by ambulatory blood pressure monitoring, but these methods have not been assessed for accuracy in operation away from the hospital environment. We have used the Oxford system for intra-arterial ambulatory blood pressure monitoring as the standard against which the indirect techniques can be compared. We evaluated self-recorded blood pressure, the Remler M2000, and the Avionics 1978 Pressurometer. In addition we have assessed how well self-recorded blood pressures (as measured by epidemologists) on awakening and on going to bed reflected the daytime blood pressures. We have also compared the recorded reductions during trials with anti-hypertensive agents.

Methods

Each method of non-invasive measurement was assessed separately.

Department of Cardiology and Divisions of Bioengineering & Clinical Sciences, Northwick Park Hospital & Clinical Research Centre, Harrow, Middlesex, HA1 3UJ, U.K.

Home blood pressures

Fifty-seven patients with essential hypertension were recruited but two were unable to learn the technique of self-recorded blood pressure measurements; 35 were on no medication. The group consisted of 17 females and 38 males with a mean age of 51.8 years (range 23–70).

The patients attended a special session of the Hypertension Clinic where an indirect measurement was recorded using the Hawkesley random zero sphygmomanometer (Gelmam Ltd). There were taught the technique of self-recording using a calibrated anaeroid gauge, standard techniques of measurement (1) and phase V for diastolic pressure. The patients' recordings were checked using a double-listening stethoscope but none were excluded from the study on the grounds of inaccurate recordings. Home blood pressures were recorded after five minutes rest in the sitting position, four times daily at 8–9 a.m., 1–2 p.m., 5–7 p.m., and at bedtime, for ten days.

During this period intra-arterial ambulatory blood pressure monitoring was undertaken. Patients were freely ambulant in their normal environment and over two days (2) only attended hospital at 12-h intervals for calibration and equipment checks. During these visits indirect recordings of blood pressure were made by the physician using a random zero sphygmomanometer, followed by a check on the patient's technique using a double listening stethoscope.

The intra-arterial tape recording was marked with an event signal whenever an indirect reading was taken, both at home and in the hospital. Indirect measurements were made on the dominant arm and intra-arterial recordings on the contra-lateral arm. The pressure difference between the arms was assessed by two observers recording the pressure in each arm simultaneously. One random zero sphygmomanometer was connected to two blood pressure cuffs. A series of paired readings on each arm were recorded and repeated after switching the cuffs providing a total of eight paired readings.

Remler M2000

Twenty-eight patients volunteered to wear the Remler M2000 for one day in addition to the Oxford system for ambulatory intra-aterial recording. There were 7 females and 21 males with a mean age of 50 years (range 23–67). ten patients were receiving antihypertensive therapy.

Simultaneous readings of intra-arterial, clinic and Remler M2000 pressures were recorded on three occasions in the hospital. The Remler M2000 was linked via a Y connector to a random zero sphygmomanometer and the clinic pressure auscultated using a standard stethoscope in the usual position. Thus simultaneous clinic and Remler pressure were recorded from the same arm whilst intra-arterial pressures were recorded from the contra-lateral arm. Pressures were recorded hourly at home in the sitting position and the intra-arterial tape was marked with an event signal.

Avionics 1978 Pressurometer

Twenty patients were recruited from those undergoing intra-arterial recording. The only difference in the protocol from that for the Remler was that a standard mercury sphygmomanometer was used in place of the random zero sphygmomanometer, which could not be used with the Avionics Pressurometer as this instrument "searched" for the systolic pressure.

Morning and evening self-recorded blood pressures

Fourteen patients additionally measured their blood pressures in the supine position on awakening (defined as morning pressures) and in the supine position on going to bed (defined as evening pressures).

Self-recorded blood pressures during a clinical trial with verapamil and prazosin

Ten patients who were undergoing a clinical trial with the calcium ion antagonist verapamil were asked to record their blood pressures as described, before and after treatment with verapamil. A further 12 patients who were undergoing a clinical trial with prazosin also recorded their pressures.

Data analysis

A hybrid computer was used to compute hourly mean intra-arterial blood pressure (3) and also a one min average systolic and diastolic pressure at each selected time marked by the event signal. Analysis was divided into assessment of pressures recorded away from hospital and clinic pressures recorded whilst attending hospital. A system to mark events on the intra-arterial tape was added mid-way through the home blood pressure study, enabling 27 patients to have clearly identifiable event marks corresponding to the exact time they recorded their blood pressure at home. In the laboratory, event marks were initially produced by disconnecting the intra-arterial transducer from the tape-recorder for a short period immediately prior to the indirect measurement.

The analyses of the Remler and Avionics recorders followed similar lines. Three pressures were selected at random from the home recordings and the corresponding one min mean intra-arterial pressure was digitised using the computer. The scope of this paper limits us to presenting data from the first of these three recordings. For each comparison the following information was calculated: mean and standard deviation of measurements by each method; mean, standard deviation and frequency distributions of between-method differences (the mean difference is referred to as the mean discrepancy). Only the lines of identity are shown on the scatter plots; regression lines and correlation coefficients are not presented. These are a measure of association only and by definition the different methods of recording the blood pressure must by associated. Correlation gives no measure of the agreement of the different methods of blood pressure measurement nor information on precision or accuracy, and if misused may give misleading results (4). Differences between two methods were also assessed by Student's paired "t" test.

Similary, morning and evening self-recorded blood pressures were compared to mean daytime self-recorded and to intra-arterial blood pressures. The reductions in blood pressure as recorded by patients, the physician and intra-arterial measurement were similarly assessed.

Results

Analysis of the inter-arm differences showed that no patient had a mean difference greater than 10 mmHg and most had differences less than 5 mmHg. In order to assess our methods of validation (i.e. the use of a one minute mean intra-arterial pressure) we took records from 28 patients and for each patient a single reading was randomly selected. The systolic and diastolic points which were marked on the intra-arterial trace corresponded with the first Korotkoff sound and the point of disapperance of Korotkoff sounds. These intra-arterial pressures were then compared with the average intra-arterial pressure over one min from which they were selected. The mean discrepancy was -2/2 mmHg (Table 1).

Clinic blood pressure – intra-arterial blood pressure

The mean discrepancy for this comparison was -13/1 mmHg (Table 1). The scatter plot (Fig. 1) showed that the majority of systolic points lay above the line of identity whilst the diastolic points were more evenly distributed.

Table 1. Comparison of home, clinic and intra-arterial blood pressures.

	Mean	SD	Mean Diff. A−B	SD of Diff.	P	N	Fig No.
Systolic							
A. IABP (l'mean)	162	28.7	− 2	2.9	<0.001	28	–
B. IABP (Beat to beat)	164	28.8					
A. Clinic BP	156	25.6	−13	16.2	<0.001	55	1
B. IABP	169	26.6					
A. Home BP	164	37.8	0	23.0	>0.9	27	2
B. IABP	164	32.6					
A. Patient BP	171	34.3	− 2	5.9	>0.5	31	3
B. Clinic BP	173	35.2					
Diastolic							
A. IABP (l'mean)	88	15.4	− 2	2.1	<0.001	28	–
B. IABP (beat to beat)	90	15.2					
A. Clinic BP	95	17.7	1	13.0	>0.5	55	1
B. IABP	94	13.0					
A. Home BP	97	14.4	3	16.7	>0.2	27	2
B. IABP	94	16.5					
A. Patient BP	103	21.6	2	7.0	>0.1	31	3
B. Clinic BP	101	19.4					

IABP = Intra-arterial blood pressure; SD = standard deviation.

N.B. Mean values have been rounded to whole number thus difference between mean values in column 1 may not correspond exactly with mean difference in column 3.

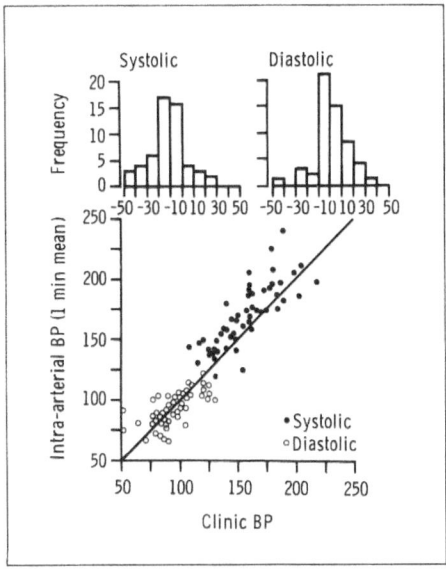

Fig. 1: Scatter plot and frequency histogram of clinic BP – intra-arterial BP (1 min mean). Frequency histogram: Systolic BP: 36% within ± 10 mmHg of the intra-arterial BP. Diastolic BP – 65% within ± 10 mmHg.

Home blood pressure

Blood pressure recorded by patients at home (home BP-intra-arterial BP) compared to simultaneous intra-arterial blood pressure gave a mean discrepancy value of 0/3 mmHg (Table 1). The plot of home BP – intra-arterial (Fig. 2) showed a wide scatter of points. The number of patients included in this analysis was limited to 27 due to the late addition of the event marking sytems.

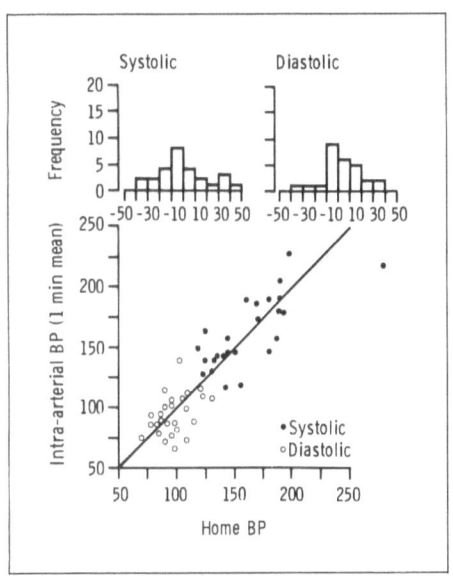

Fig. 2: Scatter plot and frequency histogram of home BP – intra-arterial BP (1 min mean). Systolic BP: 47% within ±10 mmHg: Diastolic BP: 55% within ± 10 mmHg.

Comparison of the physician and patient recorded pressure (using a double listening stethoscope and anaeroid gauge) showed very good agreement with a mean dicrepancy value for patient BP – clinic BP of -22/2 mmHg (Table 1) confirmed by the scatter plot (Fig. 3).

Fig. 3: Scatter plot and frequency histogram of patient recorded BP – clinic BP. Systolic BP: 93% within ± 10 mmHg. Diastolic BP: 83% within ± 10 mmHg.

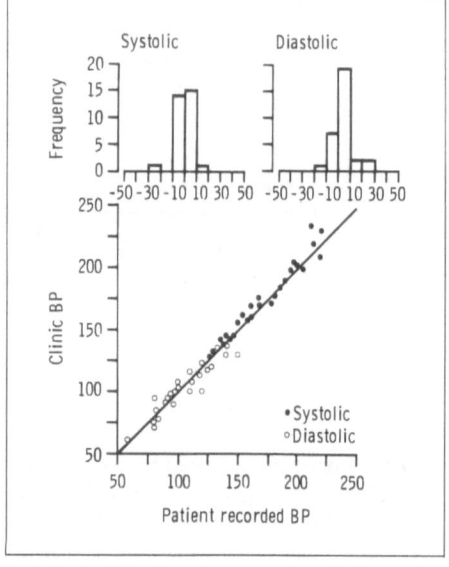

Fig. 4: Scatter plot and frequency histogram of Remler M2000 – intra-arterial BP. Systolic BP: 54% within ± 10 mmHg. Diastolic BP: 78% within ± 10 mmHg.

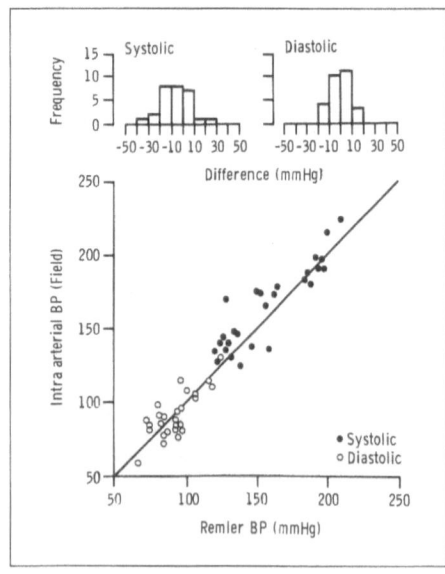

Away from the hospital environment the mean discrepancy of intra-arterial BP – Remler was 1/2 mmHg (Table 2). The scatter plot (Fig. 4) showed wide deviation of the points from the line of identity but diastolic points were distributed more evenly. The mean discrepancy for clinic BP – Remler was -2/4 mmHg (Table 2). The plot was similar to Fig. 4 and showed modest scatter around the line of identity with the majority of diastolic points lying below the line.

Table 2. Comparison of Remler M2000, Avionics 1978 Pressurometer and intra-arterial blood pressure.

	Mean	SD	Mean Diff. A–B	SD of Diff.	P	N	Fig. No.
Systolic							
A. IABP	159	31.2	– 1	15.5	>0.5	28	4
B. Remler	158	32.6					
A. Clinic BP	163	27.8	– 2	9.9	>0.05	28	–
B. Remler	163	30.3					
A. IABP	148	25.7	– 2	15.9	>0.05	18	–
B. Avionics	150	28.0					
A. Clinic BP	165	28.2	3	12.6	>0.1	18	–
B. Avionics	162	32.3					
Diastolic							
A. IABP	93	22.4	2	11.6	>0.2	28	4
B. Remler	92	17.8					
A. Clinic BP	99	15.6	4	5.9	<0.001	28	–
B. Remler	95	14.1					
A. IABP	88	17.6	–11	12.3	<0.01	18	–
B. Avionics	99	18.1					
A. Clinic BP	102	13.2	8	18.3	>0.05	18	–
B. Avionics	94	16.9					

IABP = Intra-arterial blood pressure; SD = standard deviation.

Avionics 1978 Pressurometer

The Pressurometer over-estimated intra-arterial diastolic pressures at home with mean discrepancy values of -2/-11 mmHg (Table 2). The scatter plot which was similar to Fig. 4 showed even distribution of the systolic points around the line of identity but diastolic points lay above the line of identity indicating higher Avionic recorded diastolic pressures.

The Pressurometer over-estimated indirect pressures. Table 2 shows that the mean discrepancy of the Avionics Pressurometer BP – clinic BP was 3/8 mmHg. The scatter plot was silmilar to Fig. 3 and showed fairly close grouping but there were 2 systolic and 3 diastolic points which deviated widely.

Morning and evening pressure

The scatter plot (Fig. 5) and data (Table 3) demonstrated that the mean differences for morning supine home BP and evening supine home BP compared with mean daytime home blood pressure were not accurately reflected as far as the individual was concerned.

Table 3. Means and mean differences of morning and evening supine home blood pressures.

	N	Mean	SD	Mean Difference	SD of Differences	P
a. Morning supine						
Systolic						
Morning	14	153	27.2	5	19.0	>0.2
HBP (mean of day)		147	19.5			
Morning	14	153	27.2	−9	21.6	>0.2
IABP (mean daytime)		162	27.4			
Diastolic						
Morning	14	92	12.7	0	10.9	>0.9
HBP (mean of day)		92	15.9			
Morning	14	92	12.7	7	11.1	<0.05
IABP (mean daytime)		85	11.4			
b. Evening supine						
Systolic						
Evening	10	149	20.0	0	13.3	>0.9
HBP (mean of day)		149	24.8			
Evening	10	149	20.0	−12	17.8	>0.05
IABP (mean daytime)		161	29.6			
Diastolic						
Evening	10	88	16.7	−3	7.9	>0.2
(mean of day)		91	18.2			
Evening	10	88	16.7	6	12.1	>0.1
IABP (mean daytime)		82	12.3			

HBP = Home blood pressure; IABP = Intra-arterial blood pressure; SD = standard deviation.

Self-recorded pressures during a clinical trial of anti-hypertensive agents

Generally there was poor agreement between different methods of blood pressure measurement in individual patients but as far as the group was concerned generally good agreement was observed (Fig. 6 and Table 4).

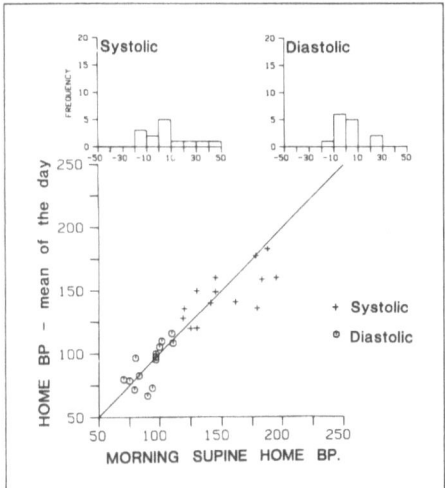

Fig. 5: Scatter plot and frequency histogram of morning supine blood pressure – home blood pressure (mean of that day). Systolic BP: 50% within ± 10 mmHg. Diastolic BP within ± 10 mmHg.

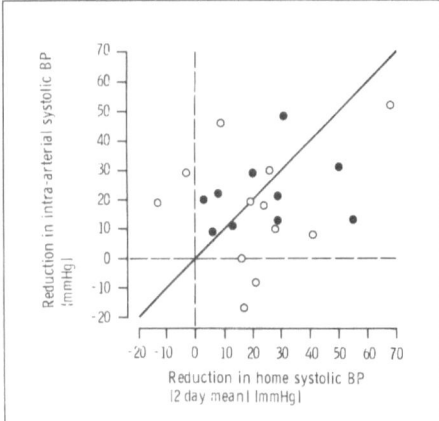

Fig. 6a: Scatter plot of systolic blood pressure changes recorded by home BP (2 day mean) v intra-arterial BP (mean daytime) during studies with verapamil (●) and with prazosin (○).

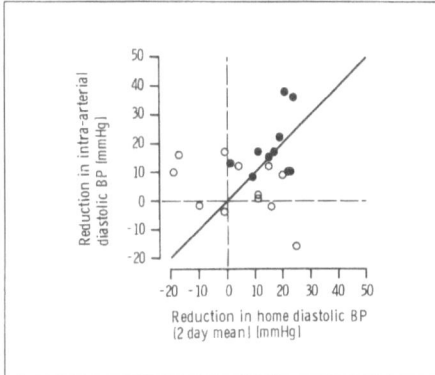

Fig. 6b: Scatter plot of diastolic blood pressure changes recorded by home BP (2 day mean) v intra-arterial BP (mean daytime) during studies with verapamil (●) and with prazosin (○).

17

Table 4. Changes in blood pressure recorded by different methods after treatment with Verapamil (n = 10) and with Prazosin (n = 12).

	Verapamil		Prazosin	
	Mean change	SD	Mean change	SD
Intra-arterial	23/19	112.3/10.1	18/5	19.2/9.6
Clinic BP	38*/20	13.6/10.1	28/18**	21.5/8.5
Home BP	24/16	17.9/7.3	21/6	20.5/13.7

$* p < 0.05$; $** p < 0.01$; SD = Standard deviation.

Discussion

Despite the limited information concerning the accuracy of the indirect methods of ambulatory blood pressure monitoring, these methods are being increasingly advocated (5,6). In the study of self-recorded blood pressure measurements no patients were excluded and only two patients were unable to master the technique. There was a wide variation in the accuracy of self-recorded blood pressures compared with intra-arterial recordings with occasional individual differences of nearly 50 mmHg. There was no difference in the relationship between self-recorded and clinic blood pressure measurements when compared to intra-arterial ambulatory blood pressures. There was good agreement of both indirect techniques as has been noted previously (5, 7, 8).

The Remler M2000 and Avionics 1978 Pressurometer both showed a similar relationship to intra-arterial pressures when compared with self-recorded pressures. The comparison of Remler – clinic BP showed less scatter than did the similar comparison of Avionics – clinic BP. The Avionics Pressurometer when compared to intra-arterial blood pressure also over-estimated the diastolic pressure to a greater degree than the similar comparison for the Remler M2000.

These data show that indirect methods provide estimates of the intra-arterial pressure which may be inaccurate by as much as 50 mmHg. Of the three methods, self-recorded pressures showed the closest agreement with standard indirect pressures, indicating that automated machines provide little advantage over self-recorded home blood pressure measurements. Self-recorded pressures recorded by patients on awakening and on going to bed (as used by epidemiologists (7)) do not relate well to mean daytime pressure, and serial measurements are therfore advised. The reduction in self-recorded blood pressures during clinical trials agreed well with intra-arterial pressures as far as a group of patients was concerned, but showed variable accuracy in each individual. This method is a useful tool for the assessment of the efficacy of anti-hypertensive agents in a group of patients.

All indirect ambulatory methods are subject to the same inaccuracies as clinic (office) measurements. An accurate method for assessing blood pressure variability remains to be described.

References

1. Kirkendall WM, Burton AC, Epstein FH, Freis ED: Circulation 36: 980–988 (1967).
2. Millar-Craig MW, Hawes D, Whittington J: Med Biol Eng & Comput 16: 727–731 (1978).

3. Cashman PMM, Stott FD, Millar-Craig MW: Med & Biol Eng & Comput 17: 629–635 (1979).
4. Altman DG: Br Med J 2: 1473–1475 (1980).
5. Julius S, Ellis CN, Pascaul AV, Matice M, Hansson L, Hunyor SN, Sandler LN: J Am Med Assoc 229: 663–666 (1974).
6. Laughlin KD, Fisher L, Sherrard DJ: Am Heart J 98: 629–634 (1979).
7. Joossens JV, Brems-Heyns E, Claessens J: In: Kesteloof W (ed) Commission of the European Communities Biological Sciences – Medical Research. Methodology and standardisation of non-invasive blood pressure measurement in epidemiological studies. Proceeding of a workshop in Leuven (Belgium), Commission of the European Communities, Directorate General "Research and Education" (1976).
8. Laughlin KD, Sherrard DJ, Fisher L: J Chron Dis 33: 197–206 (1980).

Address for correspondence:
Dr. E. B. Raftery,
Department of Cardiology,
Northwick Park Hospital,
Harrow, Middlesex, HA1 3UJ, U.K.

Can short-term recording of blood pressure in supine patients replace ambulatory blood pressure monitoring

D. L. Clement, F. Colardyn, L. Packet, and G. O. Van Maele

Summary: In this study, blood pressures were recorded in 29 patients with mild to moderate hypertension using three different monitoring techniques. Casual blood pressures were measured while the patients were seated using a standard mercury sphygmomanometer. The Arteriosonde or the Dinamap blood pressure recorder was used in each patient to measure blood pressure for 3 hours at 5 minute intervals while the patients remained in the supine position. In addition, blood pressure was recorded in ambulatory patients during 12 hours at 30 minute intervals using the Portometer (Remler). The averages of blood pressures obtained with the various techniques were compared. Casual blood pressure was significantly higher than blood pressure measured by the semiautomatic devices; however, data from the Portometer and Arteriosonde were found to be very close to each other. The histograms of blood pressure averages obtained using both monitoring techniques do largely overlap. Casual blood pressure was localized on the 85° percentile of the histograms.

From these data it can be concluded that casual blood pressure is far from ideal for identifying the patients' blood pressure level. Three hours of blood pressure recording in supine patients may be a convenient and cheap alternative to ambulatory blood pressure monitoring in the assessment of the blood pressure level in hypertensive subjects.

Introduction

It has long been shown both by invasive and non-invasive techniques that large differences exist between office readings of blood pressure and ambulatory recordings (1). In most of these studies only the means obtained with both techniques are compared and the differences listed; it is in most cases impossible to determine whether the office readings are part of the spectrum of blood pressures recorded during ambulatory monitoring and if so, where they are localized on the histogram. Therefore, in the present work, office blood pressure readings were compared to the data obtained in the same patients by two non-invasive semi-automatic blood pressure recording devices: the Portometer for ambulatory recordings and either the Arteriosonde or Dinamap for supine recordings. In fact, the Arteriosonde and Dinamap were included to investigate the relationship between blood pressures derived from the ambulatory device and those recorded during quiet relaxed conditions. The use of the latter techniques allows recording of blood pressure under standardized conditions. However, the relationship between blood pressures obtained under these conditions and those obtained during ambulatory recordings has not yet been established.

Department of Cardiology, University of Gent, Belgium.

21

Patients and methods

29 patients with mild to moderate arterial hypertension were studied. Blood pressure was found to have been elevated in these patients for at least two years. ECG revealed no left ventricular hypertrophy or left ventricular hypertrophy without strain. Eye fundi showed changes grade I or II according to Keith-Wagener and Barker criteria.

Casual blood pressure was recorded in the office in the sitting position three times consecutively, at one minute intervals.

To record blood pressure and heart rate in the patients' normal environment, the Portometer (Remler M 2000) was used. This apparatus was developed by Hinman and associates (2); it has been extensively tested and widely used by Sokolow and co-workers (3, 4, 5).

The reliability of this technique was determined in 50 patients. The data recorded on tape and those measured simultaneously using a sphygmomanometer were compared. A very close correlation between both measurements of systolic and diastolic blood pressures was found ($r^2 = 0.99$, $p < 0.001$), confirming earlier findings (6, 7); only at higher levels of pressure were small differences documented.

In the present work, Portometer recordings were performed for 12 hours at 30 minute intervals.

In the same patients, recording of blood pressure was performed in the supine position, using either the Arteriosonde or Dinamap, for 3 hours at 5 minute intervals. The accur-

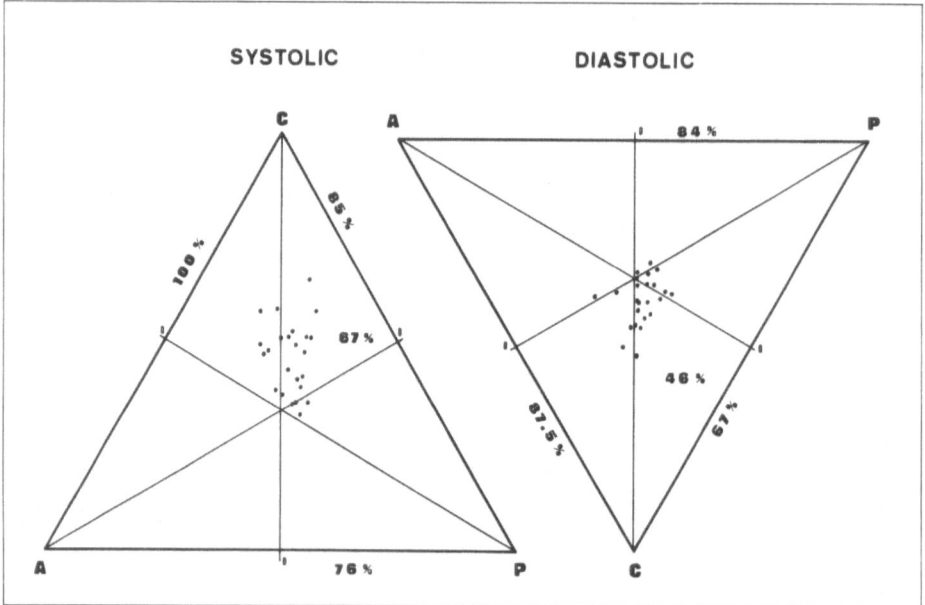

Fig. 1. Comparison of casual blood pressure (C) with Arteriosonde (or Dinamap) recordings (A) or Portometer recordings (P). A point is situated at the zero line when both techniques yield the same result; the data for every comparison are given on each side of the triangle; the numbers indicate how many times (in percentage) one technique gives higher results than the other.

acy of both these techniques has been assessed previously (8). The Portometer, Arteriosonde and Dinamap have been used for many years in our department in the evaluation of blood pressure variability (8, 9, 10, 11). Performance of the techniques was recently further documented (J. Hypertension, in press).

Results and discussion

As could be expected, office readings were significantly higher ($p < 0.01$) than the mean of values obtained by portometer (169/103 versus 146/94 mmHg); this closely corresponds to earlier well documented findings with the same technique (1). Surprisingly, Portometer recordings were only slightly higher than Arteriosonde readings (139/89 mmHg, $p < 0.01$). Means and limits of 2e and 3e quartile of the measurements were only slightly different. Portometer readings of highest and lowest systolic blood pressures were higher and lower respectively than those obtained using Arteriosonde-Dinamap recordings. Diastolic blood pressure readings were not different. These findings contrast with the general belief that blood pressure recorded in quiet and relaxed conditions is markedly lower than that obtained in ambulatory patients.

Office readings of systolic blood pressure were higher than Portometer readings in 85% of the cases, and higher than Arteriosonde readings in 100% of the cases; Portometer readings were higher than Arteriosonde in 80% of the cases (Fig. 1).

For diastolic blood pressure, office (casual) blood pressure was higher than Arteriosonde in 87,5% of the cases and higher than Portometer in 67% of the cases. For systolic blood pressure, the median of the differences between casual blood pressure and Arteriosonde or Dinamap was respectively 24 and 26 mmHg; the largest difference was 72 and 56 mmHg respectively. For diastolic blood pressure, the median of the differences was 16 and 10 mmHg, with the largest difference being 24 and 26 mmHg.

The practical importance of these large differences could be derived from the observation that values which were frankly hypertensive in the office were found to be within normal limits with the semi-automatic recording devices. This occurred in 10 patients with Arteriosonde and in 7 patients with Portometer.

It is clear that the definition of hypertension might have to be re-evaluated in the light of these and similar data.

Although there is a positive and significant ($p < 0.001$) correlation between the office readings and the non-invasive recordings for the group as a whole, which is better for systolic than for diastolic values, the individual blood pressures for either Portometer or Arteriosonde cannot be predicted from the office readings (Fig. 2).

When the histograms derived from both the methods are compared, a surprisingly marked overlap is found for systolic and for diastolic blood pressure.

That the casual blood pressure is far from ideal for identifying the patients' blood pressure is illustrated by its localization on the histograms, where it can be found around the 85° percentile.

These data illustrate again the large differences existing between office readings and ambulatory recordings of blood pressure; the most unexpected finding was the very close relationship between ambulatory recordings and those performed during three hours, in relaxed conditions but with a larger number of measurements. It can be speculated that, to plot the histogram, one needs a large enough number of points regardless of whether

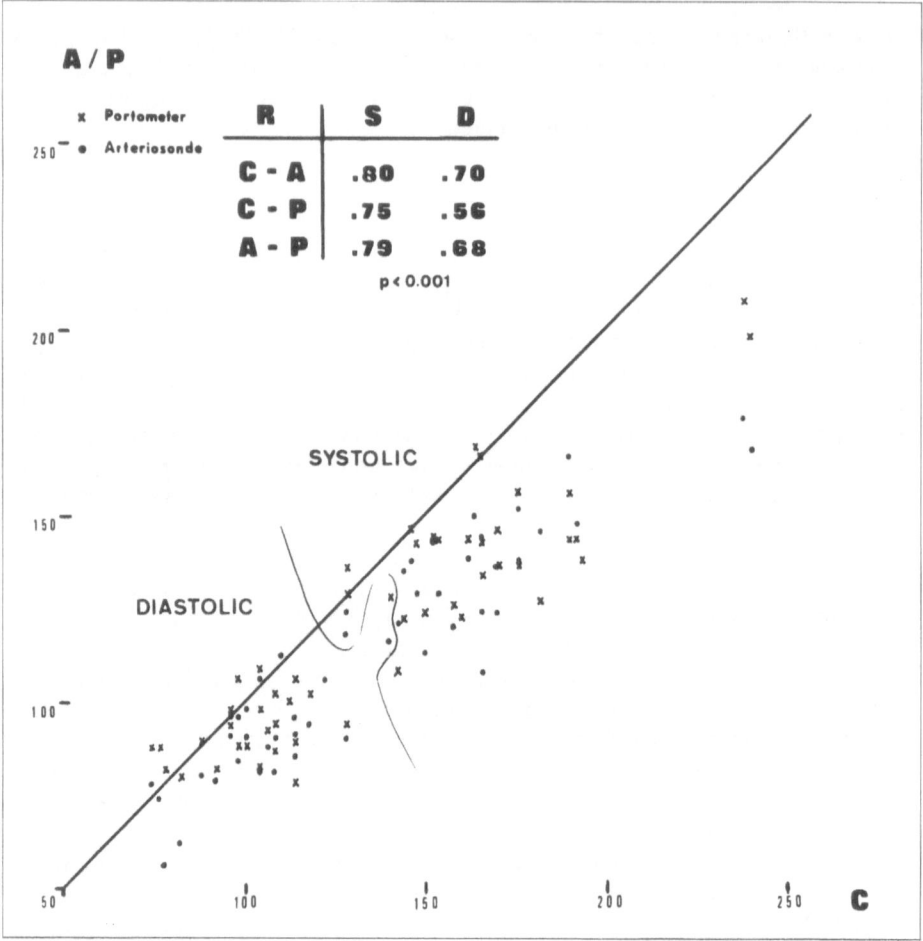

Fig. 2. Correlation of Arteriosonde/Dinamap readings (A) to casual blood pressure (C). Note that both for systolic and diastolic blood pressure the vast majority of casual pressures is higher than the semi-automatic readings. Upper left in the figure are the correlation coefficients for systolic (S) and diastolic (D) blood pressure. There is a significant correlation between any of the data studied (p < 0.001).

these have been recorded over 12 hours of 3 hours, and regardless of whether recordings were made ambulatory or in the supine position. These observations, if confirmed, could have important consequences for the daily measurement of blood pressure. Casual blood pressure gives only a glimpse of the blood pressure profile; Portometer recordings largely expand on this matter. Recordings in the supine position provide a convenient and cheap method for the assessment of blood pressure and, as the data show, the blood pressure level measured in this way is surprisingly similar to data obtained in ambulatory patients.

24

References

1. Perloff D, Sokolow M, Cowan R: Clinical relevance of ambulatory blood pressure measurements. Biotelemetry Patient Monitg 8: 67–80 (1981).
2. Hinman AT, Engel BT, Bickford AF: Portable blood pressure recorder: accuracy and preliminary use in evaluating intradaily variations in pressure. Am Heart J 63: 663–668 (1962).
3. Kain H, Hinman AT, Sokolow M: Arterial blood pressure measurements with a portable recorder in hypertensive patients: I. Variability and correlation with "casual" pressures. Circulation 30: 882–892 (1964).
4. Sokolow M, Werdegar D, Kain HK, Hinman AT: Relationship between level of blood pressure measured casually and by portable recorders and severity of complications in essential hypertension. Circulation 34: 279–298 (1966).
5. Sokolow M, Perloff D, Cowan R: The value of portably recorded blood pressures in the initiation of treatment of moderate hypertension. Clin Sci Mol Med 45: 195s (1973).
6. Cowan RM, Sokolow M, Perloff D: Methodological consideration in determining the accuracy of an indirect blood pressure recorder. In: Stott FD, Raftery EB, Gould L (ed). ISAM: pp 241–245 (1979).
7. Bachmann K, Bäuerlein G: Ambulatory monitoring of arterial blood pressure. Comparison between blood pressure measurements obtained with the Remler M–2000 portable recorder and by radiotelemetry under laboratory conditions and during everyday activities. Biotelemetry Patient Monitg 8: 47–55 (1981).
8. Clement DL: Blood pressure variability in hospitalized patients. Acta Clin Belg 32: 163–167 (1977).
9. Clement DL, Bogaert MG, Pannier R: Effect of beta-adrenergic blockade on blood pressure variation in patients with moderate hypertension. Europ J Clin Pharmacol 11: 325–327 (1977).
10. Clement DL: Effect of sympathetic nervous activity on blood pressure variability. Blood Pressure Variability, pp. 43–48 MTP Press (1979).
11. Clement DL, Cardon E, Castro M, De Pue N, Packet L, Van Maele GO: Effect of metoprolol and of guanfacine on ambulatory blood pressure and its variations. Br J Clin Pharmacol 15: 471S–478S (1983).

Address for correspondence:
Professor Denis L. Clement
University Hospital
Department of Cardiology
185, De Pintelaan
B–9000 Gent
Belgium

Ambulatory blood pressure monitoring: methods to assess severity of hypertension, variability and sleep changes

R. A. Reeves, A. M. Johnson, A. P. Shapiro, Y. M. Traub, and R. Jacob

Summary: Twenty-four hour non-invasive ambulatory blood pressure-heart rate monitoring was performed on 4 normotensive subjects, 30 patients with essential hypertension, and 4 patients with renovascular hypertension. Division of systolic and diastolic blood pressure (BP) and heart rate (HR) measurements into day and night (asleep) points and expression of variability as coefficient of variation (std.dev. x 100%/mean) revealed that age, sex, level of blood pressure, and antihypertensive treatment with diuretic with or without beta-adrenergic blocking agents did not alter variability, which averaged 11% for BP and 13% for HR. Decreases in BP and HR with sleep (respective means 13% and 14%) were universal, and unaffected by the above factors.
A method of assessing total 24-hour exposure to hypertension by use of a computer-generated "area under the curve" of degree of BP elevation multiplied by time of elevation is described, which has proved useful in following treatment success and may be helpful in predicting cardiovascular risk from hypertension.

Introduction

Although the existence of variability in blood pressure (BP) and heart rate (HR) has been known for some time (1), methods to quantify this variability and to assess its significance are still being improved upon (2). Many antihypertensive medication regimens currently employed include late-evening dosing even though it is well known that BP routinely falls, and in some patients considerably so, with sleep (3). Quantification of these sleep changes, studies of the importance of night BP levels, and attempts to correlate "real-world" measures of BP elevation with subsequent morbidity from cardiovascular events are still evolving (4).

In this study we present results of a retrospective examination of 24-hour non-invasive ambulatory BP-HR monitoring in an attempt to clarify some of these methodological considerations.

Methods

Subjects

Forty-four consecutive patients underwent 24-h ambulatory BP-HR monitoring by an automatic inflatable cuff and electrocardiographic method (Del-Mar Avionics, Irvine,

Division of Hypertension and Clinical Pharmacology
Department of Medicine
University of Pittsburgh School of Medicine
Pittsburgh, Pennsylvania
Supported in part by NHLBI Grants Nos. HL20724 and HL27159

Calif.) for evaluation of hypertension. BP and HR were recorded automatically every 15 or 30 min. All antihypertensive medications were continued during monitoring. Four records were judged technically unsatisfactory and were excluded, as were 2 donc on patients with cardiac transplants who are part of another report (11).

Patients were classified clinically by etiology (essential or proven reno-vascular) and severity of hypertension (normotensive, mild, moderate, severe).

Data analysis

Each record was divided into a day (awake) and night (asleep) period based on a patient diary. The mean, standard deviation and coefficient of variation (CV = 100% x std. dev./mean) of systolic BP (SBP), diastolic BP (DBP) and HR were calculated by computer for day and night periods separately. The percent. changes of mean SBP, DBP and HR with sleep were then computed.

A measure of total daily BP elevation was calculated as follows: for SBP and DBP individually, the amount of BP elevation in mmHg above 140/90 was multiplied by the time spent there in hours, and this pressure-time area was then integrated by trapezoidal methods over the recording period and adjusted to a standard 24-h record length. The systolic and diastolic areas (in mmHg x h) were then printed on a computer-generated SBP and DBP vs time graph, and the "area under the curve" was hatched in by the plotter to make it more visible.

Results

Table 1 shows the mean day and night BP's and HR and the mean ages for the diagnostic subgroups. The more severely hypertensive patients tended to be older.

Table 1. Blood Pressure and Heart Rate: Day and Night Means by Group.

Group	N	Age	Day		Night	
			BP	HR	BP	HR
Normal:	4	44	109/74	80	94/65	66
(SEM		7.7	1.8/1.8	5.8	3.8/1.4	6.7)
Essential Hypertension Patients:						
Mild	8	40	124/84	76	110/72	64
(SEM		4.3	2.3/1.4	3.5	2.4/2.4	3.0)
Moderate	14	47	132/94	77	112/79	69
(SEM		3.5	1.9/1.0	2.3	2.7/1.6	1.9)
Severe	8	52	164/104	82	145/90	67
(SEM		5.1	9.8/4.0	5.0	7.9/3.9	4.0)
R–V HyT	4	41	165/109	69	142/93	61
(SEM		8.2	16/12	3.6	10/12	2.8)

N = number of subjects in the group. BP in mmHg, HR in beats/min.
SEM = Standard error of the mean.
R–V HyT = Renovascular hypertension patients.

Sleep changes

Fig. 1 demonstrates that BP and HR are approximately 15% lower at night, and that these sleep decreases were similar in all groups. All individuals decreased both BP and HR with sleep. The degree of these BP sleep decreases was little influenced by antihypertensive treatment (Fig. 2), and was unrelated to age (Fig. 3) or gender (data not shown).

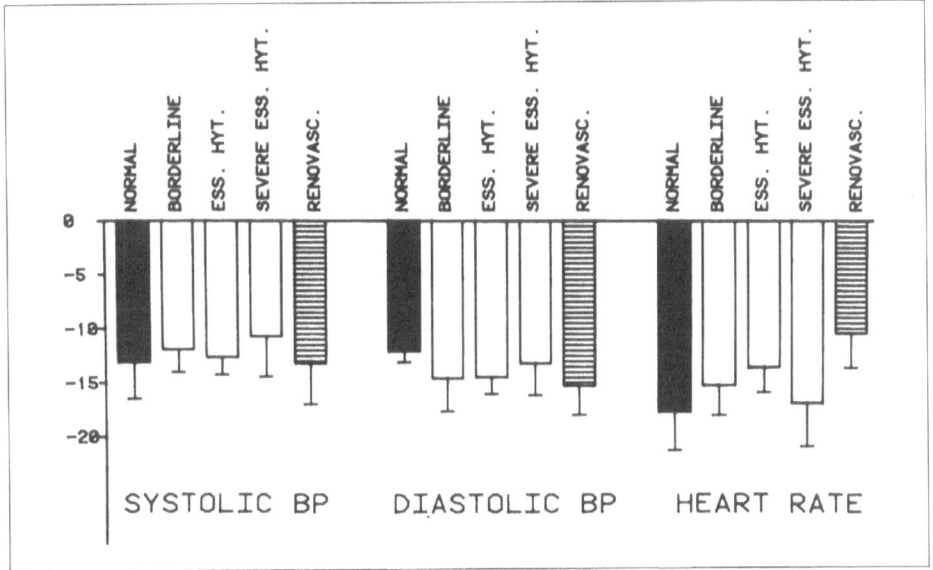

Fig. 1. Percent. fall in blood pressure and heart rate with sleep. By analysis of variance, no differences are significant between patient groups.

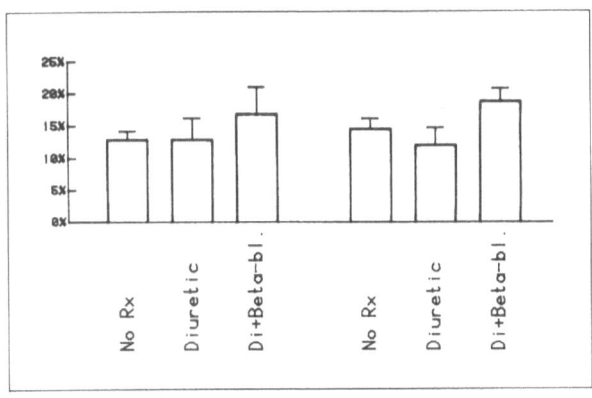

Fig. 2. Percent. fall in blood pressure with sleep: relation to antihypertensive treatment. By analysis of variance, no differences are significant between treatments.

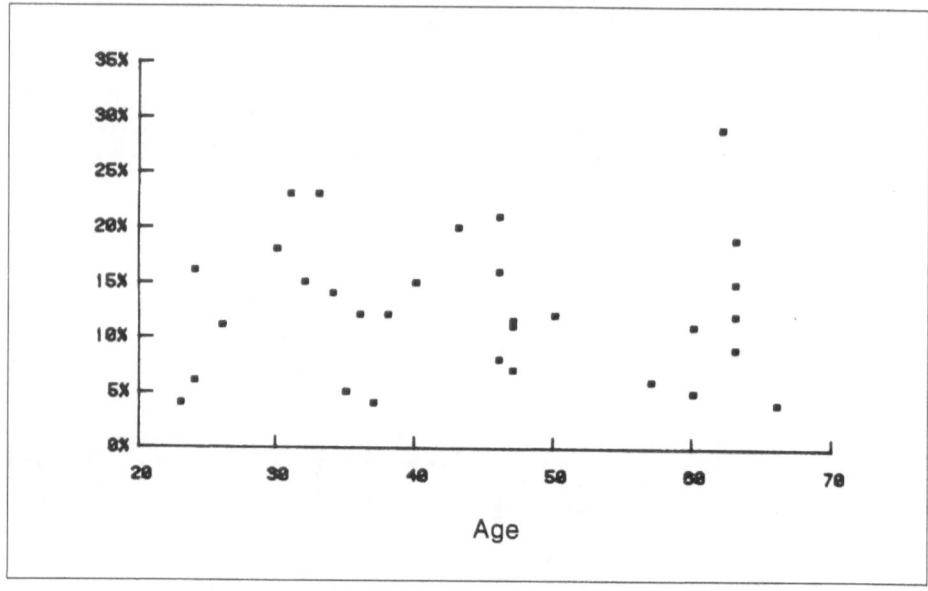

Fig. 3. Percent. fall in systolic blood pressure with sleep: relation to age.

Variability

Neither presence of diuretic or diuretic plus beta-blocker antihypertensive therapy nor severity of hypertension appeared to influence CV of day SBP (Fig. 4); the CV for DBP and HR (not shown) were similarly stable.

In Fig. 5, the CV of BP and HR at night are shown to be similar to the waking values (here, the 4 normal subjects and the 30 essential hypertensive patients are considered together).

Fig. 4. Coefficient of variation of daytime systolic blood pressure: relation to antihypertensive treatment and hypertension severity. No differences are significant.

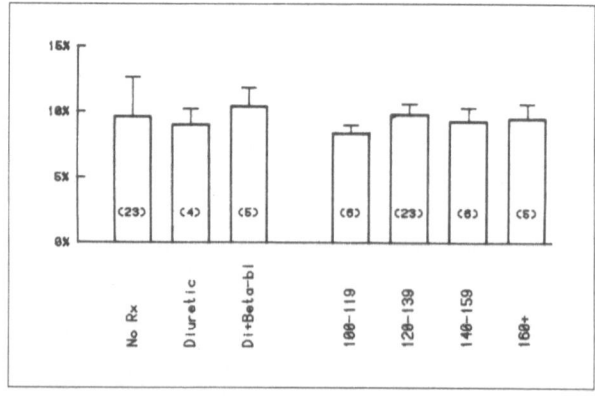

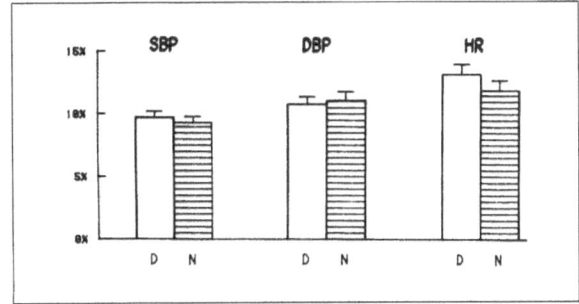

Fig. 5. Coefficients of variation of day and night systolic and diastolic blood pressures and heart rate for 4 normal and 30 essential hypertensive patients: differences day vs night are not significant.

No correlation was found between CV and age, sex, or mean HR (data not shown).

A subgroup of 13 essential hypertensive patients who had their monitoring done as in-patients in hospital was analyzed separately. The CV of SBP, DBP and HR were respectively $12 \pm 1.1\%$, $13 \pm 1.2\%$ and $13 \pm 1.7\%$ for the day, and $9 \pm 0.9\%$, $14 \pm 1.6\%$ and $10 \pm 1.4\%$ for the night periods, similar to the above results. In this subgroup with restricted activity, age appeared to be positively correlated with CV of day DBP ($r = 0.64$) but not with day SBP ($r = 0.13$), and with day HR ($r = 0.41$) and night HR ($r = 0.47$). No definite decision could be made concerning whether the older subjects slept less well in hospital.

Total BP elevation

Two examples of the "area under the curve" method to evaluate the total exposure to hypertension over 24 h are shown in Figs. 6 and 7. They are:

Fig. 6: A 27 year old female with essential hypertension. Although considerable hypertension is seen during the day, with systolic and diastolic BP elevation x time areas of 107/158 mmHg x h, this patient's BP falls to 120/75 with sleep, and no exposure to BP greater than 140/90 is recorded.

Fig. 7: "Fixed" hypertension in a 64 year old male. The areas show systolic and diastolic elevations of 939/463 mmHg x h, respectively, indicating considerable exposure to hypertension. However, BP falls to 130/80 during sleep.

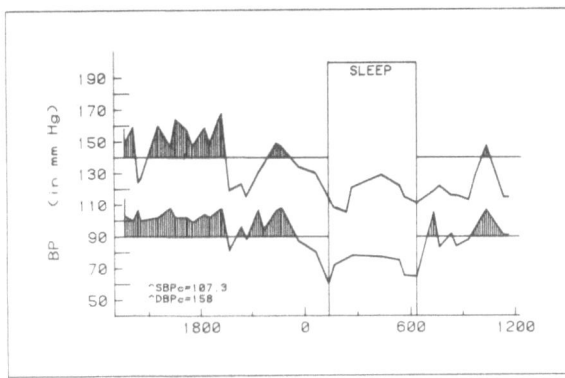

Fig. 6. Young essential hypertensive patient. Plot of systolic and diastolic BP versus time in hours (0 = midnight). Shading indicates time and degree of elevation above 140 systolic and 90 diastolic. SBPc and DBPc are areas of shading in mmHg x hrs corrected to a standard 24-h recording period.

Fig. 7. Older essential hypertensive patient. For explanation, see legend to Fig. 6.

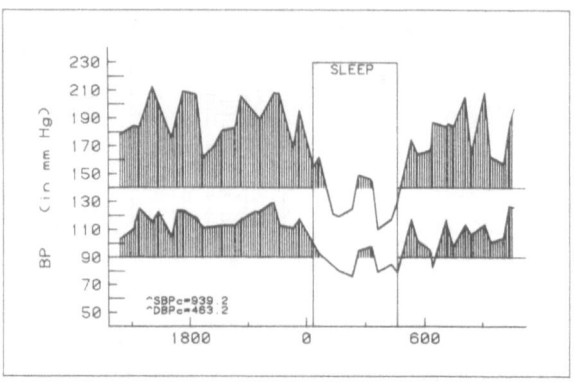

Discussion

Variability

Our results indicate a constancy of blood pressure variability when this parameter is corrected for the level of pressure, i.e., when it is expressed as coefficient of variation. In our 38 subjects, variability was independent of gender, age, level of BP, antihypertensive treatment, and whether hypertension (when present) was essential or renovascular in origin.

Sleep changes

During sleep, a relatively constant lowering in BP and HR was observed which occurred in all patients studied. Only patients with autonomic insufficiency (5), recipients of (denervated) cardiac transplants (11) and possibly those with malignant hypertension seem to be exceptions to this rule.

The methodologic point to be made is that these changes with sleep cause the BP and HR distributions to be bimodal, and thus measures of "variability" which are based on 24-h records reflect not only the true variability around the two (sleep and awake) means, but also the resetting of the mean that occurs with sleep. One solution is to evaluate only the minute-to-minute variability (2); within the limits of non-invasive technology, however, a simple division into day and night periods is sufficient to demonstrate the relative "stability of variability" or slight decrease with sleep (2, 6) which intra-arterial techniques also show. One refinement involves separating the data (based on the patient diary) according to level of physical activity at the time of recording, since SBP and HR increase with energy demand. We have tried this, and although such subdivision does further decrease and stabilize the estimated CV somewhat, it is obviously a cumbersome procedure.

One conclusion of this and other reports showing that CV is stable despite BP level may be that the concept of "labile hypertension" should be abandoned (7, 8). Such patients, like normal individuals and more severe hypertensives, have BP's which vary above and below the mean for that subject. While measuring change from an arbitrary level, such as 140/90, will reveal the presence of this variability, this does not mean that it is greater than normal. Furthermore, although a "hyperadrenergic" and perhaps hypervariable subpopulation of early essential hypertension patients may exist, any pathogenetic importance of such an increased variability remains unproved.

Where variability may prove to be of importance, however, is in its impact on the maximum BP during the day. High variability will be likely to result in higher peak pressures for any given level of mean pressure. If peak SBP during the day proves to be a determinant of end-organ damage, and hence is prognostically important (4), then lower variability could be desirable.

In this regard, the "area under the curve" method described should be helpful. Firstly, this method provides an easy way of assessing and of visually communicating the degree to which 24-h BP has exceeded a therapeutic goal (here, 140/90). We have employed this method to assess responses to therapy, although there is a possibility that a training effect after repeated wearing of the device will lead to lower measured pressures. Secondly, the possibility that this method might provide better prognostic information than the 24-h mean pressure, the peak SBP during work (4), the casual clinic BP (9) or several home BP readings (10) remains to be explored by longitudinal studies.

Finally, the possibility that level of night BP may be prognostically important, or conversely that the normal decrease in BP with sleep may mean that night-time medication for hypertension is unnecessary or even ill-advised, are questions that remain to be explored through 24-h monitor methods. Clearly, the area under the BP-time elevation curve depends on the duration of sleep, and this fact provides a rationale for the sleep treatment of hypertension used by Russian clinicians.

In summary, we have presented data indicating that variability of BP and HR when expressed as coefficient of variation is relatively stable, and that the sleep decrease in BP and HR should be taken into account in computing variability and in assessing therapy of hypertension. The "area under the curve" method presented is useful in quantifying severity of hypertension, and may prove to have prognostic importance.

References

1. Pickering GW: High Blood Pressure. (2nd ed). p. 46. Grune & Stratton (New York 1968).
2. Mancia G, Ferrari A, Gregorini L, Parati G, Pomidossi G, Bertinieri G, Grassi G, di Rienzo M, Pedotti A, Zanchetti A: Blood pressure and heart rate variabilities in normotensive and hypertensive human beings. Circ Res 53: 96–104 (1983).
3. Raftery EB, Millar-Craig MW, Mann S, Balasubramanian V: Effects of treatment on circadian rhythms of blood pressure. Biotelemetry Patient Monitg 8: 113–120 (1981).
4. Devereux RB, Pickering TG, Harshfield GA, Kleinert HD, Denby L, Clark L, Pregibon D, Jason M, Kleiber B, Borer JS, Laragh JH: Left ventricular hypertrophy in patients with hypertension: importance of blood pressure response to regularly recurring stress. Circulation 68: 470–2 (1983).
5. Mann S, Altman DG, Raftery EB, Bannister R: Inverted daily blood pressure pattern in autonomic impairment. Proceedings of the 9th Annual Meeting of the International Society of Hypertension (Mexico City, 2/82) No. 267 (1982).
6. Semplicini A, Pessina AC, Palatini P, Mormino P, Casiglia E, Ventura E, Dal Palu C: Computer analysis of continuous blood pressure recordings in essential hypertension. Biotelemetry Patient Monitg 8: 100–105 (1981).

7. Julius S: Borderline hypertension: significance and management. Cardiovasc Clin 9: 31–41 (1978).
8. Horan MJ, Kennedy HL, Padgett NE: Do Borderline hypertensive patients have labile blood pressure? Ann Int Med 94: 466–8 (1981).
9. The Hypertension Detection and Follow-up Program: Reduction in mortality of persons with high blood pressure including mild hypertension. JAMA 242: 2572–80 (1979).
10. Sokolow M, Werdegar D, Kain HK, Hinman AT: Relationship between level of blood pressure measured casually and by portable recorders and severity of complications in essential hypertension. Circulation 34: 279–98 (1966).
11. Thompson M, Shapiro AP, Johnsen A, Itzkoff, J. Ginchereau, E., Griffith B, Hardesty R, Bahnson, H, McDonald, R: New onset hypertension following cardiac transplantation. In: Transplantation Proceedings, 15 (Suppl 1): 2573–2577 (1983) (Presented at Transplantation Symposium, Houston, June, 1983 et Council of High Blood Pressure Research meeting, Cleveland, Oct. 1983)

Address for correspondence:
Dr. A.P. Shapiro
1183 Scaife Hall
University of Pittsburgh School of Medicine
Terrace and DeSoto Streets
Pittsburgh, Pennsylvania 15261

Interfacing the Del Mar Avionics Model 1978 PIII system with the Apple IIe computer

Kennith G. Bolen*, Leland Ramsey**, Ray W. Gifford*, Jr.

Summary: Permanent data storage and retrieval and also data analysis have been areas of concern for many users of the Del Mar Avionics Model 1978 Pressurometer. Unless the user has the Del Mar Avionics Model 1981 Pressurometer Data Analysis System available, all data handling is done manually. Storage of the data without the 1981 Analysis System is by hard copy only.

At The Cleveland Clinic Foundation, the Del Mar Avionics Model 1978 has been interfaced with the Apple IIe Computer. All necessary software to accomplish data transfer, data analysis, and data storage/retrieval has been developed. A floppy disk is used for data storage and retrieval. Graphic capabilities are provided by way of the commercially available software package VISITREND/VISI-PLOT. Analysis of data and reporting of data obtained during a typical 24-hour collection period can be accomplished in 5 to 10 minutes actual time.

This development offers a convenient alternative to the Pressurometer Data Analysis System.

Introduction

Ambulatory blood pressure monitoring is now often used in the evaluation and treatment of hypertensive patients. The multiple blood pressures obtained using such monitoring systems usually are summarized as means and standard deviations of all data, or they are graphically displayed in relation to the actual time of the blood pressure measurement. At present, only a few computer programs are available for the evaluation of data obtained during long-term ambulatory blood pressure monitoring.

In this paper, we present a new hardware and software program which can be used to retrieve data from the Del Mar Avionic Pressurometer III system. In addition, the program presented here will allow the user to edit data and to perform statistical and graphical analysis using an Apple IIe computer system.

Method

The interface between the Apple computer and the Del Mar Avionics Pressurometer III Ambulatory Blood Pressure Monitor was designed using information obtained from the service manuals for each of the two components. The hardware required to accomplish the interfacing was built from commercially available materials. The software to support

---

* Department of Hypertension and Nephrology
** Department of Biomedical Engineering
  The Cleveland Clinic Foundation

the system interface was then developed and tested by us at The Cleveland Clinic. Testing the system involved repetitive data transfers and data manipulation using both the Del Mar Avionics Blood Pressurometer Charter, Model 1979, and the interface developed at The Cleveland Clinic. Ten sets of raw data were transferred using both systems: first, the Del Mar Model 1979 and secondly, the interface designed by us. After the transfers were made, all data sets were compared for possible error in our software design. The same ten sets of data were then used to test our program designed to manipulate the data once it was transferred into BASIC. The software was designed to do standard deviations, means, and counts on the total 24-hour data collection. We ran our program using these data sets and then compared these results with manually calculated results. Our program was also designed to accomodate data storage and retrieval to and from a floppy disk. The program was run to test these functions for possible data losses.

Graphic displays of analyzed data were made possible by providing the ability to structure files compatible with the commercial package VISITREND/VISIPLOT.

Technical Discussion

System Hardware

The Del Mar Avionics PIII contains its own on-board microprocessor, an RCA 1802. The PIII accumulates data from the ambulatory pressure measurements in a solid state memory which is maintained by an auxilliary battery when the PIII is turned off or the main battery removed. The auxilliary battery loses charge during times when the PIII is turned off and the data are lost after 24 to 48 hours if they are not recovered within this time.

The blood pressure data can be recovered, however, by any computer with an appropriate parallel interface. Software in the PIII will respond to requests from the host computer and transfer the data. At The Cleveland Clinic, we used an off-the-shelf parallel interface card made for the Apple II series computers. A second card was farbricated in-house which contains buffers to protect the PIII outputs and also allows for interconnection of the Apple and the PIII. A block diagram of the system is shown in Figure 1. The entire interface could be easily built onto a single interface card if the loss of two slots in the Apple is not possible in a given installation.

System Software

A machine language program handles the actual transfer of data from the PIII to the Apple. This part of the software generates the required 'handshaking' or communications signals for the transfer. From the first 'byte' of information transferred from the PIII, the program determines how many data sets are available, transfers the appropriate number of bytes from the PIII, and stores the data in the Apple II memory. The data transferred includes the systolic and diastolic pressures, the heart rate, and the time the reading was made. The time is given by a number that indicates the amount of time passed since the PIII was last reset.

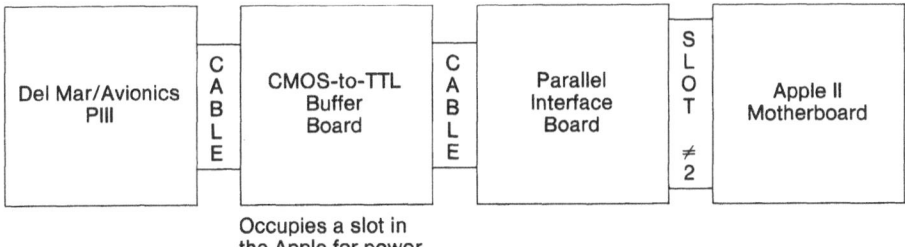

Occupies a slot in
the Apple for power.

Fig. 1. Apple II/Avionics PIII Interface, Block Diagram.

The most important part of the program is written in Applesoft BASIC. This program recovers the data from the storage area of the machine language program, allows calculations and manipulation of the data, and stores the data onto floppy disk for more permanent storage. The BASIC program is compiled to provide greater speed of execution than is possible for an uncompiled Applesoft program.

The program Main Menu (Fig. 2), shows the options available to the operator of the program. When first started, the study name, edit number, and patient name will be empty. The study name will be filled in if the data acceptance parameters are changed from the default values. The edit number is changed when data from the PIII is edited. The patient name is filled in after data is loaded from the PIII or if data is loaded from an existing disk file. When data is to be loaded from the PIII, the operator is asked the starting date and time of the data collection and the number of data sets collected each hour. After data has been transfered from the PIII, the patient demographic data and information about the equipment used is collected (Fig. 3). The statistics are calculated using the current acceptance parameters and the program stores the data to disk.

Fig. 2. Main Menu

```
              Program Main Menu

          Ambulatory blood pressure analysis
          (1) Load data from pressurometer
          (2) Edit acceptance Parameters
          (3) Edit pressure data
          (4) Load pressure data from disk
          (5) Print report
          (6) Create VISIPLOT files
          (7) Edit demographics information
          (8) Print demographics catalog

          (0) Exit program

       Study: _____      Edit number _____

       Patient: _____

          Enter your selection by number _____
```

Fig. 3. Patient Demographics.

```
                    Demographic Screen
                Patient demographic information
            Last name  _____
            First name  _____
        Clinic number  _____
                  Age  _____
                  Sex  _____

    Monitor number  _____        Cuff Number  ____
            Cable  _____

    Battery number  _____      Voltage in   ____
                                   Voltage out  ____
```

The acceptance parameters for the statistical analysis of the data may be changed using Menu Option 2 (Fig. 4). A study name is given to each revision of the acceptance parameters and those parameters stored to disk. The revised parameters may be called into the program at any time using the study name. The minimum and maximum acceptable values for the systolic, diastolic, and pulse pressures and heart rate may be altered as desired. A heart rate of exactly zero may be allowed, which can be used to accept data taken without the ECG cable. The Marker feature allows data within the range specified on the screen to be marked on the report of the data. If data is present in the program, statistics are recalculated using the new acceptance parameters and the statistical results may be stored to disk if desired.

Our program allows the actual data from the PIII to be altered by selecting Option 3 in the Main Menu. This is useful in eliminating artifactual data before creating the VISI-PLOT compatible files used for generating graphics. Data edited by this option is marked in the report and is stored on disk as a new file, the actual data from the PIII is never lost.

Fig. 4. Acceptance Parameters.

```
                Data Acceptance/Marker Screen
                  Data acceptance parameters

                    Acceptance      Markers
                    min    max      min    max

    Systolic        50__   255      0____  0____
    Diastolic       30__   150      0____  0____
    Heart rate      30__   220      0____  0____
    Allow heart rate = 0:  yes

    If syst. ≥ 100 then pulse press.       12__
    If syst. ≤ 100 then pulse press.       6__

    Study name: _____

    Edit or enter return for next field
```

Option 4 loads pressure data from the disk when given the patient name, study name, and edit number. This data can then be edited, new reports run, and new statistics calculated just as with data loaded from the PIII. A report from the program is shown in Figure 5. The report includes the maximum, minimum, and mean for pressures and heart rate and the standard deviations for the data set. A listing of the pressure data is provided that includes marking of data that is considered artifactual under the present acceptance parameters. In future reports the marker system described above will be implemented. In addition, frequency histograms for the data will be available as well.

Graphics are provided for by creating files that may be used by the VISIPLOT program available from VisiCorp. The pressures, heart rate, and the histogram data (when available) are incorporated into a file that can be read by the VISIPLOT program. Presently, the VISOPLOT file can contain only 150 data sets which must appear at regular inter-

---

Cleveland Clinic Foundation
Department of Hypertension and Nephrology

Report of Ambulatory Blood Pressure Monitoring

Report Date: 11–17–83

Name: AAVO PUUSSAAR
Clinic number: 1–158–439–0
Age: 46
Sex: male

Diagnosis:

Monitoring began at 11:20 hrs on 11–16–83, and lasted 24 hours and 17 minutes.

95 pressure readings were satisfactory out of 101 attempted.

Readings were taken each 15 minutes.

Systolic Pressures:
The lowest systolic pressure occurred at 3:54 hrs, when the BP was 67/54.
The highest systolic pressure occurred at 11:58 hrs, when the BP was 160/84.
The mean systolic pressure was 110.46 ± 16.66 (S.D.)

Diastolic pressures:
The lowest diastolic pressure occurred at 3:40 hrs, when the BP was 72/49.
The highest diastolic pressure occurred at 15:12 hrs, when the BP was 132/108.
The mean diastolic pressure was 78.79 ± 10.69 (S.D.)

Heart Rate:
The lowest rate occurred at 3:54 hrs. The rate was 60, the BP was 67/54.
The highest rate occurred at 13:43 hrs. The rate was 125, the BP was 139/86.
The mean heart rate was 81.98 ± 11.97 (S.D.)

Is Diurnal Fluctuation Normal? _____

Comments:

Technician _____   Physician _____

Fig. 5. Report of BP Analysis.

vals. This means that data collection must be adjusted so that all the data for analysis will be contained within 150 data sets or that data must be dropped from the beginning or end of the collection. Our program drops data from the first hour and from the end of the collection if there is more data than can be accomodated by VISIPLOT. The histogram graphics data will never contain more than 150 points so that the entire collection is represented in the histogram plot. A sample of the graphics output from VISIPLOT is shown in Figure 6.

All of the demographic information is collected in a simple file on each disk by our program. Option 7 allows the demographic information to be edited if required and Option 8 will print a catalog of the patient data available on a single disk.

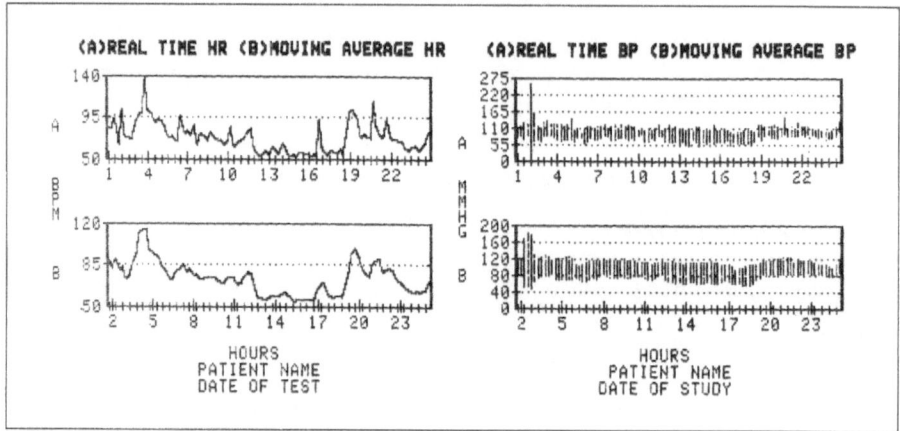

Fig. 6. VISIPLOT graphic Representation

Discussion

The purpose of this interface and supportive software development has been to provide users of the Del Mar Avionics PIII System an alternative method of more fully analyzing collected data. The interface we have developed is a definite addition due to the easy to use software that supports it. The ten data sets we tested initially allowed us the ability to detect major as well as minor changes necessary in the software, and further development continues. Our software allows the user to transfer data with ease and accuracy from the PIII to the Apple computer. Other functions provided for are: first, editing of data points; second, editing demographic data on each file; third, changing editing parameters for acceptance or rejection of data; fourth, storage of a data file to disk; fifth, retrieving a data file from disk; and sixth, creating a VISIPLOT file. By providing the community of blood pressure investigators with yet another alternative method of rapidly accessing raw data to the computer for analysis, we feel that anyone wishing to do serious studies of blood pressure can be accommodated with adequate equipment at moderate expense. This also provides an easy method of sharing data with coleagues by simply sharing floppy disks loaded with the data. Another advantage we have experienced since the development is that of faster report generation to the physician. What took us several hours to accomplish in the past, now takes us approximately 15–20 minutes. The present and future advancement of hypertensive study and research at The Cleveland Clinic has benefited greatly by this interface development.

Technical bibliography

Apple Computer, Inc.: Apple II Reference Manual. Apple Computer, Inc. (Cupertino, Calif. 1981).
Apple Computer, Inc.: Apple IIe Reference Manual. Apple Computer, Inc. (Cupertino, Calif. 1982).
Apple Computer, Inc.: Applesoft Reference Manual. Apple Computer, Inc. (Cupertino, Calif. 1981).
Del Mar Avionics, Inc.: Preliminary Service Manual, Pressurometer III System. Del Mar Avionics, Inc. (Irvine, Calif. 1981).
SSM Microcomputer Products, Inc.: Users Manual, AIO-II Serial and Parallel Interface. SSM Microcomputer Products, Inc. (San Jose, Calif.).
Zaks Rodney: Programming the 6502. Sybex, Inc. (Berkeley, Calif. 1980).

Address for correspondence:
Ray W. Gifford, Jr., M.D.
Department of Hypertension and Nephrology
The Cleveland Clinic Foundation
9500 Euclid Avenue
Cleveland, OH 44106

Blood pressure fluctuation and amplitude in normal human subjects

Michael A. Weber, Jan I.M. Drayer, Eleanor R. Chard

Summary: Whole-day ambulatory blood pressure monitoring utilizing a portable non-invasive device (Pressurometer III) was performed in 34 normal subjects undertaking their usual activities at work and at home. To evaluate reproducibility, the monitoring procedure was repeated two to six weeks later in each subject. For all subjects together, the averages of the whole-day systolic or diastolic blood pressures on the two study days were not different from each other. For further analysis, each study day was divided into 12 two-hour periods; within each participant, the highest and lowest two-hour averages for systolic and diastolic blood pressures, and the times at which they occurred, were then identified. For the group as a whole, there were no differences between the two study days in the averages of the highest and lowest blood pressure values; moreover, the averages of the times at which they occurred corresponded closely. The blood pressure amplitudes, defined as the differences between the highest and lowest values during the day for each subject, were also similar on the two study days. Thus, as measured by the highest and lowest points of the circadian blood pressure fluctuations, the whole-day time-blood pressure pattern appears to be reproducible from day to day. Of interest is the fact that the amplitudes correlated closely with the standard deviations (regarded as indices of hour-to-hour variability) of the full 24-hour blood pressure averages, indicating that there might be a relationship between short-term blood pressure changes and the pattern of blood pressure for the day as a whole.

Introduction

The availability of portable non-invasive techniques for the automated repetitive measurement of blood pressure enables ambulatory monitoring to be performed in active human subjects. The potential for better understanding blood pressure patterns, and for the clinical assessment of patients with hypertension, has led to several studies that have utilized this technology. Ambulatory monitoring has been employed to assess the validity of conventional blood pressure measurements (1, 2), and to examine clinically important conditions such as left ventricular hypertrophy (3, 4) or the effects of age on the characteristics of hypertension (5). Beyond these physiologic purposes, ambulatory blood pressure monitoring has been used to evaluate the efficacy and duration of antihypertensive therapy (6, 7, 8).

Data based on normal subjects, however, has become available only recently (9). Clearly, knowledge about normal blood pressure patterns is necessary before hypertensive states can be adequately described and diagnosed. Simple and practical indices of the whole-day blood pressure pattern include the documentation of highest and lowest blood pressure values, and the differences between them (amplitude).

Section of Clinical Pharmacology and Hypertension Veterans Administration Medical Center Long Beach, California and the University of California Irvine, California

One of the major factors in assessing the validity and reliability of this technology is to test whether it is reproducible within individuals. In this study we have performed 24-hour blood pressure monitoring on two separate days, several weeks apart, in a group of normal human volunteers. We have assessed the reproducibility of the actual measurements of the highest and lowest blood pressure values throughout the day, and the times at which they occurred. We have also evaluated the reproducibility of the amplitude of the blood pressure fluctuation throughout the day, and have analyzed its relationship to other blood pressure measurements during the monitoring periods.

Methods

Ambulatory blood pressure monitoring was carried out in 34 normal male volunteers, aged 26 to 60 years. The participants in the study were all in excellent health, without history or physical findings of significant clinical abnormalities. Blood pressure, measured by a conventional mercury sphygmomanometer, was less than 140 mmHg systolic and less than 90 mmHg diastolic in the supine posture.

Automated blood pressure monitoring was carried out in each patient on two separate occasions. Measurements were carried out with a Pressurometer III (Del Mar Avionics, Irvine, California) set to measure and record blood pressure and heart rate every 7.5 min throughout a full 24 h period. The accuracy of the system was cross-checked against a mercury sphygmomanometer at the beginning of the monitoring period; a discrepancy of 5 mmHg or greater was considered unacceptable, and any necessary adjustments were made to the Pressurometer equipment so as to ensure a closer concordance between the two blood pressure measuring methods. The ambulatory monitoring was undertaken for a full day with the patient performing his usual work duties during the day and then going home in his normal fashion at night. Between two and eight weeks (average: 6 weeks) after the first full 24 h monitoring period, a second identical study was performed in each participant.

The full 24 h recording was divided into 12 consecutive two-hour periods for the purpose of analysis. For each two-hour period, the individual blood pressure and heart rate readings (usually 16 for each two-hour period) were averaged as a representation of that period. The specific analyses used in this study are described in more detail in the Results section.

Results

The average of the blood pressures for the day as a whole for each patient were obtained by calculating the mean of all twelve two-hour periods for both systolic and diastolic blood pressure. For all 34 subjects together, the average ($\pm$ S.D.) systolic blood pressure during the first study day was 122 ± 11 mmHg, which was not significantly different from the average of 120 ± 13 mmHg during the second monitoring period. Similarly, the respective values for the diastolic blood pressure, 76 ± 7 mmHg and 74 ± 9 mmHg, were not different from each other.

Within each patient, the two-hour periods during which the highest average systolic and diastolic blood pressures occurred and during which the lowest average systolic and diastolic blood pressures occurred were identified. For the 34 patients together, the averages of the highest and lowest blood pressure values during the first study day and the second study day are shown in Table 1. There were no differences between the highest values for either systolic or diastolic blood pressures between the two study days; similarly, there were no differences between the lowest systolic and diastolic blood pressures during the two study days. Thus, the average values for the highest and lowest blood pressures during the two study days appear to be highly consistent. Fig. 1 is a representation of 24 h clocks on which are indicated the average times at which the highest and lowest systolic and diastolic blood pressures occurred during the two 24 h study periods. The average time at which the highest diastolic blood pressure occurred during the second study day was just significantly different ($p < 0.05$) from that on the first study day; however, the times of the lowest diastolic blood pressures, and both the highest and lowest systolic blood pressures, were not different between the two days.

On each study day within each individual patient, the amplitude of the systolic and diastolic blood pressures was defined to be the difference between the averages of the highest and lowest two-hour periods. For all 34 patients together, the systolic blood pressure amplitude on the first study day was 36 ± 22 (SD) mmHg, which was not dif-

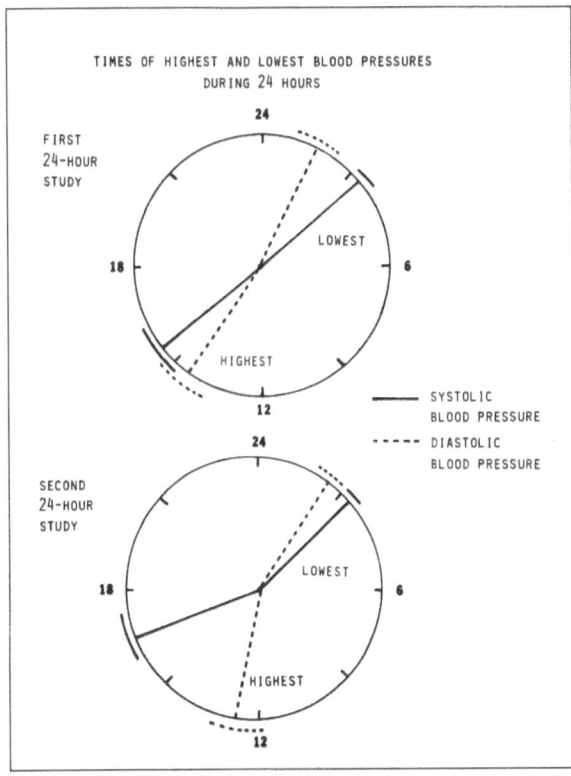

Fig. 1. The times at which the highest and lowest systolic and diastolic blood pressures occurred during two separate 24 h periods of ambulatory blood pressure monitoring in 34 normal human subjects. The values portrayed on the 24 h clocks are mean ± S.D. (shown as the short lines outside the clock faces) values. Significances of differences between the corresponding times on the two study days are given in the text.

45

Table 1: Averages of the highest and lowest blood pressure values observed during two separate days of automated blood pressure monitoring. Values are mean + S.D., n = 34.

	Systolic blood pressure		Diastolic blood pressure	
	First study day	Second study day	First study day	Second study day
Highest value (mmHg)	137 ± 14	135 ± 15	86 ± 8	86 ± 10
Lowest value (mmHg)	102 ± 10	100 ± 12	61 ± 9	58 ± 11

Table 2: Correlation coefficients (r values) between the systolic or diastolic blood pressure amplitudes (difference between highest and lowest values during the day) and various measurements of blood pressure during the 24h study day in 34 normal human subjects.

	Systolic blood pressure		Diastolic blood pressure	
	First study day	Second sudy day	First study day	Second study day
Casual	0.56***	0.49**	0.25	−0.07
24h mean	0.47**	0.34*	0.03	−0.10
Standard deviation of 24h mean	0.96***	0.96***	0.86***	0.90***
Daytime mean	0.64***	0.50**	0.26	0.08
Nighttime mean	0.01	0.01	−0.39*	−0.37*

* $p < 0.05$; ** $p < 0.01$; *** $p < 0.001$

ferent from the value of 35 ± 11 mmHg on the second study day. The respective diastolic amplitudes, of 25 ± 8 mmHg and 28 ± 8 mmHg, also were not different. Correlations between the systolic and diastolic blood pressure amplitudes and various parameters of blood pressure throughout the two study days are summarized in Table 2. For systolic blood pressure, the amplitude correlated significantly (on both study days) with casual blood pressure (as measured by a conventional mercury sphygmomanometer at the start of the ambulatory blood pressure monitoring period), as well as with the full 24 h blood pressure average, with the standard deviation of the full 24 h blood pressure average, and with the average of all blood pressures during the daytime period (6.00 a.m to 10.00 p.m). The systolic blood pressure amplitude did not correlate, however, with the average of blood pressure during the nighttime period (10.00 p.m. to 6.00 a.m.). For diastolic blood pressure, the amplitude did not correlate with the casual blood pressures, or with the full 24 h blood pressure average or the daytime blood pressure average. It did correlate directly, however, with the standard deviation of the 24 h blood pressure average, and it also correlated significantly (but inversely) with the average of the nighttime blood pressures during the two 24 h monitoring periods. The relationship between the systolic and diastolic blood pressure amplitude and the standard deviations of the full 24 h blood pressure averages are shown graphically in Fig. 2 and 3. Additionally, in Fig. 4 (for the first study day only), are shown the relationships between the systolic blood pressure amplitude and the average of the daytime systolic blood pressures, and also between the diastolic blood pressure amplitude and the average of the nighttime diastolic blood pressures.

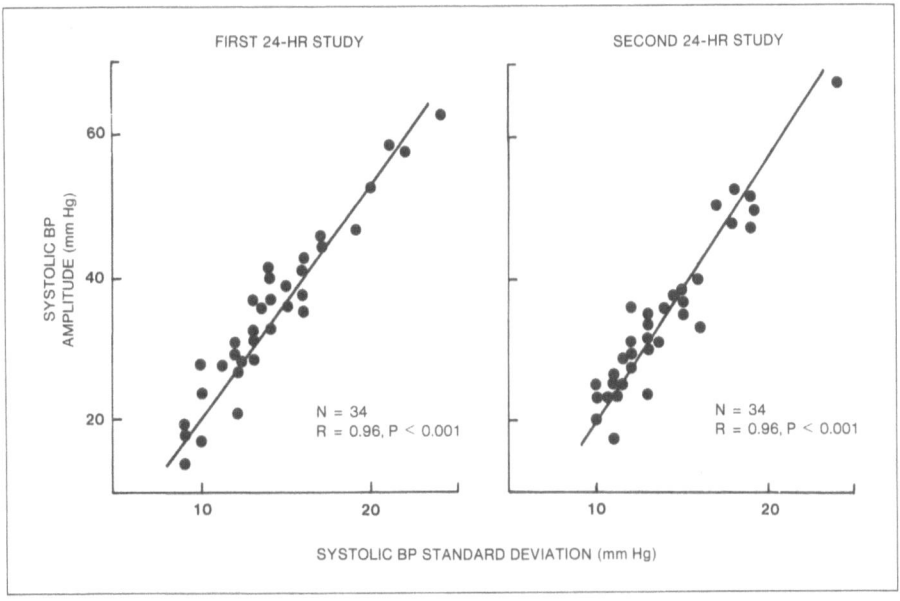

Fig. 2. Relationships between the standard deviations of the 24 h systolic blood pressure averages and the systolic blood pressure amplitudes (differences between highest and lowest values during the day) in 34 normal subjects undergoing whole-day ambulatory blood pressure monitoring on two separate study days.

Discussion

In a previous communication (10) we reported on the reproducibility of blood pressures measured in hypertensive patients during full 24 h monitoring periods in a controlled in-hospital setting. In the small group of patients studied, the average blood pressures on the two monitoring days, as in the present study, were closely similar, but there was variability between patients. Some individuals tended to have blood pressure averages during the two study days that were closely similar, but in others there ap-

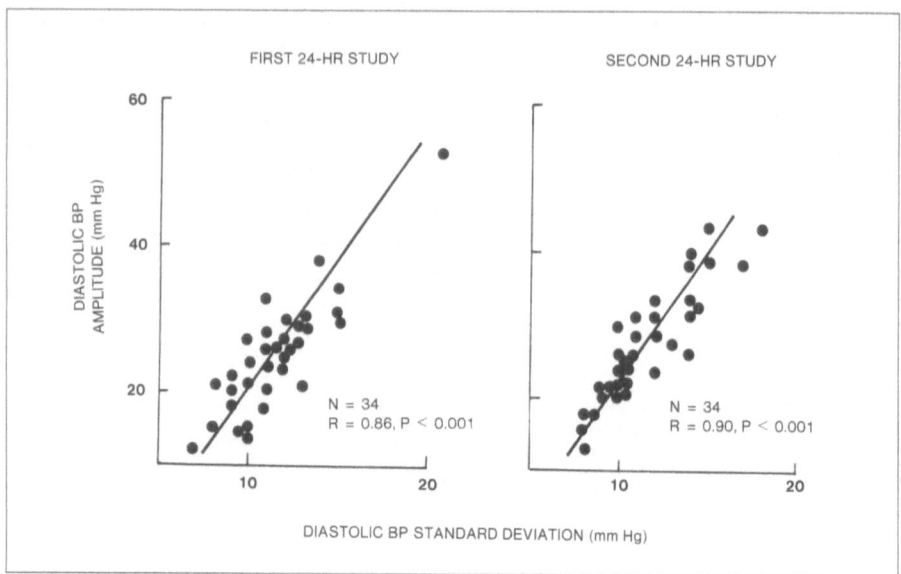

Fig. 3. Relationship between the standard deviations of the 24 h diastolic blood pressure averages and the diastolic blood pressure amplitudes (differences between highest and lowest values during the day) in 34 normal subjects undergoing whole-day ambulatory blood pressure monitoring on two separate study days.

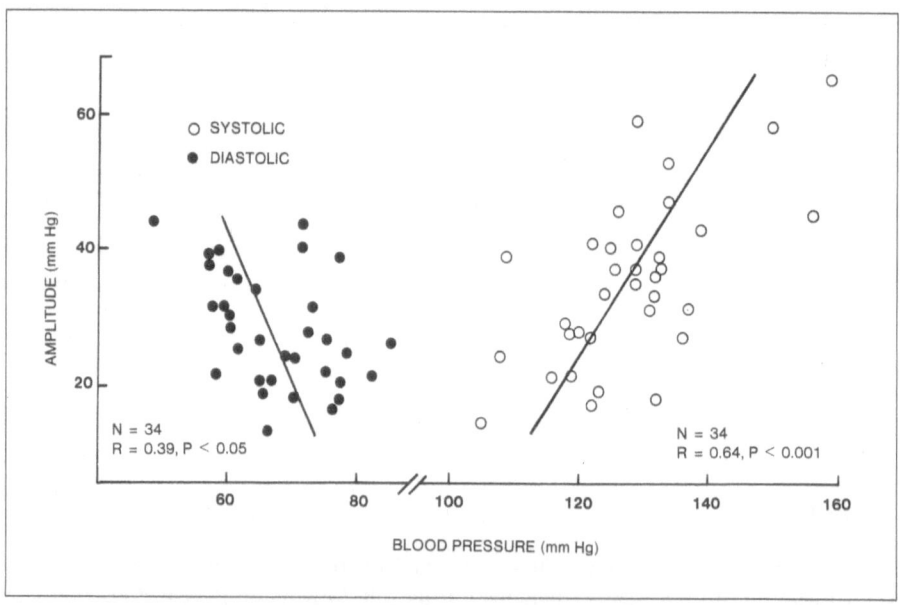

Fig. 4. Relationships between the systolic blood pressure amplitudes (differences between the highest and lowest values during the whole day) and the averages of the daytime (6.00 a.m. to 10.00 p.m.) systolic blood pressures, and between the diastolic blood pressure amplitudes and the averages of the nighttime (10.00 p.m. to 6.00 a.m.) diastolic blood pressures. Data are shown for 34 normal subjects undergoing whole-day ambulatory blood pressure monitoring.

peared to be marked differences. There were not sufficient patients, however, to adequately test the reproducibility of the blood pressure pattern itself by examining criteria such as highest or lowest blood pressure values or amplitudes.

In the present investigation, which was based on ambulatory normal volunteers, the overall systolic and diastolic blood pressure averages for the two study days were also closely similar. Moreover, the averages of the highest and lowest blood pressure values were reproducible for the patients as a whole. This applied both to the actual values of the highest and lowest blood pressure measurements as well as to the times of day at which they occurred. Using this simple analytic approach it is reasonable to conclude that one of the key characteristics of the circadian blood pressure pattern, the extremes of the blood pressure values and the times of day at which they occurred, were consistent from one monitoring period to another. This finding not only helps validate the technology used for obtaining the blood pressure data, but also suggests that qualitative characteristics of the blood pressure contour might be sufficiently well defined to allow for future classification techniques that could be based upon the shape of the time-blood pressure curve itself.

In this study, the amplitudes of the blood pressures were defined simply as being the differences between the highest and lowest two-hour systolic and diastolic blood pressure averages during the full 24 h periods. For both systolic and diastolic blood pressures, the average amplitudes were consistent from one study day to the next, confirming the findings with the highest and lowest blood pressure readings. Of particular interest is the fact that the systolic blood pressure amplitude correlated significantly with the full 24 h blood pressure average, as well as with the casual blood pressure readings and the daytime readings. These three indices of blood pressure have been shown previously by us to be quite closely related to each other (5, 11), and it is thus not surprising that there was only a minimal difference between the correlations linking each of them and with systolic blood pressure amplitude. It is of interest, however, that the correlation between the systolic amplitude and the nighttime readings was very weak, and suggests that a factor linking the systolic amplitude and the other indices of blood pressure might be based, at least to some extent, upon the greater variability of blood pressure that occurs during the waking hours. In contrast, the diastolic blood pressure amplitude did not correlate significantly with any of the blood pressure measurements that had been significant for the systolic blood pressure amplitude. In fact, the diastolic blood pressure amplitude was related solely to the nighttime blood pressure average, where the correlation coefficient actually was negative. This suggests that the diastolic blood pressure amplitude is influenced primarily by nighttime diastolic readings; in particular, the lower these values are at night, the greater is the amplitude of diastolic blood pressure for the day as a whole. This differs from the systolic blood pressure, where the positive correlation with the daytime readings indicates that the greatest systolic blood pressure amplitudes are caused by systolic blood pressure readings during the daytime hours. Although highly speculative, it might be possible to consider the idea that systolic and diastolic blood pressures throughout the day may be influenced by differing factors that are operative at separate times of the day.

For both the systolic and diastolic blood pressure amplitudes, there was a strong and highly significant correlation with the standard deviation of the full 24 h blood pressure mean. The standard deviation was derived from the mean of all blood pressures throughout the day, and thus represents an index of minute-to-minute blood pressure variability throughout the day. Thus, the findings of close relationships between the standard deviations and the blood pressure amplitudes suggests that the variability of blood pressure, on a comparatively short-term basis, is highly predictive of the spread of blood pressure observations for the day as a whole. Although the full physiological significance of this finding is not clear, it does suggest that short-Term blood pressure variability might be a determinant of the overall blood pressure pattern.

References

1. Floras JS, Jones JV, Hassan MO, Osikowska B, Sever PS, Sleight P: Cuff and ambulatory blood pressure in subjects with essential hypertension. Lancet 1: 107 (1981).
2. Sokolow M, Werdegar D, Kain HK, Hinman AT: Relationship between level of blood pressure measured casually and by portable recorders and severity of complications in essential hypertension. Circulation 34: 279 (1966).
3. Drayer JIM, Weber MA, DeYoung JL: Blood pressure as a determinant of cardiac left ventricular muscle mass. Archives Int Med 143: 90–92 (1982).
4. Devereux RB, Pickering TG, Harshfield GA, Sachs I, Jason M, Hollis DK, Laragh JH: Relation of hypertension left ventricular hypertrophy to 24-hour blood pressure (abstract). Circulation 64 (suppl. II): 321 (1981).
5. Drayer JIM, Weber MA, DeYoung JL, Wyle FA: Circadian blood pressure patterns in ambulatory hypertensive patients. Am J Med 73: 493–499 (1982).
6. Drayer JIM, Weber MA, DeYoung JL, Brewer DD: Long-term blood pressure monitoring in the evaluation of antihypertensive therapy. Archives Int Med 143: 898–901 (1983).
7. Millar-Craig MW, Mann S, Kenny D, Raftery EB: The effect of once daily atenolol on ambulatory blood pressure. Br Med J 1: 237 (1979).
8. Gould BA, Mann S, Kieso H, Subramanian VB, Raftery EB: The 24-hour ambulatory blood pressure profile with verapamil. Circulation 65: 22 (1982).
9. Kennedy HL, Horan MJ, Sprague MK, Padgett NE, Shriver KK: Ambulatory blood pressure in healthy normotensive males. Am Heart J 106: 717–722 (1983).
10. Weber MA, Drayer JIM, Wyle FA, DeYoung JL: Reproducibility of the wholeday blood pressure pattern in essential hypertension. Clin. Exp. Hypertension A4: 1377–1390 (1982).
11. Weber MA, Drayer JIM, Wyle FA, Brewer DD: A representative value for the whole-day blood pressure. JAMA 248: 1626–1628 (1982).

Address for correspondence:
Michael A. Weber, M.D.
VA Medical Center (W130)
5901 East Seventh Street
Long Beach, California 90822
USA

Accuracy and reproducibility of ambulatory blood pressure recorder measurements during rest and exercise

Ann Ward and Peter Hanson

Summary: Blood pressure (BP) readings obtained by an Avionics ambulatory BP monitoring device (ABPM) were compared with values obtained simultaneously by auscultation (AUSC) in 14 non-hypertensive individuals on two separate days during the following standardized conditions: (1) 15 minute supine rest (SU), (2) 2 minute standing rest (ST), (3) 90 second isometric handgrip at 50% max. (HG), (4) submaximum bicycle exercise at 50, 75, 100, and 125 Watts (BEX). Pearson product moment correlations between ABPM and AUSC on Day 1 for systolic pressures (SBP) ranged from 0.92 to 0.96 during SU, ST and HG and was 0.92 during BEX, while diastolic pressures (DBP) were 0.74 to 0.93 during SU, ST, and HG and 0.60 during BEX. Correlations between ABPM and AUSC on Day 2 were similar to Day 1. The correlations between Day 1 and Day 2 for SBP measured by ABPM were 0.68 to 0.80 during SU, ST and HG and 0.89 during BEX and were similar to the reproducibility of AUSC readings (SU, ST and HG = 0.70 to 0.76, BEX = 0.93). The correlations between Day 1 and Day 2 for DBP during SU, ST and HG were 0.53 to 0.59 for ABPM and 0.63 to 0.79 for AUSC. During BEX correlations for DBP were 0.61 for ABPM and 0.28 for AUSC. In conclusion, these data indicate an overall high level of accuracy and reproducibility for ABPM at rest and during moderate levels of activity.

Introduction

Ambulatory blood pressure monitoring (ABPM) has recently been utilized for evaluation of patients with suspected hypertension (1–4) and to document the efficacy of antihypertensive therapy (5). This method provides a detailed record of average blood pressure (BP) and BP variation during activities of daily living and avoids observer error and transient BP elevations which are well known sources of measurement error in casual BP recorded during clinic visits (l).

Previous reports have shown good correlation between ABPM and standard auscultatory BP measurements at rest and low levels of exercise (6–8). However, the accuracy and reproducibility of ABPM has not been studied over a wide range of physical activities which occur in patients during monitoring conditions.

In this report we compare ABPM to auscultatory readings (AUSC) during standardized conditions of supine and orthostatic rest, isometric handgrip and submaximum bicycle exercise on two sequential days.

Cardiology Section Department of Medicine University of Wisconsin Medical School Madison, Wisconsin

Supported by funds from the Department of Medicine Research Committee

Methods

Recorder characteristics

The Del Mar Avionics Pressurometer III Model 1978 (ABPM) is a battery-powered, portable, non-invasive device which measures and records systolic blood pressure (SBP), diastolic blood pressure (DBP) and heart rate (HR) in programmed intervals of 7.5, 15 or 30 min over a 24 h period. The recording system includes a pressure transducer positioned over the brachial artery and standard pneumatic cuff wrapped snugly around the arm and transducer. A bipolar electrocardiogram (ECG) (CM$_5$ lead configuration) is used for HR and also provides a gating signal for appropriate filtering of pressure transducer signals.

Subjects

Fourteen nonhypertensive individuals (6 males and 8 females), aged 25.7 ± 2.6 years, participated in this investigation. The mean height and weight for these subjects were 171.7 ± 9.1 cm and 63.7 ± 10.3 Kg, respectively. No individuals exhibited contraindications to exercise as defined by accepted guidelines (9).

Protocol

Reproducibility of BP recordings by ABPM was tested in each subject twice within one week at approximately the same time of day. All subjects were instructed not to exercise prior to the evaluation and not to eat, drink coffee, or smoke for at least three hours prior to the evalution.
After ABPM was connected to the subject, the accuracy of the monitor was checked by measuring BP by AUSC concurrently with ABPM with an in-line mercury manometer. With the instrument in the test mode the ABPM pump inflates the cuff, but deflation rate is controlled by the deflation valve manually. Differences of 5 mm Hg or less between AUSC and ABPM for two BP values while sitting and two BP values while standing were considered acceptable.
After calibration, BP was measured simultaneously by ABPM and AUSC using the in-line manometer under the following standardized conditions:
1. Supine rest (SU): 15 min
2. Standing rest (ST): 2 min
3. Isometric handgrip (HG): 90 s at 50% maximum grip strength
4. Bicycle exercise (BEX): The third min at each of four submaximal workloads (50, 75, 100 and 125 Watts).
Auscultatory pressures were determined according to American Heart Association Guidelines (10). Systolic pressure was recorded as the first of successive audible sounds. Phase 5 was recorded as DBP for SU, ST, and HG. During BEX, phase 4 was used if phase 5 became indeterminant. Except for three subjects, all blood pressures were measured by one observer.

Data analysis

Time, BP, and HR were printed in a digital record from the Pressurometer by a Model 1979 Blood Pressurometer Charter (Del Mar Avionics). Artifactual BP readings by the ABPM were determined and rejected according to the following criteria:
1) DBP ≥ 120 mm Hg
2) SBP ≤ 80 or ≥ 240 mm Hg
3) Pulse pressure < 20 mm Hg (SBP-DBP)
Pearson product moment correlation coefficients were calculated for SBP and DBP for the following rest and exercise conditions:
1) Day 1: AUSC vs ABPM
2) Day 2: AUSC vs ABPM
3) AUSC: Day 1 vs Day 2
4) ABPM: Day 1 vs Day 2

Results

Figures 1–4 show the comparison between AUSC and ABPM on Day 1. The correlations for SBP were 0.96 during SU, 0.94 during ST, 0.92 for HG and ranged from 0.76 to 0.86 during BEX. The overall correlation for SBP during BEX across workloads was 0.92. The correlations for DBP were 0.93 during SU, 0.74 during ST, 0.88 during HG and ranged from 0.65 to 0.91 during BEX. The overall correlation for DBP across BEX workloads was 0.60.

Similar comparisons were made between AUSC and ABPM on Day 2. The correlations and standard errors were similar to those for Day 1 and thus are not listed here.

The reproducibility of ABPM and AUSC on Day 1 and Day 2 is shown in Table 1. The correlations for ABPM were 0.78 during SU, 0.68 during ST, 0.80 during HG and 0.89 during BEX. The correlations for DBP during these conditions ranged from 0.53 to 0.61.

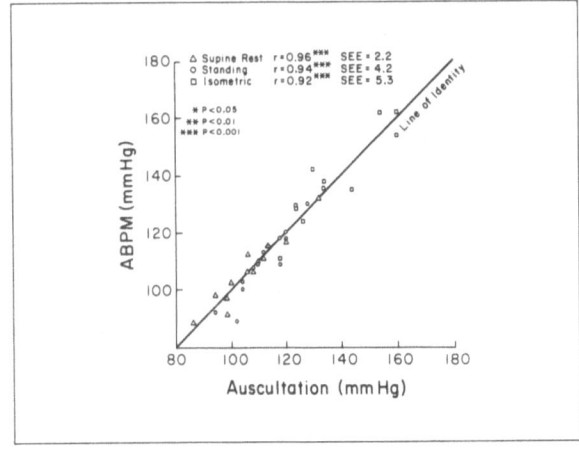

Fig. 1. Relationship between SBP measured simultaneously by auscultation and ABPM during supine rest, standing and isometric exercise.

Fig. 2. Relationship between DBP measured simultaneously by auscultation and ABPM during supine rest, standing and isometric exercise.

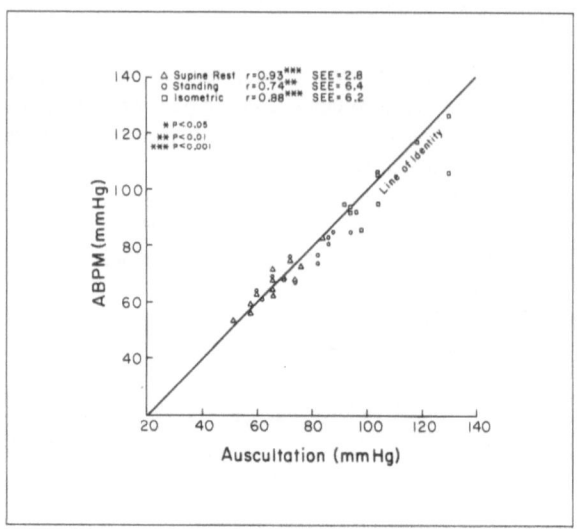

Fig. 3. Relationship between SBP measured simultaneously by auscultation and ABPM during bicycle exercise.

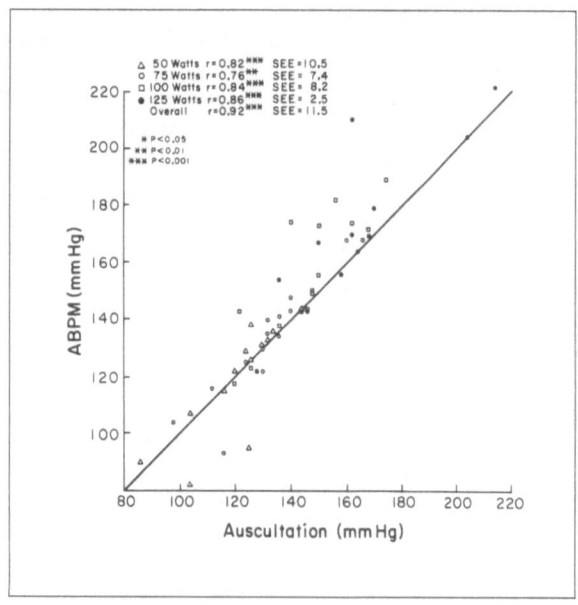

The reproducibility of AUSC for SBP was similar to that of ABPM. These correlations ranged from 0.70 to 0.93. The correlations of AUSC for DBP were higher than those for ABPM except during BEX.

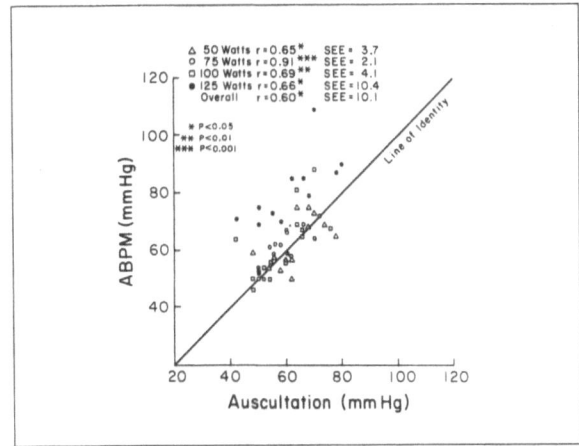

Fig. 4. Relationship between DBP measured simultaneously by auscultation and ABPM during bicycle exercise.

Table 1: Comparison between blood pressures measured by ABPM and auscultation on day 1 and day 2

Method	Condition			
	Supine Rest	Stand	Isometric	Bicycle
ABPM-SBP				
r	0.78**	0.68*	0.80**	0.89**
SEE	6.0	8.2	8.9	11.5
AUSC-SBP				
r	0.70*	0.76**	0.73**	0.93***
SEE	6.3	7.3	9.7	8.7
ABPM-DBP				
r	0.53	0.57	0.59	0.61
SEE	7.5	8.6	9.5	9.5
AUSC-DBP				
r	0.77**	0.79**	0.63*	0.28
SEE	6.7	7.1	7.8	7.2

r = Pearson product moment correlation
SEE = standard error of estimate
* $p < 0.05$
** $p < 0.01$
*** $p < 0.001$

Discussion

Long term ambulatory pressure monitoring can aid in the diagnosis and treatment of hypertension. However, the validity and reliability of the equipment must be determined under the conditions of its use. Harshfield et al found that the Del Mar Avionics Pressurometer provided valid readings compared with a mercury sphygmomanometer during sitting, standing, reclining and walking in place (6). When the reproducibility of whole-day BP pattern was examined in six hypertensive patients in a quiet in-hospital setting, good agreement was found in some patients, while in other patients there were significant differences between baseline and repeat measures (11).

In this study, we compared the Del Mar Avionics Pressurometer with auscultatory pressures over a wider range of activities. Also, we compared the reproducibility of the Pressurometer values on sequential days with the reproducibility of auscultatory pressures during standardized periods of rest and activity.

Our data show that the correlation for SBP between ABPM values and AUSC pressures were excellent during SU, ST and HG and were moderate to good during BEX. The correlations for DBP between ABPM and AUSC during the rest and exercise conditions were moderate to good.

The reproducibility of SBP readings by ABPM from Day 1 to Day 2 was moderate to good during rest and exercise conditions and were similar to the reproducibility of SBP by AUSC. The reproducibility of DBP by ABPM was low during all conditions while the reproducibility of DBP by AUSC was moderate during SU, ST and HG, but very poor during BEX.

In conclusion, these data indicate an overall high level of accuracy and reproducibility for SBP by ABPM at rest and during moderate levels of activity and a moderate level of accuracy and reproducibility for DBP.

References

1. Pickering TG, Harshfield GA, Kleinert HD, Blank S, Laragh JH: Blood pressure during normal daily activities, sleep and exercise. JAMA 247: 992–996 (1982).
2. Littler WA, Honour AJ, Pugsley DJ, Sleight P: Continuous recording of direct arterial pressure in unrestricted patients: Its rôle in the diagnosis and management of high blood pressure. Circulation 51: 1101–1106 (1975).
3. Irving JB, Brush HM, Kerr F: The value of ambulatory monitoring in borderline and established hypertension. Post Grad Med J 52 (Suppl. 7): 137 (1976).
4. Horan MJ, Kennedy HL, Padgett NE: Do borderline hypertensive patients have labile blood pressure? Ann Intern Med 94: 466–468 (1981).
5. Drayer JIM, Weber MA, DeYoung JL, Brewer DO: Longterm BP monitoring in the evaluation of antihypertensive therapy. Arch Intern Med 143: 898–901 (1983).
6. Harshfield GA, Pickering TG, Laragh JH: A validation study of the Del Mar Avionics ambulatory blood pressure system. Ambulatory Electrocardio 1(4): 7–12 (1979).
7. Kennedy HL, Padgett NE, Horan MJ: Performance reliability of the Del Mar Avionics noninvasive ambulatory blood pressure instrument in clinical use. Ambulatory Electrocardio 1(4): 13–18 (1979).
8. Sheps SG, Elveback LR, Close EL, Kleven MK, Bissen C: Evaluation of the Del Mar Avionics automatic ambulatory blood pressure-recording device. Mayo Clin Proc 56: 740–743 (1981).
9. American College of Sports Medicine. Guidelines for Exercise Testing and Training. 2nd Ed. Lea and Febiger (New York 1980).
10. American Heart Association: Recommendations for human blood pressure determination by sphygmomanometer. Hypertension 3(4): 510A (1981).
11. Weber MA, Drayer JIM, Wyle FA, DeYoung JL: Reproducibility of the whole-day blood pressure pattern in essential hypertension. Clin and Exper Hyper A4(8): 1377–1390 (1982).

Address for correspondence:
Dr. Peter Hanson
Cardiology Section University of Wisconsin Clinical Science Center
600 Highland Avenue
Madison, WI 53792

Adaptation to non-invasive continuous blood pressure monitoring

A. C. Pessina, P. Palatini, G. Sperti, L. Cordone, E. Ventura, C. Dal Palù

Summary: In this study, the Pressurometer III (Del Mar Avionics) was used to monitor blood pressure on two occasions in 17 ambulatory hypertensive patients. In 9 patients a placebo was administered between the first and the second monitoring. In the remaining 8 patients, placebo administration was discontinued prior to the first monitoring period.

Casual blood pressure and heart rate were lower during the day of the second blood pressure monitoring in both groups of patients. Similarly, average daytime and nightime blood pressures were lower during the second monitoring in both groups of patients. The differences in daytime or nighttime blood pressures between the two monitoring periods were similar for patients who received a placebo and those who had discontinued placebo therapy prior to the first monitoring period.

The results suggest that hypertensive patients may adapt to monitoring of blood pressure. Blood pressures observed during repeated ambulatory monitorings follow the pattern of casual blood pressures; blood pressures being lower during the second observation. This tendency was observed in the presence as well as in the absence of a placebo. Thus, administration of a placebo does not enhance the adaptation of hypertensive patients to repeated monitoring of blood pressure.

Introduction

A blood pressure response to placebo administration has been shown to occur in hypertensive patients (1, 2, 3). However, a downward trend in blood pressure has also been noted with repeated visits without placebo (4, 5). In both cases the mechanism is probably the same, that is the adaptation to the procedure of blood pressure measurement so that pressures may be raised at first due to the defence reaction (6), and subsequently decrease with the patient becoming more familiar with the physician and the setting. Either procedure has been recommended before starting any drug therapy, especially in subjects diagnosed as mild hypertensives at first contact. In fact many of these subjects are likely to be normotensive after the placebo and/or at the second and third visit.

In the last few years both invasive and non-invasive 24-hour continuous ambulatory blood pressures monitoring techniques have been used which provide much more information on the blood pressure trend of a given patient. The number of blood pressure values which can be obtained is far greater than with the standard sphygmomanometers and blood pressure is not influenced by the presence of the doctor since patients are freely ambulant. For these reasons it has been suggested that these techniques make the administration of placebo or repeated visits unnecessary.

Clinica Medica I, University of Padua

Indeed Gould et al. (7) showed that while casual pressure significantly falls after placebo, corresponding average 24-hour intra-arterial pressure does not. On the other hand Kain et al. (8), using the Remler non-invasive semiautomatic recorder on three successive days, reported a reduction in average 12-hour blood pressure between the first and second day, indicating that adaptation had occurred by the second day. These authors did not give a placebo to their patients. We have recently started using the non-invasive automatic Del Mar Avionics ambulatory recorder which differs in many ways from the Remler and, more importantly in this context, the patient is not required to inflate the cuff at preset time intervals. The reliability of this apparatus compared with that of the Riva-Rocci sphygmomanometer and the intra-arterial Oxford method have been reported elsewhere (9). The aim of the present study is to verify whether the administration of placebo has any effect on average 24-hour blood pressure and on blood pressure variability in patients wearing this equipment and, if it has, whether it merely reflects adaptation to the procedure of blood pressure monitoring.

Patients and methods

17 mild to moderate essential hypertensive patients aged between 19 and 55 years were included in the study. At the onset of the trial all antihypertensive medications were discontinued for at least two weeks. A first group of 9 patients (Group 1) entered a double blind cross-over trial for assessment of the hypotensive effect of once daily administration of two long-acting betablockers. The study design included a 15 day wash-out period at the end of which a 24-hour ambulatory blood pressure monitoring was performed. Patients were then given a placebo tablet in a single morning dose for the following 15 days, after which time they underwent a second ambulatory blood pressure monitoring. Since we observed in these patients a reduction of average 24-hour blood pressure after the placebo, in another group of 8 patients (Group 2) we decided to perform the first ambulatory monitoring at the end of a 15 day placebo period and the second at the end of the following 15 days without placebo. This would have allowed us to know whether the effect of placebo on average 24-hour pressure was simply due to the adaptation to the procedure of blood pressure monitoring.

Before starting the recordings casual blood pressure in each patient was taken as the mean of three consecutive readings. The measurements were made by a physician using a mercury sphygmomanometer connected through a test-jack with the transducer of the monitoring system. With this procedure the reliability of the monitoring apparatus was also verified in each patient.

Blood pressure recording apparatus

The Del Mar Avionics Pressurometer III was used. This is a protable system which operates by automatic inflations and deflations every 7.5 minutes. It consists of a pressurometer provided with a transducer and an inflating pump, an auscultatory cuff and microphone, a five lead electrode system for ECG recording and a tape recording unit.

The tapes are analysed by a scanner which provides a trend of both blood pressure and heart rate and also a digital read-out of each blood pressure value.

Data analysis and statistics

Hourly blood pressure averages were calculated for each recording and the patient's 24-hour blood pressure profile was drawn. In addition average day and night time pressures, calculated from 111.5 ± 18.1 and 57.0 ± 12.9 number of measurements respectively, and their standard deviations, as an index of blood pressure variability (10), were calculated. The results are reported for the two groups separately. To test whether casual and average day and night time pressures recorded after the wash-out period were different from those recorded after placebo, Student's t test for paired data was used.

Results

Group 1: wash-out followed by placebo

A mean fall of systolic casual pressure of 11.4 ± 19.2 mmHg ($p < 0.05$) and of diastolic casual pressure of 6.8 ± 6.9 mmHg ($p < 0.01$) (from 157.0 ± 15.8 / 102.1 ± 8.0 to

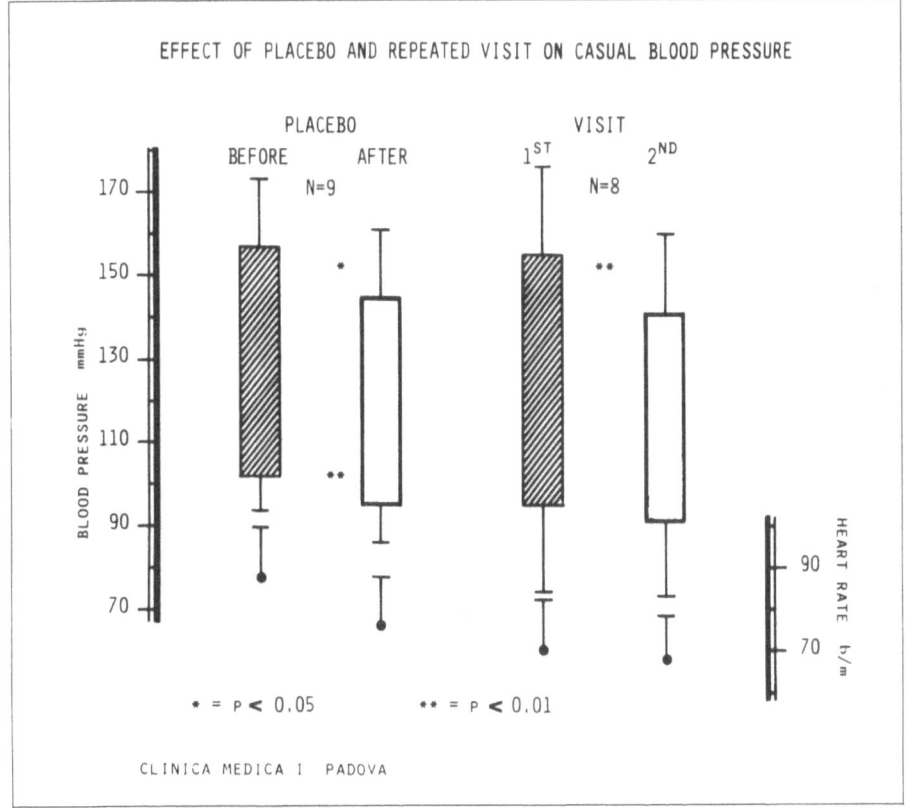

Fig. 1. Fall in casual pressure and heart rate caused by placebo (left) and the repetition of blood pressure measurement (right).

145.6 ± 16.5 / 95.3 ± 9.1 mmHg) was observed in response to placebo (Fig. 1). Heart rate tended to decrease (from 80.6 ± 12.8 to 76.9 ± 11.4 beats/min) but the change was not statistically significant.

Average day time pressure fell by 0.9 ± 7.0 mmHg systolic (N.S.) and by 4.6 ± 3.1 mmHg diastolic (p < 0.05) (from 145.4 ± 11.7 / 92.9 ± 9.6 to 144.6 ± 14.2 / 88.2 ± 9.2 mmHg).

Average night time pressure fell by 0.1 ± 10.2 mmHg systolic (N.S.) and by 8.2 ± 6.7 mmHg diastolic (p < 0.05) (from 126.2 ± 15.0 / 80.7 ± 13.2 to 126.1 ± 16.1 / 72.4 ± 8.8 mmHg) (Fig. 2).

Heart rate tended to decrease during both day and night time (from 81.9 ± 14.3 to 80.1 ± 10.6 beats/min day and from 65.1 ± 8.7 to 64.4± 8.3 beats/min night) but the change did not reach statistical significance. No change in blood pressure variability, as judged by the standard deviation from the mean day and night time pressures, was observed.

Group 2: placebo followed by wash-out

Comparison between the end of placebo administration and the end of wash-out period showed a mean fall of systolic casual pressure of 15.9 ± 18.9 mmHg (p < 0.01) and of diastolic casual pressure of 3.1 ± 6.9 mmHg (N.S.) (from 155.8 ± 21.3 / 94.9 ± 21.1 to 141.0 ± 19.6 / 91.2 ± 18.7 mmHg), as a result of the adaptation to blood pressure measurement (Fig. 2). Heart rate fell from 71.0 ± 11.9 to 68.2 ± 11.4 beats/min (N.S.).

Fig. 2. Mean day time and night time blood pressure and heart rate changes with placebo.

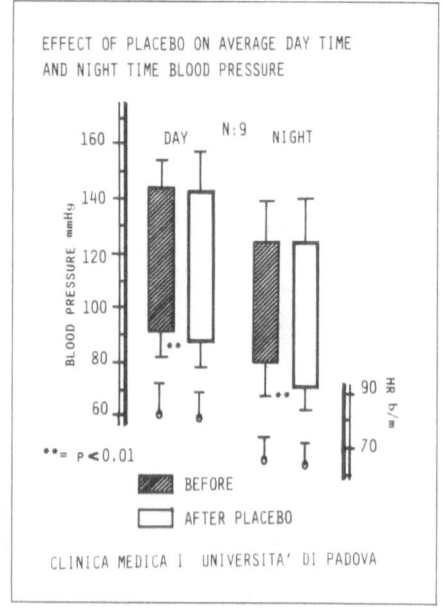

Average day time systolic and diastolic pressure fell by 6.1 ± 5.7 mmHg (p < 0.05) and 2.7 ± 4.3 mmHg (p < 0.05) respectively (from 145.4 ± 17.4 / 91.2 ± 15.5 to 139.7 ± 16.1 / 88.5 ± 14.6 mmHg). Average night time systolic and diastolic pressures decreased by 9.3 ± 11.4 mmHg (p < 0.05) and 2.1 ± 4.2. mmHg (N.S.) (from 131.2 ± 12.4 / 80.8 ± 16.4 to 121.9 ± 18.0 / 79.7 ± 14.5 mmHg) (Fig. 3).

Heart rate remained practically unchanged (from 72.3 ± 7.8 to 73.4 ± 8.3 beats/min day and from 57.4 ± 5.5 to 58.5 ± 5.2 beats/min). As in Group 1 patients, blood pressure variability was unmodified.

Discussion

Our data clearly show that a fall of both casual and to a lesser extent of mean day and night time pressures occur between the first and second time of wearing the non-invasive blood pressure recorder, irrespective of whether the patients had received a placebo.

Two considerations may be made from these results. The first concerns the placebo effect. As the reduction in blood pressure with placebo is similar to that obtained by re-measuring blood pressure, the placebo effect must simply be due to adaptation of the procedure of blood pressure measurement.

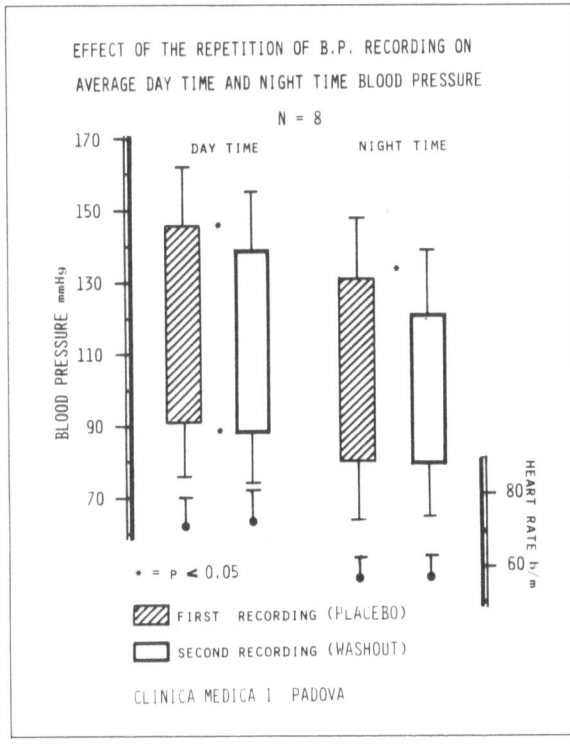

Fig. 3. Mean day time and night time blood pressure and heart rate changes with repetition of blood pressure monitoring.

The second consideration is that this adaptation not only affects casual pressure but also average 24-hour blood pressure.

The obvious explanation for this finding is that, contrary to intra-arterial methods, non-invasive ambulatory monitoring techniques operating through a cuff do induce a defence reaction when they are in operation for the first time. This hypothesis is supported by the observations that the greatest differences in blood pressure between the first and second recording were seen during the first five hours from the application of the apparatus, presumably, as a reaction to the novelty of the equipment, and at night due to the fact that patients could not sleep properly on the first night they were wearing the cuff (Fig. 4).

In conclusion our data show a difference in results between the first and second recordings. However, this difference is relatively small so that it is unlikely to have much relevance for the use which is currently made of this apparatus.

Average blood pressure and blood pressure variability are the two parameters most frequently used to diagnose hypertension, and to predict the risk and check the effectiveness of treatment when continuous blood pressure monitoring techniques are employed. A difference in average day time blood pressure of only 3.3 / 3.6 mmHg and night time pressure of 4.3 / 5.0 mmHg (n = 17) as a result of the adaptation phenomenon, without changes in blood pressure variability, is unlikely to distort this information. Apart from the intra-arterial method, which however is seldom applicable more than once in the same patient, this non-invasive method remains in our opinion the best tool in our hands to obtain these data.

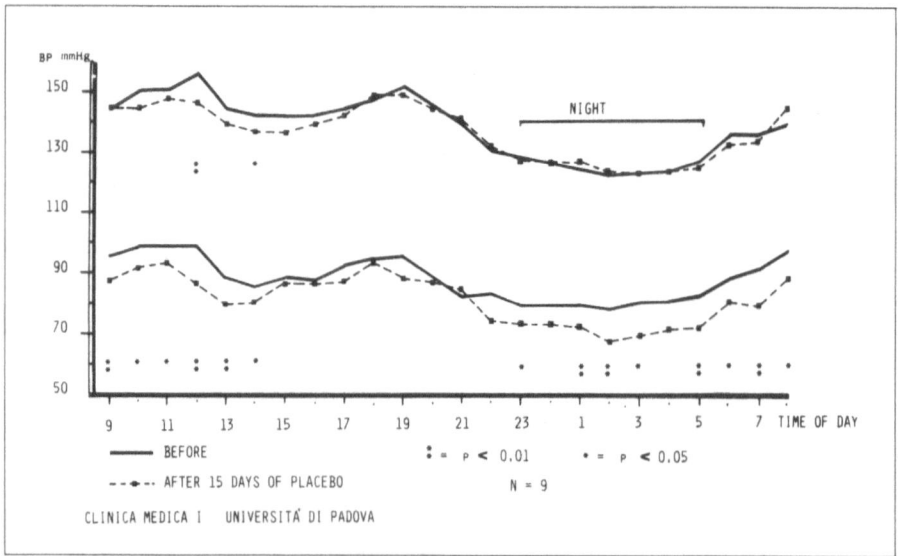

Fig. 4. Difference between the first and the second time of wearing the non-invasive equipment on 24-hour blood pressure profile.

References

1. Report of Medical Research Council Working Party on Mild to Moderate Hypertension: Randomized controlled trial of treatment of mild hypertension design and pilot trial. Br Med J i: 1437–1440 (1977).
2. Martin MA, Phillips CA, Smith AJ: Acebutolol in hypertension – A double blind trial against placebo. Br J Clin Pharmacol 8: 351–356 (1978).
3. Pugsley DJ, Nassim M, Armstrong BK, Beilin L: A controlled trial of labetalol (Trandate) propranolol and placebo in the management of mild to moderate hypertension. Br J Clin Pharmacol 7: 63–68 (1979).
4. Untreated Mild Hypertension: A report by the Management Committee of the Australian Therapeutic Trial in Mild Hypertension. Lancet i: 185–191 (1982).
5. Ambrosio GB, Bugaro L, Gabaldo S, Pigato R, Zamboni S, Dal Palù C: Blood pressure and its spontaneous variations in a northern Italian population. Clin Sci Mol Med 51: 669s–671s (1976).
6. Pickering GW: High blood pressure. 2nd Edition. Churchill (London 1968).
7. Gould BA, Mann S, Davies AB, Altman BG, Raftery EB: Does placebo lower blood pressure? Lancet ii: 1377–1381 (1981).
8. Kain HK, Hinman AT, Sokolow M: Arterial blood pressure measurements with a portable recorder in hypertensive patients. Variability and correlation with "casual" pressures. Circulation 30: 882–892 (1964).
9. Palatini P, Pessina AC, Sperti G, Mormino P, Agnoletto V, Ventura E, Semplicini A, Dal Palù C: Comparison between an indirect and a direct method of ambulatory blood pressure monitoring. In: Stott FD (ed) ISAM 81, pp 499–503. Academic Press (London 1982).
10. Littler WA, West MJ, Honour AJ, Sleight P: The variability of arterial pressure. Am Heart J 95: 180–185 (1978).

Address for correspondence:
A. C. Pessina,
Clinica Medica I, Policlinico,
Via Guistiniani 2,
I-35100 Padova, Italy

Probetto Finalizzato
Medicina Preventiva
Sottoprobetto
Malattie Degenerative

Accuracy, reproducibility and usefulness of ambulatory blood pressure recording obtained with the Remler system

Bernard Waeber, Bertrand Jacot des Combes, Marinette Porchet,
Hans R. Brunner

Summary: The Remler M2000, a portable semi-automatic blood pressure recorder, was used to measure ambulatory blood pressure during customary daily activities of normotensive and hypertensive subjects. Systolic and diastolic pressures measured simultaneously by this device and by the conventional auscultatory method were closely related throughout the day, after an acute physical exercise as well as at rest. In unselected, untreated subjects, the average of the recorded pressures was most often lower than pressures measured in the office, but ambulatory pressures could not be predicted from office readings. There was a highly significant correlation between pressure levels determined at a 3 to 4 month interval with both the conventional auscultatory method in the office and the Remler system. In hypertensive patients who were either untreated or treated chronically with beta-blocking agents, diuretics or a combinaton of both drugs, a clear diurnal variation of blood pressure was revealed by the ambulatory recordings, the lowest levels being reached in the early afternoon. Neither this diurnal variation nor blood pressure variability was influenced by antihypertensive therapy. The Remler system was also used to evaluate blood pressure outside the physician's office in untreated subjects considered by their physician to be hypertensive. The average of blood pressures recorded during the usual daily activities of the subjects were > 140 mmHg for the systolic and > 89 mmHg for the diastolic in only 39% and 44% of them, respectively. Thus, the Remler system provides accurate, reproducible blood pressure profiles in the ambulatory state which are not predictable based on office blood pressure measurements. It seems particularly useful for identifying those patients who, although hypertensive in the physician's office, remain normotensive during usual daily activities.

Introduction

For the practising physician it is often difficult to decide on the basis of office blood pressure readings whether a given patient needs antihypertensive therapy. This decision is important for the patient since treatment will most probably last for the rest of his life. It now appears that therapy is frequently initiated even though blood pressure is elevated only when taken at the physician's office. For this reason, it appears desirable in examining a patient with high blood pressure to take into account blood pressure measured during usual daily activity.

Today, the Remler M2000, a portable semi-automatic blood pressure recorder, makes it possible to measure by a non-invasive method numerous ambulatory pressures during customary daily activities (1). In this report we summarize our experience with this device both in normotensive volunteers and in hypertensive patients.

Division of Nephrology and Hypertension University Hospital, Lausanne, Switzerland

Instrumentation

The Remler M2000 (Remler Corp., San Francisco, Calif.) consists mainly of a standard, subject-inflatable arm cuff, a microphone, a pressure transducer and a tape recorder. The latter two are contained in a case weighing 0.7 Kg which is attached to a belt. In all the subjects we studied, the recorder was fitted by an experienced nurse between 7.30 and 8.30 a.m. In the clinic, 3 blood pressure readings in the sitting position were determined simultaneously with the recorder and by direct auscultation, via a mercury column temporarily connected to the inflation system. Alter leaving the clinic, the subjects were asked to record their blood pressure at 30 min intervals for 12 h. On the next morning, the recorder was brought back and the blood pressure levels were read from the magnetic tape using a decoding unit (Remler M3000, Remler Corp., San Francisco, Calif.). Diastolic blood pressures measured by auscultation with a stethoscope as well as with the portable recorder corresponded to the fifth Korotkoff's sound. The Remler system was used according to the recommendations established previously (2, 3).

Accuracy of Blood Pressure Readings Obtained with the Remler System

The accuracy of blood pressure readings taken by the Remler M2000 was assessed in 12 normotensive volunteers (4). In these subjects blood pressures were simultaneously determined with the recorder and by direct auscultation in the morning before leaving the clinic as well as in the evening prior to taking off the device. In addition, early in the afternoon, each subject ran up and down 3 flights as quickly as possible. Immediately before and after this physical exercise, one blood pressure reading was concomitantly obtained by the recorder and the conventional auscultatory method.
In all situations tested, blood pressures measured by the two different methods in the normotensive volunteers were closely related (r > 0.95 and r > 0.85 for respectively the systolic and diastolic pressure, p < 0.001). Most of the time, the difference between the two sets of pressure readings was within –4 and +4 mmHg.

Unpredictability and Reproducibility of Blood Pressure Recordings Obtained with the Remler System

We investigated in 101 unselected, untreated subjects whether blood pressure levels measured by a physician at his office are representative of those recorded in the ambulatory state (4) and whether these determinations are reproducible in time. For this purpose, the subjects were examined by the same physician at a 3 to 4 month interval. At each visit 3 blood pressures (2 in sitting and 1 in upright position) were measured. Within 2 weeks after the initial visit, the subjects were required to wear the portable recorder during their customary daily activities for a total of 12 h. In 84 subjects, ambulatory blood pressure recordings were also obtained within 2 weeks after the last office visit.
In each subject, the 3 blood pressure readings taken on the first visit at the office as well as all blood pressures determined during the first recording were averaged. The difference between the mean office and the mean ambulatory blood pressure was then calculated. In Fig. 1 the relationship between this parameter and the office blood pressure both for the

systolic (left panel) and the diastolic (right panel) is illustrated. No correlation was observed between the two sets of values. Ambulatory systolic and diastolic pressures were lower than corresponding office blood pressures by an average of 11 ± 11 (p < 0.001, mean ± SD) and 10 ± 10 mmHg (p < 0.001). Recorded pressures were higher than those measured in the office in less than 20% of the subjects.

There was a close correlation between office blood pressures (r = 0.82/0.79, p < 0.001 for systolic and diastolic respectively) as well as between ambulatory recorded blood pressures (r = 0.8/0.78, p < 0.001) obtained in 84 subjects at a 3 to 4 month interval.

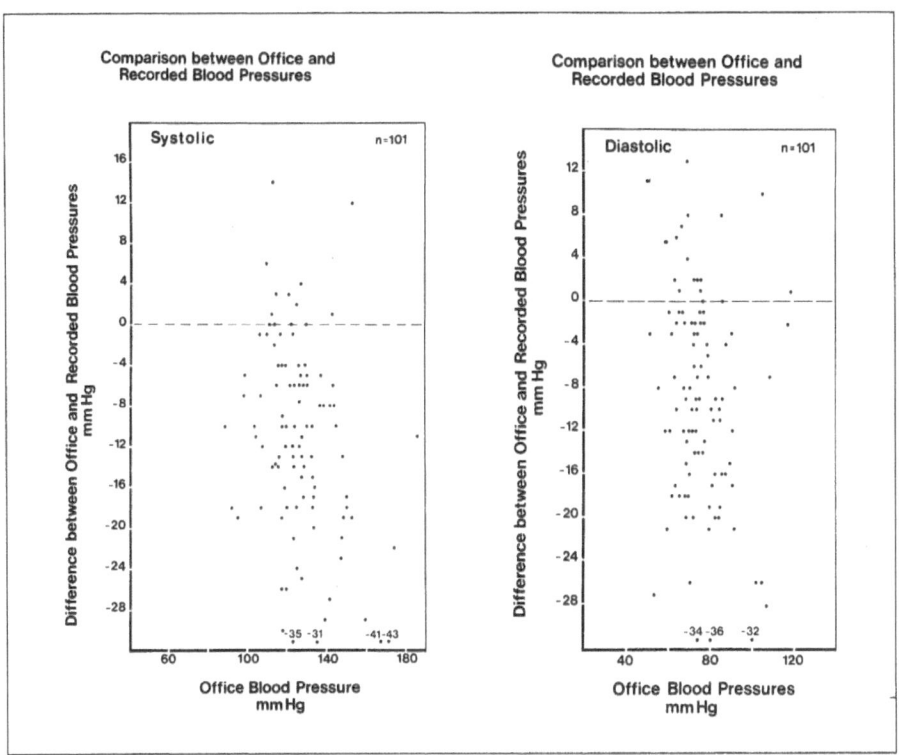

Fig. 1. The office blood pressure is on the abscissa; on the ordinate, the difference between the office blood pressure and a whole day's average of recorded pressures is depicted. The left panel describes the relationship of systolic and the right of diastolic pressures. From Jacot des Combes et al. (4).

Evaluation of Blood Pressure Variability by the Remler System

Diurnal blood pressure profiles were recorded in ambulatory hypertensive patients who were either untreated (n = 55) or treated chronically with beta-blocking agents (n = 28), diuretics (n = 42) or a combination of both drugs (n = 75) (5). The selection of untreated patients was based on clinic measurements (2 to 3 repeated blood pressures > 140/89 mmHg). Each antihypertensive drug was given at a dose generally assumed to be sufficient to lower blood pressure throughout the day.

The mean of systolic and diastolic pressures averaged in all patients over the whole day did not differ significantly among the groups, ranging from 134 to 141 mmHg for the systolic and from 84 to 98 mmHg for the diastolic. In all groups, blood pressure was highest in the morning, lowest early afternoon and tended to rise again in the late afternoon. The variability of blood pressure, reflected by the difference between the average of the 3 highest and 3 lowest values of the day, was not different between the 4 groups and ranged from 41 to 51 mmHg for the systolic and from 30 to 34 mmHg for the diastolic pressure.

Usefulness of the Remler System to Detect Patients who need Antihypertensive Therapy

Ambulatory blood pressure recordings were obtained with the Remler system in 245 untreated subjects referred to our outpatient clinic for evaluation of high blood pressure (6). In all of them, systolic blood pressures of > 140 mmHg and/or diastolic pressure levels of > 89 mmHg had been measured on at least 3 different occasions by a practising physician with the patient in the sitting position.

For all patients taken together, blood pressure levels during the day were $139/87 \pm 21/16$ mmHg. Only 39% of the patients were found to have a mean of systolic pressure levels above 140 mmHg and 44% of diastolic pressure levels above 89 mmHg throughout the day. Out of the 245 patients, only a minority of 28% had at the same time systolic and diastolic pressures higher than 140 and 89 mmHg respectively.

Comments

In our experience as well as that of other investigators (1–3), the Remler system gives accurate blood pressure profiles throughout the day, without requiring restriction of physical activity. Our findings also confirm that ambulatory pressures are generally lower than those measured in the physician's office (2). It has to be stressed, however, that basal blood pressure levels during customary daily activities differ, in the individual subject, in a highly unpredictable manner from the blood pressure readings taken at the physician's office. It is of note that monitoring of intra-arterial pressure has also shown lower pressures outside the clinic, and the level of this parameter cannot be extrapolated from office readings (7). Blood pressure recording by a non-invasive method appears therefore to be very helpful for the physician in recognizing patients who really need antihypertensive therapy because of the persistence of high blood pressure levels outside the office.

In our hypertensive patients, a diurnal variation of blood pressure was evidenced by the ambulatory recordings. Blood pressure was highest in the morning, lowest early afternoon and tended to rise again thereafter. These blood pressure variations were not modified by antihypertensive drugs such as beta-blocking agents and/or diuretics. The same drugs had no influence either on the marked blood pressure variability observed in our patients. Interestingly, despite the impressive blood pressure changes occurring during the day, both office and ambulatory blood pressures were proven to be well reproducible at a 3 to 4 month interval. This suggests that during long term follow-up of an individual subject, a single Remler recording makes it possible to judge with some confidence whether an office blood pressure is representative of basal blood pressure or whether it rather over- or underestimates this parameter.

To date there is strong evidence that blood pressure profiles obtained with the Remler system enable to discriminate better than office blood pressures between hypertensive patients at high risk and those at low risk for developing cardiovascular complications (8). Accordingly, ambulatory blood pressure monitoring with a non-invasive method seems preferable to office blood pressure measurement to decide in an individual patient on the need and the aggressiveness of antihypertensive therapy.

Acknowledgement

We thank Ms. A.-F. Stalé and Ms. A. Campiche for typing the manuscript. This study was supported in part by grants Nr. 3.914–0.80, Nr. 3.224–0.81 and Nr 3.730–0.81 of The Swiss National Science Foundation.

References

1. Hinman AT, Engle BT, Bickford AF: Portable blood pressure recorder : Accuracy and preliminary use in evaluating intradaily variations in pressure. Am Heart J 63: 663–668 (1962).
2. Kain HK, Hinman AT, Sokolow M.: Arterial blood pressure measurements with a portable recorder in hypertensive patients. I: Variability and correlation with "casual" pressures. Circulation 30: 882–892 (1964).
3. Sokolow M, Wardegar D, Kain HK, Hinman AT.: Relationship between level of blood pressure measured casually and by portable recorders and severity of complications in essential hypertension. Circulation 34: 279–298 (1966).
4. Jacot des Combes B, Porchet M, Waeber B, Brunner HR: Ambulatory blood pressure recordings: Reproducibility and unpredictability. Hypertension (In press).
5. Jacot des Combes B, Brunner HR, Waeber B, Porchet M, Biollaz J.: Blood pressure variability in hypertensive patients: Effect of beta-blocking agents and/or diuretics. J Cardiovasc Pharmacol (In press).
6. Waeber B, Jacot des Combes B, Porchet M, Biollaz J, Schaller M-D, Brunner HR: Ambulatory blood pressure recording to identify hypertensive patients who truly need therapy. J Chron Dis 37: 55–57 (1984).
7. Floras JS, Jones JV, Hassan MO, Osikowska B, Sever PS, Sleight P: Cuff and ambulatory blood pressure in subjects with essential hypertension. Lancet ii: 107–109 (1981).
8. Perloff D, Sokolow M, Cowan R: The prognostic value of ambulatory blood pressures. JAMA 249: 2792–2798 (1983).

Address for correspondence:
H.R. Brunner, MD
Division of Nephrology
and Hypertension
C H U V
1011 Lausanne
Switzerland

Reproducibility of ambulatory blood pressure recordings

Desmond J. Fitzgerald[1]), Kevin O'Malley[1]), Eoin T. O'Brien[2])

Summary: Reproducibility of ambulatory blood pressure recordings was assessed in 19 untreated hypertensive subjects over a six month period. Ambulatory blood pressure was recorded using a semiautomatic portable blood pressure recorder (Remler M2000) from 900 h until retiring. The mean ($\pm$ SEM) number of days on which recordings were made in each patient was 5.1 ± 0.31, the period between recordings being 2–6 weeks. Parameters derived from these recordings were the peak, trough and mean of all daily recordings, and the standard deviation and coefficient of variation of these recordings were derived as indices of blood pressure variability. Analysis of variance of the first 3 days of ambulatory blood pressure recordings showed no change in any of these parameters over time. The coefficients of variation within patients of the mean, peak and trough blood pressures were less than 11%. In comparison, the coefficients of variation of the parameters of blood pressure variability were greater than 20%. Analysis of variance of the first three ambulatory recording days (all patients had at least three) showed that the within-patient variance was significantly less than between-patient for the mean, peak and trough systolic and the mean and trough diastolic blood pressures but not for the peak diastolic pressure or parameters of blood pressure variability. In conclusion, ambulatory blood pressure measurements are reproducible. The poor reproducibility of the standard deviation and coefficient of variation negates their usefulness as measures of blood pressure variability.

Introduction

Repeated indirect recordings of blood pressure in hospital have proven reproducible from day to day when hourly averages or the means of recordings for the whole day are compared (1, 2) while measures of blood pressure variability are poorly reproducible (2). However, patients are restricted in hospital, and increasingly portable blood pressure recorders are being used to assess ambulatory blood pressure behavior outside hospital during normal daily activities (3). Ambulatory monitoring can only be considered a practical method of assessing blood pressure behavior if results are reproducible over a prolonged period. Other investigators have examined reproducibility of ambulatory recordings. However, these studies were either in hospital (4) or over 2–3 days within a short period of each other (5, 6, 7). In this study, the reproducibility of non-invasive ambulatory recordings is assessed over a 6 month period in non-hospitalized ambulant patients.

Methods and patients

Ambulatory recordings were performed repeatedly on 19 hypertensive subjects using the Remler M2000 semi-automatic recorder (8) at intervals of 2–6 weeks over a 6 month

---
[1]) The Blood Pressure Clinic Charitable Infirmary Jervis St. Dublin and

[2]) Dept. of Clinical Pharmacology Royal College of Surgeons in Ireland St. Stephen's Green Dublin.

period. None of the subjects were on drug treatment during the study. The mean age of the study group (7 men, 12 women) was 43.9 ± 2.1 with a range of 29–60 years. Patients attended the hospital in the morning where the recorder was attached. For the remainder of the day patients carried out their normal activities while recording their blood pressure every 30 min. A successful day-recording was defined as one in which 10 or more recordings were decodable. Day-recordings with fewer than 10 decodable individual recordings were not included in the analysis.

Reproducibility of five parameters was assessed; the peak, trough, mean, standard deviation and coefficient of variation of daily ambulatory recordings. The coefficient of variation within subjects was derived for each parameter and compared against that for between subjects. Time-related changes in recording parameters were assessed from the first three successful day-recordings (all patients had at least three) by two-way analysis of variance.

Results

The mean ($\pm$ SEM) number of successful day-recordings over the period of study was 5.1 ± 0.31 (range 3–7). Mean, peak, and trough systolic pressures, and mean and peak diastolic pressures tended to fall between the first (R_1) and third (R_3) days of recording (Table 1). However, these differences were not statistically significant. Over the same period clinic blood pressure for the group as a whole (mean $\pm$ SEM) remained unchanged ($160 \pm 3.9/96.3 \pm 1.7$ Vs $160 \pm 4.1/96.8 \pm 3.2$) although mean clinic pressure at the first clinic visit which occurred 4 weeks before the study began had been slightly higher ($163 \pm 3.5/99 \pm 1.6$).

Coefficients of variation of blood pressure parameters were less within patients than between patients, with the exception of measures of blood pressure variability (Table 2). Similarly, the two-way analysis of variance of the first three successful ambulatory recordings in all 19 subjects showed that between-patient variance was significantly greater than within-patient variance for systolic peak (F 5.6, P < 0.05), trough (F 13.5, P < 0.001) and mean pressures (F 16.4, P < 0.001) and for diastolic mean (F 11.5, P < 0.01) and trough pressures (F 7.4, P < 0.01). However, variance of diastolic peak pressure and of the standard deviations and coefficients of variation of systolic and diastolic pressures were not greater between than within patients.

Table 1: Comparison of First Three Remler (R) Ambulatory Blood Pressure Recordings.

	Systolic			Diastolic		
	R_1	R_2	R_3	R_1	R_2	R_3
Mean BP (mmHg)	151.4 ± 3.1	149.7 ± 3.6	148.8 ± 3.7	98.3 ± 2.3	97.7 ± 3.1	95.8 ± 3.0
Peak BP (mmHg)	174.6 ± 3.6	172.3 ± 4.02	170.7 ± 4.1	113.7 ± 2.6	112.9 ± 3.1	108.6 ± 3.6
Trough BP (mmHg)	130.5 ± 3.2	130.9 ± 3.9	128.1 ± 4.2	80.6 ± 4.9	81.2 ± 4.1	81.6 ± 3.2
SD (mmHg)	11.9 ± 0.67	11.8 ± 0.72	12.4 ± 0.63	7.4 ± 0.42	8.1 ± 0.33	7.5 ± 0.52
CV (%)	8.3 ± 0.57	8.5 ± 0.52	8.3 ± 0.5	7.9 ± 0.6	8.8 ± 0.58	7.3 ± 0.38

SD = standard deviation; CV = coefficient of variation

Table 2: Comparison of Coefficients of Variation Between and Within Subjects for Different Parameters of Non-invasive Ambulatory Blood Pressure.

	Systolic		Diastolic	
	Within patients	Between patients**	Within patients	Between patients
Mean BP (%)	4.8* (1.0–12.1)	8.8–10.7**	5.9* (1.4–12.5)	10.2–14.4**
Peak BP (%)	6.4 (2.8–13.2)	9–10.5	6.4 (1.3–13.7)	10.1–11.9
Trough BP (%)	7.9 (3.4–16.8)	10.8–14.3	10.7 (3.8–16.6)	17.2–26.7
SD (%)	21.1 (8.8–38.4)	22.3–26.7	20.1 (6.9–32.5)	17.6–30.7
CV (%)	22.8 (9.4–38.3)	25.6–30.5	21.8 (1.1–35.0)	22–32.9

* Mean within-patient coefficient of variation for all subjects (range).
** Range of between-patient coefficient over the first three ambulatory recordings.
SD = standard deviation; CV = coefficient of variation of all recordings through the day.

Discussion

This study fails to confirm previous findings of a significant fall in ambulatory blood pressure during repeated ambulatory non-invasive blood pressure recordings (4, 6). Conway (4) demonstrated a fall of 18 mmHg and 9 mmHg in mean ambulatory systolic and diastolic pressures respectively between the first and third day of ambulatory recording in hypertensive subjects. However, their patients had been hospitalized for the study so that this change may partly reflect the fall in blood pressure which occurs during hospitalization of hypertensive subjects (9). Kain et al (6) noted a more modest fall between the first and third successive day of ambulatory recording. The fall in systolic pressure which was about 5–6 mmHg occurred largely in the early part of the day. This resembles the fall found between successive recordings in our study. However, the significance of this may have been exaggerated by multiple paired comparisons. Direct ambulatory blood pressure monitoring using the Oxford recording system in 8 patients showed no mean difference in blood pressure levels on two successive days of recording (5) in agreement with the findings of this study.

Of greater importance than a mean change in blood pressure is the variability of parameters used to describe ambulatory blood pressure behavior. Van Maele and Clements (7) compared Remler ambulatory blood pressure recordings made on two separate days and found that of the measured parameters, including mean blood pressure, only the variance of daily recordings was reproducible. This was determined for each patient from the ratio of the variances of the recordings for each day. However, with a mean of 24 recordings in a day, within-patient variance would have to change by 50% before a significant difference could be shown between two days of recordings in a single patient. The present study showed that the mean of daily systolic and diastolic recordings were highly reproducible in most subjects. Furthermore, peak and trough blood pressure recordings were also reasonably reproducible in comparison with the between-subject variability of these parameters. However, indices of blood pressure variability, the standard deviation and coefficient of variation, were poorly reproducible in all but a few patients for both systolic and diastolic blood pressure when compared with between-patient variability. Similar results have been shown for repeated recordings of blood pressure in hospitalized patients using an automatic blood pressure recorder (2). The differences in variability between subjects or between days in the same subject may represent within-patient variation only. Thus, in drug studies the variation in these parameters within subjects must be considered before an effect, or more importantly the lack of an effect, is attributed to a drug.

In conclusion, the peak, trough and mean blood pressure recorded using the Remler ambulatory blood pressure recorder are reproducible over a period of several months whereas indices of blood pressure variability derived from such recordings are not.

Acknowledgement

We acknowledge gratefully grants from the Royal College of Surgeons in Ireland and Ciba Laboratories.

References

1. Athanassiadas D, Draper GJ, Hanow AJ, Cranston WI: Variability of automatic blood pressure measurements over 24-hour periods. Clin Sci 36: 147–156 (1969).
2. Weber MA, Drayer JM, Wyle FA: Consistency of the 24-hr. blood pressure profile (abst.). Clin Res 30: 24A (1982).
3. Horan MJ, Padgett NE, Kennedy HL: Ambulatory blood pressure monitorings: recent advances and clinical applications. Am Heart J 101: 844–847 (1981).
4. Conway N, Rubenstein D, Ervanwel R, Gibbons D: Measurement of blood pressure using a portable recorder operated by the patient. Cardiovasc Res 4: 537–544 (1970).
5. Mann S, Millar-Craig MW, Balasubramanian U, Cashman PMM, Raftery EB: Ambulant blood pressure: reproducibility and the assessment of interventions. Clin Sci 59: 497–500 (1980).
6. Kain H, Hinman AT, Sokolow M: Arterial blood pressure measurements with a portable recorder in hypertensive patients 1. Variability and correlation with 'casual' pressures. Circulation 30: 882–892 (1964).
7. Van Maele GO, Clements DL: Reproducibility of blood pressure measurements obtained with semi-continous recording devices. ISAM, 1981. Proceedings of the Fourth International Symposium on Ambulatory Blood Pressure Monitoring and the Second Gent Workshop in Blood Pressure Variability. Ed. Stott, FD, Raftery EB, Clement DL, Wright SL: 589–595 Academic Press (London, 1982).
8. Fitzgerald DJ, O'Callaghan WG, O'Malley K, O'Brien ET: Accuracy and reliability of two indirect ambulatory blood pressure recorders: Remler M2000 and Cardiodyne Sphygmolog. Br Heart J 48: 572–579 (1982).
9. Hossman V, FitzGerald GA, Dollery CT: The influence of hospitalization and placebo therapy on blood pressure and sympathetic function in essential hypertension. Hypertension 3: 113–118 (1981).

Address for correspondence:
Dr. Eoin T. O'Brien
The Blood Pressure Clinic
Charitable Infirmary
Jervis Street
Dublin 2

Blood pressure measurement in an ambulatory setting

Nemat O. Borhani, Frances LaBaw, Signe Dunkle

Summary: Errors in blood pressure measurement can be significantly reduced by consideration and control of sources of error such as inadequate physical setting, equipment failure and poor technician performance. Inadequate setting and equipment failure can be ameliorated with the administration of rigorous quality control measures based on the knowledge of optimum standards. Technician performance is dependent on effective training and testing in the standard methodology, followed up with periodic re-testing and continuous supervision. Reducing measurement error greatly enhances the dependability of results obtained in an ambulatory setting.

Introduction

Importance of accurate monitoring

Elevated arterial blood pressure is a powerful risk of mortality and morbidity. The association between the level of blood pressure, both systolic and diastolic, and mortality, as well as morbidity, from cardiovascular diseases and stroke, is a positive graded association. That is, the rate of morbid events is related numerically to the level of blood pressure. Unfortunately, level of blood pressure, like other biological quantitative variables, is subject to variation.

There are two important sources of variation in blood pressure measurement, the biological variation and the measurement error variation. Since the former is subject to only minimal control, and indeed the object of ambulatory blood pressure monitoring, the latter demands scrupulous attention.

Sources of measurement errors in ambulatory blood pressure monitoring

Measurement errors are derived from three sources. The first is an inadequate setting, such as unsuitable furnishings, lack of privacy or too much noise. Secondly, faulty equipment is a frequently overlooked source of error resulting from poor selection, maintenance and repair. The third and most important source of error is erroneous technical performance of the standard blood pressure measurement methodology due to inadequate initial training or insufficient supervision.

Department of Community Health School of Medicine University of California, Davis, California 95616

Physical setting

Ambulatory blood pressure measurements are performed in a variety of settings. Technicians may have difficulty properly positioning the equipment or the subject. Settings may work against the need for barriers to protect the subject's privacy and maximize the technician's concentration. Finally, the acoustic suitability of a setting may be compromised.

Equipment

Sphygmomanometers and stethoscopes are fixtures which frequently escape the attention of otherwise conscientious practitioners. A thoughtful look around many offices and screening sites will reveal equipment problems. The recently introduced automatic blood pressure measurement equipment demands especially rigorous attention.

Technician performance

Blood pressure measurement methodology training and experience varies widely from technician to technician (the term technician refers to anyone, physician, nurse or lay volunteer who undertakes the standardized technique of blood pressure measurement). Technicians may have received inadequate training in methodology, may have performed faulty technique without correction for many years and may find it difficult to change habits, or may not understand the potential for error and the importance of accuracy in blood pressure measurement. Rarely is inaccurate measurement the result of malicious technician intent.

Common errors include improper preparation and positioning of the subject, selection of incorrect cuff size, inadequate application of the cuff, and failure to use the premeasurement palpatory blood pressure determination to accurately define the level to which the cuff should be initially inflated for proper measurement.

Another set of problems occur on the technician's subconscious level; these are the triple threat of terminal digit preference, observer bias and inattention.

Terminal digit preference is the tendency a person has to select a particular number, say the number four, repeatedly rather than the number actually encountered. Observer bias is seen when the observer believes a person such as an obese, middle-aged, black female or an athletic, young white male should have blood pressure in a particular range. Dramatic examples of bias occur when the results of the blood pressure measurement will determine the need for treatment of an individual; i.e., all people with a DBP of 95 mmHg or greater will be placed on a medication known for its side effects. The technician's unconscious bias may result in readings of 92 mmHg and 94 mmHg in excess of the actual occurrence of these readings. Terminal digit preference and observer bias compromise the goal of accurate blood pressure monitoring. The chief contributor to these two measurement errors and inaccurate measurement in general is inattention.

An examination of monitoring sites, blood pressure measurement equipment and technician performance in the plethora of ambulatory blood pressure monitoring programs currently existent will reveal problems enough to make any thoughtful person doubt the usefulness of the data being gathered. The cost in incorrect detection and treatment may be monumental.

Technical quality assurance

Physical setting management

A great deal of thought and attention must go into the physical setting in which blood pressure is measured. The site can vary from a meager private home with little furniture, to a clinic with inadequate space, to a community screening site in a noisy shopping center.

Forethought must be exercised to ensure blood pressures can be accurately measured despite the limitations of the setting.

The first consideration is the position of the equipment and the subject. The need to position each correctly demands that adequate furniture be available and in some cases cushions or pads to support the subject's feet or arm.

The need for a subject's privacy and the technician's attentiveness can become a serious obstacle in open screening sites such as shopping malls or station-to-station screening in large clinic settings. Care should be taken to provide some form of privacy barrier, at a minimum curtained screens or hinged panels. In those cases when subjects must remove clothing to bare their arms for blood pressure measurement, privacy barriers are essential.

Finally, noise control is of utmost importance. It is assisted by the use of privacy barriers, but requires further attention. When blood pressure measurements are planned in high-traffic areas, noise control should be provided. Thought should be given to re-routing the activities surrounding the screening site. Pads should be placed under equipment to reduce the noise created when equipment is moved on the desk or table. Sites should be rejected if noise cannot be controlled.

Equipment selection, maintenance and repair

The equipment includes sphygmomanometers, a complete selection of arm cuff sizes, and stethoscopes of good quality. The difference in reliability versus utility between mercury and aneroid sphygmomanometers bears serious consideration before a choice is made. If the sphygmomanometers are to be used to collect data for clinical studies the mercury sphygmomanometers should always be selected.

Equipment maintenance should be handled both on a routine and on an as needed basis. Each piece of equipment should be numbered and logs should be established for routine equipment inspection, calibration and maintenance. Equipment should be rotated among technicians according to a documented schedule. Technicians are initially trained to inspect all blood pressure measurement equipment before use and should be encouraged to maintain interest in and attention to the condition of the equipment they use.

Repair procedures should be established when equipment is initially put in use. The resources for repair should be established and all of the resource contact information should be at hand.

Of particular importance in maintenance and repair is the handling of mercury that may escape from the mercury sphygmomanometers. All technicians should be trained to avoid touching loose mercury, but it is the responsibility of the supervisor to guarantee the correct clean-up and disposal of loose mercury. Clear instructions for mercury clean-up procedures should be prominently displayed and the supervisor should be completely familiar with the instructions including the telephone numbers of the appropriate hazardous waste disposal resource and the emergency services agency. All mercury spills should be fully documented.

Methodology training procedures

Health professional training

To establish a program of blood pressure measurement proficiency begin by training a core group of health professionals. Train health professionals first in the basic blood pressure measurement methodology. Then continue on to preparation for the instruction and supervision of technicians. Health professionals, so prepared, can train and supervise technicians who may otherwise have little experience or few skills in the health care field. The blood pressure measurement training for health professionals should be taught by a person who is proficient in the technique, having successfully completed one of the approved methodology certification programs (e.g., the AHA programs), and who has substantial academic and practical experience to act as a bona fide specialist in hypertension and blood pressure measurement methodology. Without these accoutrements of credibility the professionals undergoing training may not be sufficiently motivated to adhere to the methodology, especially in the case that adherence may dictate abandonment of deeply ingrained habits and attitudes.

Instructor / supervisor training

The individual who undertakes the instruction and supervision of technicians should undergo further training specific to the task. The instructor/supervisor candidate should be thoroughly trained in all aspects of methodology, including a review of the history, anatomy, physiology and physics of blood pressure measurements; the evaluation, monitoring, maintenance and repair of blood pressure equipment; effective adult education strategies for technical training and verification; and ambulatory screening supervision and management.

Technician training

Persons with little or no background in health care require a training program tailored to their needs. All technician-trainees should be screened to ensure their hearing, sight and manual dexterity are equal to the requirements of the blood pressure measurement technique. Technicians should only be trained by adequately trained instructors. All programs of technician training should have, as ready resources, experts in the field of hypertension. It is not necessary nor is it desireable to include lectures on anatomy, physiology, epidemiology or treatment of hypertension in the technician training program. If a trainee is interested in pursuing more information about high blood pressure measurement or hypertension, encourage them with a selected bibliography and an invitation to discuss the material, on an individual basis at another time, any reading they may complete from the bibliography.

Testing

Four methods of testing are commonly used for verification of blood pressure measurement technique proficiency. The first test method is the instructor-trainee blood pressure measurement practicum using a stethoscope with one diaphragm/bell and two headsets which allow simultaneous readings; this is usually termed the double stethoscope or Y tube test. Written tests, usually multiple choice and fill-in type, are frequently employed. Finally, audiotape and videotape/films of blood pressure measurement sequences may be used for testing. Of the four methods of testing, the double stethoscope test must be used in all blood pressure measurement technique verification. The trainee's performance is judged during the double stethoscope test both on adherence to technique and comparability of readings between the instructor and the trainee.

The written test is optional. It can be used as a pre- and post-test and should never be used to disqualify a trainee. It serves as a vehicle of emphasis for specific details of technique.

The audiotape and videotape/film tests each have their proponents and seem to be used to the exclusion of one another. Each, in truth, serves quite different purposes. The audiotape tests encourage and refine the technicians' skills in listening to the nuances of the Korotkoff sounds. The videotape/films are a more practical test of the audiovisual coordination required in reading blood pressures. Trainee preformance on the videotape/film blood pressure sequences is most indicative of the trainee's level of attentiveness. Both the audio and video blood pressure sequences are useful as training or as testing materials.

It is important when testing trainees to present the testing in a well organized fashion. A set of written instructions should accompany each test, the criteria by which trainees will be graded should be articulated. All trainees should be assisted to review, practice and retest at each step of the testing plan until they complete the test successfully. Every effort should be made to allay trainee anxiety while motivating them to the highest level of competency.

Re-testing/re-training

To assure continued technician competency, a program of re-testing, usually every six months and no less than once a year, should be conducted. Technicians should be alerted in advance of the re-testing.

A complete series of re-testing should always include the double stethoscope performance and reading comparability test. Technicians who fail any portion of the re-testing should suspend their blood pressure measurement duties and begin a program of review, re-training, practice and re-testing until they successfully complete the re-test series.

References

WA Baum Company: Baumanometer service manual. Copiague (New York 1973).

NC Taylor Instruments: Before using your new tycos mercurial. Arden (1967).

World Health Organization: Guidelines for the Treatment of Mild Hypertension: Memorandum from World Health Organization/International Society of Hypertension Meeting, September 27–29, 1982. Bulletin of the World Health Organization 61 (No. 1): 53–56 (1982).

Curb D, LaBarthe DR, Cooper, SP, Cutter, GR, Hawkins, CM: Training and certification of blood pressure observers. Hypertension 5: No. 4: 610–614 (1983).

Hypertension Detection and Follow-Up Program Cooperative Group: Variability of blood pressure and the results of screening in the hypertension detection and follow-up program. J Chron Dis 31: 651–667 (1978).

Kirkendall WM, Feinleib M, Mark AL: American Heart Association Recommendations for human blood pressure determination by sphygmomanometer. Booklet No. 70-019-B (1980).

Manning DM: Correspondence, avoiding sphygmomanometer-cuff hypertension. New Engl J Med 306: 109 (1982).

Massachusetts Department of Public Health: Mercury and the hazards of vacuum cleaning. New Engl J Med February 13: 369 (1975).

National Institutes of Health: Guidelines for Educating Nurses in High Blood Pressure Control. NIH Publication No. 82-1141 (December 1981).

National Institutes of Health: Resources for Educating Nurses in High Blood Pressure Control. NIH Publication No. 81-2208 (June 1981).

Shepard DS: Reliability of blood pressure measurements: implications for designing and evaluating programs to control hypertension. J Chron Dis 34: 191–209 (1981).

U.S. Department of Health and Human Services: The 1980 Report of the Joint National Committee on Detection, Evaluation and Treatment of High Blood Pressure. NIH Publication No. 82-1088 (December 1981).

Workshop on Improving Clinical and Consumer Blood Pressure Measuring Devices: Problem-solving technology: reaching a consensus on diagnostic technology for hypertension. Clin Eng 7: No. 4 (July–August 1979).

List of blood pressure measurement training manuals and audiovisual materials

Rober J. Brady Company: How to Measure Blood Pressure. Prentice-Hall (Bowie, Maryland 1974).

Chicago Heart Association: Blood Pressure Measurement: A Handbook for Instructors (Chicago 1979).

High Blood Pressure Information Center: National High Blood Pressure Coordinating Committee: A Review of Techniques and Training Programs for Measurement of Blood Pressure (1978).

Hypertension Detection and Follow-Up Program: HDFP Manual for Training and Certification of Observers. National Heart Lung and Blood Institute, Bethesda, Maryland.

Indiana School of Nursing: Blood Pressure Measurement. Indiana University Audiovisual Center (1978).

LaBarthe D, Poizner SB, Cutter GR, Casey B: Measurement of blood pressure: A manual for training and certification of observers. Hypertension Detection and Follow-Up Program, Besthesda, Maryland: National Heart, Lung and Blood Institute (1981).

Maryland Affiliate, American Heart Association. Blood Pressure: Its Control and Measurement, 2nd. Edition (1980).

McCarthy D, Poi K, Leventhal H, Safer M: Blood Pressure Measurement Program: Nurse Instructor Manual. American Heart Association, Wisconsin Affiliate (Milwaukee, Wisconsin 1980).

Prineas RJ: Blood Pressure Sounds: Their Measurement and Meaning. Gamma Medical Products Corporation (1978).

Address for correspondence
Nemat O. Borhani, M.D.
Professor and Chairman
Department of Community Health
School of Medicine
University of California, Davis
Davis, California 95616

Home and office blood pressures. Clinical observations and hemodynamic mechanisms

Fetnat M. Fouad, Carolyn Nemec, Robert C. Tarazi, Stephen C. Textor, Emmanuel L. Bravo

Wide fluctuations in arterial pressure have long been recognized as a feature in many hypertensive patients and have consistently been a major difficulty in decisions for treatment and understanding of pathophysiology. It is only in the past decade that more precise estimates of the degree of diurnal variations could be obtained by ambulatory 24-hour recordings of blood pressure from intra-arterial catheterization (1) or non-invasive methods (2–3). In the absence of these methods, it is still possible to avoid the pitfalls associated with sole dependence on office blood pressure levels by asking the patients to measure their own pressures at home or at work. This was the method used for over forty years in our center; it had many advantages that could outweigh its limited number of daily observations. Blood pressure could be followed over long periods of time and not be limited to one day; the patients developed a greater sense of participating in their follow-up and came to recognize their pressure fluctuations as a physiolgoical variable analagous to changes in daily weight.

Patients are taught to measure their own blood pressure by an experienced nurse. They measure their own blood pressure twice daily at home both in the sitting and standing positions. A regular log of these measurements is mailed to our center every 2–4 weeks. The accuracy of these readings is checked using a double stethoscope whenever the patients come for an outpatient visit or occasionally by a studient visiting them at home. The weekly average of these blood pressure values is then calculated and plotted (Fig. 1). In the evaluation of the patient's course, his/her office arterial pressure readings are compared with the average of home blood pressure records during the week corresponding to the office visit.

Our study of the discrepancies between home and office blood pressure records included three aspects: a) the clinical evaluation of some factors that account for these differences, b) an investigation of possible hemodynamic mechanisms, and c) a correlation of cardiac complications (left ventricular hypertrophy) with both sets of records to define which one was more closely linked with target organ damage.

Cleveland Clinic Foundation, Research Division

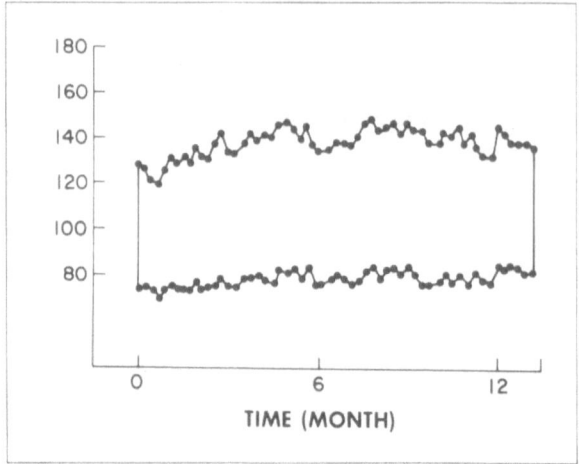

Fig. 1. The weekly average of twice daily home blood pressure values (taken by the patient) are calculated and plotted. Ordinate represents home systolic (upper line) and diastolic (lower line) blood pressure (mmHg).

Clinical evaluation

The first part of this report was based on our experience with fifty-five hypertensive patients whose records met the following conditions:

a) antihypertensive medications had been kept constant for a long enough period of time (at least one month);

b) presence of complete and uninterrupted records of twice daily home blood pressure measurements over that same period of time, and

c) the patient had at least three office visits during that period.

The group consisted of 23 women and 32 men with a mean age of 48 ± 1.4 (SEM) years. Sixteen patients were untreated; all others were taking either diuretics or beta-blockers, or a combination of beta-blockers and diuretics. A part of these data has been previously reported (4).

Figure 2 illustrates the discrepancy between home and office blood pressures. Sixty-five percent. of patients had higher office blood pressure > 10 mmHg. Indeed, using 140/90 mmHg as an arbitrary measure of borderline hypertension, 33% of patients had "normal" home blood pressures (weekly average) while the corresponding office blood pressures were elevated.

It has been previously suggested that the higher office blood pressure could be attributed to such factors as anxiety, stress, fear and unfamiliarity with the medical surroundings (5). This hypothesis, however, was not supported by our experience. We found no "telltale" clinical sign that could point to apprehension or stress; the patient appeared calm, showed no visible perspiration and was asked to relax his muscles consciously when his blood pressure was being measured. Moreover, using heart rate as an indicator of "tension", we found no correlation between office-home blood pressure discrepancy and office heart rate. Finally, a marked difference between office and home blood pressures persisted in 34 patients over a follow-up period of 12 months, irrespective of the treatment used and of the number of follow-up visits (4).

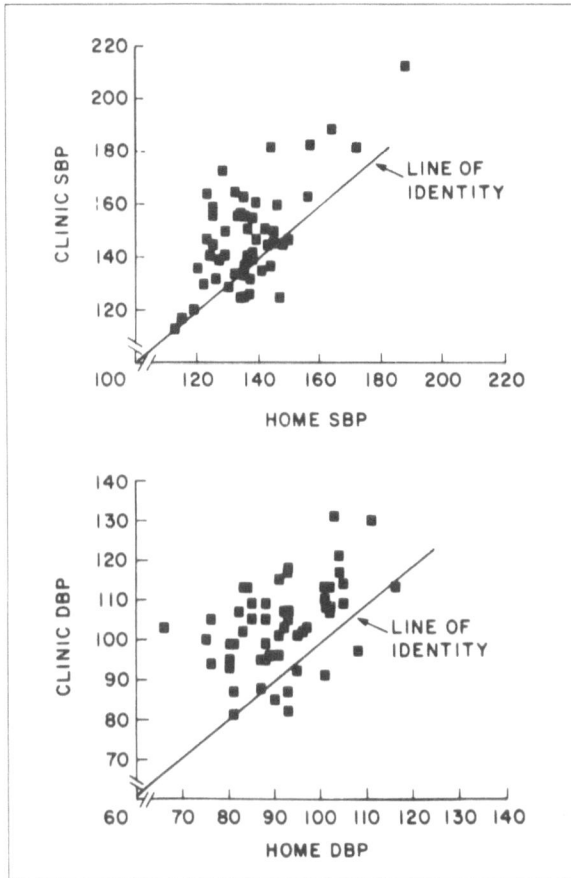

Fig. 2. Correlation between clinic and home systolic blood pressure (SBP) or diastolic blood pressure (DBP). Values are expressed in mmHg. In both instances, there was a discrepancy between clinic and home blood pressure readings in most of the patients, shown by the shift to the left of the line of identity. Based on data from Nemec et al. (submitted).

Hemodynamic investigations

We have previously reported that in adolescents undergoing invasive hemodynamic evaluation, the blood pressure recorded intra-arterially in the laboratory could be either higher or lower than the home blood pressure average for the corresponding week (6). A systematic investigation of this difference revealed no correlation with the level of cardiac output (Fig. 3). If the transient change in blood pressure provoked by the laboratory test was related to a cardiac expression of emotion, one would have expected a positive correlation between the rise in pressure and the change in output. These findings suggested that cardioadrenergic drive with its consequent hyperkinetic circulation could not be the only factor explaining the higher office or laboratory blood pressure (6).

Experience with beta and alpha adrenoceptor blockers is particularly significant in that regard. A previous study (7) of patients treated with propranolol from our laboratory showed that the occasional rise of arterial pressure during a test was related to an increase in peripheral resistance (Table 1). Others had also shown that the pressor effect of stress or pain which was related to a rise in output in untreated patients was still maintained during beta-blockade even though the increase in cardiac output was prevented (8, 9). Conversely, Andren & Hanson (10) showed that the pressor effect of noise was due to a rise in peripheral resistance in untreated subjects and that this mechanism persisted during treatment with alpha-blockers; its hemodynamic pattern was changed, however, to a rise in cardiac output.

In summary, the neural drive responsible for office hypertension could not be related to a homogenous hemodynamic pattern; it could be expressed by a rise in either cardiac output or peripheral resistance or could change from one to the other according to the type of treatment.

Clinical significance: relation to target organ damage

These findings underline the urgent need to define the appropriate blood pressure for follow-up during long-term patients' care and evaluation of antihypertensive therapy. Although epidemiologic studies and insurance mortality statistics have used office blood

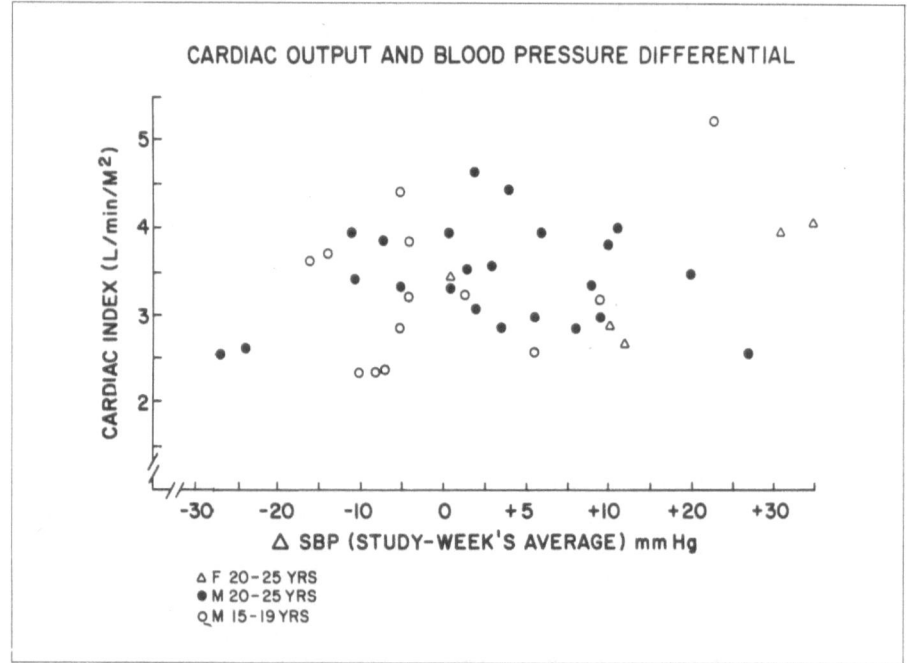

Fig. 3. Lack of correlation between cardiac index (dye dilution technique) and the difference between lab intra-arterial systolic blood pressure (BP$_{ia}$) and home systolic blood pressure pressure average for that week (BP$_{av}$) in adolescents. (With permission from Fouad et al., Am Heart J 96: 646–654 (1978) (6).

Table 1.

	Pretreatment	Propranolol therapy	
		Concordant MAP	Discordant MAP*
MAP (mmHg)			
Home average	120	108	104
During study	124	112	142
Heart rate (beats/min)	78	61	59
Cardiac index (liters/min/m²)	3.18	2.56	2.35
TPR (units) +	39.0	43.1 (+10.5%)	61.0 (+56.5%)

* MAP = mean arterial pressure, "concordant" and "disconcordant" refer to comparison of blood pressure during study with home blood pressure average at that time (see text).

+ TPR = total peripheral resistance; the increase over pretreatment values was significantly higher in the "discordant" than in the "concordant" studies, averaging + 46 percent. of the pretreatment value with a standard error of difference -11.5 (paired test = 4.00, $p < 0.02$).

(With permission from Tarazi and Dustan, Amer J Cardiol 29: 633–640 (1981) (7).

pressure (11), home blood pressure averages have been found to be more important in relation to target organ damage (12). Using left ventricular hypertrophy (LVH) as an index of target organ damage, Ibrahim, Gifford and Tarazi (13) found that electrocardiographic signs of LVH (voltage and ST-T) during antihypertensive therapy correlated much more closely with home systolic blood pressure ($r = 0.46$, $p < 0.001$) than with office systolic pressure. Table 2 illustrates an example of such changes in a single patient. Similarly, Drayer et al. (14) and Rowlands et al. (15) found that left ventricular mass determined by M-mode echocardiography correlated with 24-hour blood pressure averages but not with office blood pressure. It would seem as if the BP fluctuations during the day rather than a blood pressure level at any one point in time are more important determinants of target organ involvement.

In conclusion, office blood pressure may be higher or lower than home blood pressure. The exact mechanism of these blood pressure differences is not clear; but it could not be related solely to factors such as anxiety and environmental stress. The discrepancy be-

Table 2. EKG Follow-up in one hypertensive patient.

	1.28.75	3/21.77
Home Bp (average for week)	222/125	133/83
Office BP	226/127	180/105
EKG		
ST-T	strain	N
R + S max	48	43

tween home and office blood pressure was not influenced by the duration of follow-up nor by the type of antihypertensive medication used. Finally, it is not yet clear which blood pressure (in the office, twice daily at home, or 24-hour ambulatory average) is the more relevant in clinical follow-up, particularly in relation to target organ involvement.

References

1. Raftery EB, Millar-Craig MW: Information derived from direct 24-hour recordings. In: Clement D, ed; Blood pressure variability. Lancaster, MTP Press 67 (1979).
2. Messerli FH, Glade LB, Ventura HO, Dreslinski GR, Suarez DH, MacPhee AA, Aristimuno GG, Cole FE, Frohlich ED: Diurnal variations of cardiac rhythm, arterial pressure, and urinary catecholamines in borderline and established essential hypertension. Am Heart J 104: 109–114 (1982).
3. Weber MA, Drayer FIM, Wyle FA, Brewer DD: A representative value for whole-day BP monitoring. JAMA 248: 1626–1628 (1982).
4. Nemec CF, Tarazi RC, Textor SC, Mujais SK, Fouad FM, Bravo EL: An evaluation of discrepancy between clinic and home blood pressures in hypertensive patients. (Submitted)
5. Page IH: Hypertension – the fledgling of modern medical practice. Postgrad Med 61: 203–206 (1977).
6. Fouad FM, Tarazi RC, Dustan HP, Bravo EL: Hemodynamics of essential hypertension in young subjects. Am Heart J 96: 646–654 (1978).
7. Tarazi RC, Dustan HP: Beta adrenergic blockade in hypertension: Practical and theoretical implications and long-term hemodynamic variations. Amer J Cardiol 29: 633–640 (1972).
8. Nicotero JA, Beamer V, Montsis SE, et al: Effects of propranolol on pressor responses to noxious stimuli in hypertension. Amer J Cardiol 22: 657–666 (1968).
9. Ulrych M: Changes of general haemodynamics during stressful mental arithmetic and non-stressing quiet conversation and modification of the latter by beta-adrenergic blockade. Clin Sci 36: 453–461 (1969).
10. Andren L, Hansson L, Bjorkman M, Jonsson A: Noise as a contributory factor in the development of elevated arterial pressure. A study of the mechanisms by which noise may raise blood pressure in man. Acta Med Scand 207: 493–498 (1980).
11. Kannel WB: Role of blood pressure in cardiovascular morbidity and mortality. Progr Cardiovasc Dis 17: 5 (1974).
12. Sokolow M, Werdegar D, Kain HK, Hinman AT: Relationship between level of blood pressure measured casually and by portable recorders and severity of complications in essential hypertension. Circulation 34: 279–298 (1966).
13. Ibrahim MM, Tarazi RC, Dustan HP, Gifford RW Jr: Electrocardiogram in evaluation of resistance to antihypertensive therapy. Arch Intern Med 137: 1125–1129 (1977).
14. Drayer JIM, Weber MA, DeYoung JL: BP as a determinant of cardiac left ventricular muscle mass. Arch Intern Med 143: 90–92 (1983).
15. Rowlands DB, Ireland MA, Stallard TJ, Glover DR, McLeay RAB, Watson RDS: Assessment of left ventricular mass and its response to antihypertensive treatment. Lancet (Feb): 467–470 (1982).

Address for correspondence:
Fetnat M. Fouad, M.D.
Research 1
Cleveland Clinic Foundation
9500 Euclid Avenue
Cleveland
Ohio 44106

Home vs clinic blood pressure in essential hypertension with and without behavioral therapy

Chalemphol Thananopavarn[1], Iris B. Goldstein[2], David Shapiro[2], Michael S. Golub[1], and Mohinder P. Sambhi[1]

Summary: Behavioral treatments of relaxation alone (RL = 13) and relaxation in combination with EMG biofeedback (RL/BF = 14) were given to uncontrolled essential hypertensives (diastolic blood pressure greater than 90 mmHg) between the ages of 35 and 62. Comparisons were made between RL, RL/BF and a control condition in which patients monitored their own blood pressures (SM = 14). These three groups of patients all receiving anti-hypertensive medications were compared with a fourth un-medicated relaxation group (RL/noD = 17). Both home and clinic laboratory blood pressure were compared during 6 weeks of baseline and 10 weeks of treatment. In the baseline period, sitting quietly for 15 min in the laboratory significantly reduced the systolic blood pressure in the anti-hypertensive drug treated patients. This effect was not apparent in the un-medicated group. Relaxation and relaxation/biofeedback were equally effective in reducing blood pressure at home in the morning and evening and produced significantly greater systolic and diastolic decreases than those seen in the SM control group. Relaxation therapy in the non-drug group was significant only for morning blood pressures. Clinic blood pressures did not reflect significant differences between the groups. It is concluded that the setting (laboratory/clinic vs home) and the condition (before or after sitting quietly) under which blood pressure measurements are made may influence the effect of medications or behavioral therapy.

Introduction

In the management of uncomplicated mild essential hypertension, a non-pharmacological therapy including stress reduction has been recommended as the initial therapy in conjunction with low salt, weight reduction and exercise. Relaxation and yoga exercises has been reported to lower blood pressure in patients with moderate to severe hypertension (1). On account of variability in ambulatory blood pressure, it has been very difficult to evaluate the efficacy of behavioral therapy in patients with mild hypertension. The present study evaluated the efficacy of blood pressure reduction of behavioral therapy techniques in uncontrolled hypertension (diastolic greater than 90 mmHg) with or without antihypertensive drug therapy. Changes in blood pressure in the baseline period both at the laboratory and at home in patients on and off antihypertensive therapy were also examined.

[1]) Department of Medicine University of California, Los Angeles Hypertension Division, V.A. Medical Center, Sepulveda

[2]) Department of Psychiatry and Biobehavioral Sciences University of California, Los Angeles

This study was conducted at the Sepulveda Veterans Administration Medical Center and was supported by the American Heart Association (Greater Los Angeles Affiliate) Grant No. 701-G2-2.

89

Method

108 patients were recruited in the pre-baseline period and had diastolic blood pressure greater than 90 mmHg. Secondary hypertension and other concomitant disorders such as diabetes mellitus, congestive heart failure and renal disease were excluded. This period included 3 office/laboratory visits and daily home morning and evening BP measurements with an electronic sphygmomanometer. 24 patients were rejected because their average diastolic BP fell to less than 90 mmHg; additionally more patients were excluded because of non-compliance with home BP recordings. 58 patients were enrolled in the two week baseline period. This period included three laboratory baseline sessions. At each session patients sat quitly for 10 min, followed by three blood pressure (pre) and pulse rate measurements. After fifteen more min of quiet sitting three final determinations of BP recordings were performed (post). There were 17 patients in the non-drug group who had not taken anti-hypertensive medications for at least 6 months prior to their participation. Many had discontinued medications because of side effects. Forty patients in the drug treated group had been taking the same dose of medication for the past 6 months. The drug treated patients were divided into three groups: 1: Relaxation (N = 13); 2: Relaxation/biofeedback (N = 14); and 3: Self-monitoring (N = 14). The non-drug group (N = 17) was instructed to lower their blood pressure with the relaxation technique (2). Each group was seen in the laboratory 2 times the first week and once every two weeks for a total of 7 sessions. The relaxation groups were instructed in a progressive relaxation technique and were asked to practise this technique each evening with the aid of a tape cassette recording. Home blood pressures were recorded before and after these 20 min sessions. The RL/BF group additionally received biofeedback to reduce frontalis muscle activity during the laboratory sessions. The self-monitoring group was instructed to lower BP through awareness and to moniter BP at home. The final two weeks of home and clinic measurements were used for comparison with the 2 weeks of baseline measurements using Newman-Keuls a posteriori tests (3).

The patient profile in each study group is shown in Table 1. It is evident that the majority of the study patients were in their fifties and most of them were white males. Mean diastolic BP averaged near 100 mmHg. This was the average BP in the laboratory (pre). Other characteristics not shown here, smoking, alcohol consumption, work conditions and family history of high blood pressure, were similar in each of the groups.

Table 1. Description of patient sample.

	Relaxation	Relaxation/ Biofeedback	Self- monitoring	Relaxation/ non-drug
Mean age (yrs)	54 ± 5	52 ± 5	53 ± 7	53 ± 8
Sex	10 M, 3 F	11 M, 4 F	12 M, 2 F	13 M, 4 F
Race	12 W, 1 Blk	13 W, 1 Blk	13 W, 1 Blk	17 W
Mean BP (mmHg)	147 ± 10	145 ± 12	146 ± 14	148 ± 10
	99 ± 5	100 ± 7	99 ± 4	99 ± 6

The medications prescribed by the patients' personal physicians were maintained unchanged throughout the study. The treatment given was distributed proportionately in various groups of antihypertensive medication (Table 2).

Table 2. Anti-hypertensive medications in three drug groups.

	RL	RL/BF	SM
Diuretic	4	5	4
Beta-blocker	2	2	2
Diuretic & beta-blocker	1	1	1
Clonidine	1	0	2
Clonidine & diuretic	1	2	1
Methyldopa	1	1	1
Vasodilator & diuretic	1	1	1
Combination of 3 drugs with different actions	2	2	2

RL = Relaxation (N = 13); RL/BL = Relaxation/Biofeedback (N = 14);
SM = Self-Monitoring (N = 14).

Results

Laboratory blood pressure

Blood pressures taken in the laboratory in both drug and non-drug groups were compared before and after sitting quietly for fifteen min (pre vs post). There was no change in diastolic blood pressure in either group. Blood pressure in the drug group reduced from 99.1 ± 5.4 mmHg to 97.1 ± 5.3 mmHg (ns) whereas BP in the non-drug group reduced from 99.1 ± 5.5 mmHg to 98.4 ± 5.5 mmHg (ns). Only systolic BP significantly decreased in the drug-treated group, from 145.7 ± 10.0 mmHg to 141.4 ± 8.4 mmHg ($p < 0.01$), while the non-drug group showed a reduction of BP from 147.5 ± 10.0 to 144.7 ± 8.4 mmHg (ns).

Home blood pressure

Blood pressures in the non-drug treated group were significantly higher for morning systolic BP when compared to their evening BP (138.9 ± 9.5 vs 135.4 ± 9.7 mmHg = $p < 0.01$). A smaller and insignificant fall in systolic BP was seen in the smaller non-drug treatment group. Diastolic BP demonstrated the similar trend without significant difference in morning and evening BP.

Blood pressure changes during the study period

Added biobehavioral treatment significantly lowered both systolic and diastolic blood pressure in drug treated groups when compared to the self-monitoring group only in home blood pressure measurements (both a.m. and p.m.). No significant differences were observed in laboratory BP. Relaxation in the non-drug group did not lower BP, as much as the drug-treated group, although this difference was not statistically significant (Fig. 1).

Fig. 1. Blood pressure changes from control period. * indicates significant difference of both systolic and diastolic levels compared to selfmonitoring group.

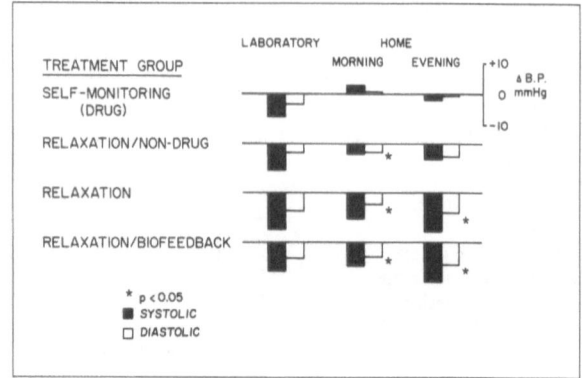

Discussion

The effects of interventions to treat hypertension are traditionally measured during a patient visit to a clinic, office or laboratory. Several studies here suggested that such casual blood pressures do not correlate well with longer periods of blood pressure measurement (4, 5). The variability of BP throughout the day may contribute to such findings. It is also reasonable that the stress of a clinic blood pressure may variably override the effect of any intervention. Mancia et al. (6) have recently reported that intra-arterial blood pressures may rise dramatically during the period of physician attendance.

The present study suggests that home blood pressures over a two week period were able to demonstrate an effect of biobehavioral interventions whereas clinic measurements did not. This results may be practically explicable by the greater number of days of measurement at home (14) than those determined in the laboratory (3). It is also possible that the home setting may avoid the stress superimposed by the clinic/laboratory setting.

Additionally, the results suggest that patients who are taking antihypertensive drugs may have an even greater difference between home blood pressure recordings and clinic recordings than those who are on no medications. The relaxation group on medications had a greater, though not statistically significant, response to this intervention than did the relaxation group not on medications. Also the medication group seemed to have a greater fall in systolic blood pressure with quiet sitting than did the smaller group not on medication. The heterogeneity of the drug treatments and the unequal group sizes make such analyses difficult, but further investigation of this question appears warranted.

Conclusion

The setting (clinic/laboratory vs home) and the condition (before or after sitting quietly) under which blood pressure measurements are made may influence the effect of medications or behavioral therapy.

References

1. Shapiro D, Goldstein IB: Biobehavioral perspectives on hypertension. J Consult Clin Psychol 50: 841–858 (1982).
2. Jacobson E: Progressive Relaxaton. University of Chicago Press (Chicago 1938).
3. Winer BJ: Statistical Principles in Experimental Design. McGraw-Hill (New York 1971) .
4. Drayer JM, Weber MA, DeYoung JL, Wyle FA: Circadian Blood Pressure Patterns in Ambulatory Hypertensive Patients: Effects of Age. Am J Med 73: 493–499 (1982).
5. Harshfield GA, Pickering TG, Kleizert HD, Blank S, and Laragh JH: Situational Variations of Blood Pressure in Ambulatory Hypertensive Patients. Psychosomatic Med. 44: 137–245 (1982).
6. Marcia G, Bertinieri G, Grassi G, Parati G, Pomidossi G, Ferrari A, Gregorini L, Zanchetti A: Effects of Blood Pressure Measurements by the Doctor on Patient's Blood Pressure and Heart rate. Lancet II: 695–698 (1983).

Address for correspondence:
C. Thananopavarn, M.D.
Hypertension Division
V.A. Medical Center
Sepulveda, Ca., 91343

Aerospace applications of ambulatory blood pressure monitoring

William Thornton, John Wallace

Introduction

The authors have been involved in the clinical testing, verification and use of the P-II and P-III "pressurometers" from their earliest days. One of the authors is in the NASA space program and as part of our investigation of the behavior of normal blood pressure in a variety of circumstances, made a series of recordings while flying high performance jet AirCraft A/C and for comparison, while a passenger in civil transport A/C. He also made a series of recordings during space flight on the NASA Shuttle. Excerpts from these are shown to illustrate an individual's BP response to the aerospace environment.

Background

Relatively little inflight data on blood pressure exists. The earliest reported measurements were those of v. Diringshofens and Belonoschkin in 1932 and 1933 (1, 2), followed by McFarland's study during trans-Pacific clipper flights in 1937 (3). Kirsch also took manual measurements during combat flights (bombers) in WWII (4). The first comprehensive inflight measurements were made by Roman (5) in specially instrumented jet fighters in which K sounds and cuff pressures were simultaneously recorded and manually correlated. This technique was also used in the Mercury and Gemini flights (6, 7) BP was taken at a fixed location on Skylab using automated K sound technique (8). There is at least one report from Italy of the use of the P-III in A/C flight (9).

Methodology

A standard P-III recorder was installed as shown in Fig. 1. Calibration readings were made immediately before and after actual use as a part of the record in TEST position using Hg manometers except on the space flights where a calibrated aneroid gauge was used. During T-38 flights the recorder was stowed in the right side map case. It was worn with the shoulder strap on civil A/C and on the ground. In weightlessness it was attached to any convenient clothing point.
Data reduction on the T-38 flights was done on a Tandy TRS-80 computer modified and programmed to our specifications, on a DMA 1981 connected via cross country Modem on the civil flights and by DMA 1981 and manual plotting on the space flight.

Hypertension Service, Dept. Medicine, UTMB Galveston, Texas

Fig. 1 Typical installation of P-III blood pressure recorder. 1 – Transducer, 2 – Cuff, 3 – Electrodes, 4 – P-III B.P. recorder, 5 – Pneumatic Hose.

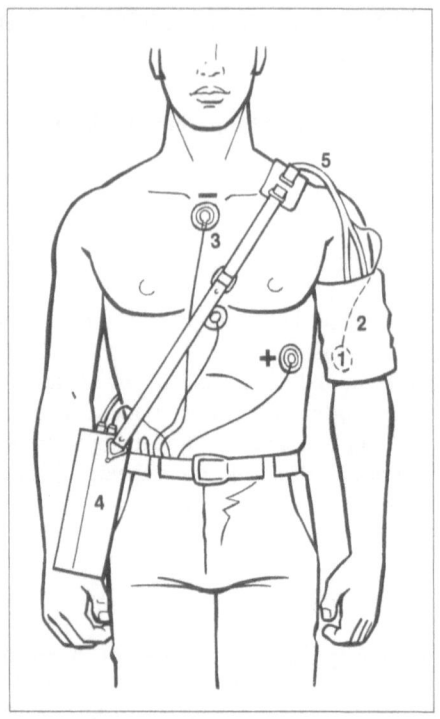

A series of fragments of the recording of the launch and first day and night of Shuttle Mission STS-8, Fig. 6, were obtained as follows. The P-III functioned well but data transfered to a special interim storage device was lost. The initial portion of this P-III data was written over during its reuse on entry. A portion of the prelaunch data was manually copied and the portion not obliterated was retrieved postflight by the 1981 processor. EKG electrodes were lost at 17.40 h and not replaced. A second P-III was used to record Misson Day-MD-5 data.

Results

All records shown were made by and from the same individual whose characteristics are given in Table 1. In the T-38 flights he was the pilot under the conditions shown on the captions of the plots and or otherwise a passenger. Six flights were made in the T-38, a two place supersonic jet used for proficiency training in the astronaut program. There were four civil flights with a total of 7 legs. On the Space Shuttle STS-8, records were made during launch and day 1, on day 5 and during re-entry. Several 24-hour records were made during normal 1 g activities during this period of inflight studies.

Fig. 2. shows a typical daily record during usual activities in 1980. There is large variability: physical exercise and emotional reaction produce the expected rise while sleep produces its normal individual fall.

96

Table 1: Subject's Characteristics.

	T-38/Civil Flights	Space Flight
Age, years	51	54
Height, inches	73	73
Weight, pounds	203	199
Max O^{*2} intake, ml kg^{-1} min^{-1}	54	44
Pilot time – T-38	2500 hrs	

Casual (Annual Physical) Blood Pressures)					
1967 - 108/70	1971 - 116/80	1975 - 118/90	1979	-	110/70
1968 - 114/76	1972 - N.R.	1976 - 118/86	1980	-	120/70
1969 - 128/80	1973 - 110/72	1977 - 110/70	1981	-	122/72
1970 - 124/80	1974 - 108/66	1978 - 110/70	1982	-	110/80
			1983	-	120/82

Laboratory				
Blood	Na^+	140 meq/l	Glucose	70 mg/dL
	K^+	4.1 meq/l	Hct.	41.3
	Cl^-	105 meq/l	RBC	4.79×10^6 cells/mm^3
	CO_2	28 meq/l	WBC	5.1×10^3 cells/mm^3
	BUN	23 mg/l		normal differential

Urine	24 h sample, 2000 ml volume
	Specific Gravity 1.022, normal micro. exam
	pH – 8.0
	Glu., Blood, Ketone, Bilirubin and Urobilin – Neg
	Alderosterone – 5 ugm/day
	PRA – 2.00 ngm/ml/24 h
	Serum Creatinine 1.2 mg/l Creatine Clear – 115 ml/min
	Protein 20 mgm/24 h

The initial T-38 flight (Fig 3) made under the bag in actual near minimum weather produced a large increase in pressures which showed a decline through the flight. Certain activities produced transient increases. An episode of anger inadvertently recorded during a phone call produced a large elevation.

Flights in civil A/C were similar to the first flight shown in Fig. 5.

Launch/first day of space flight shows a slight elevation during preflight and launch followed by decreased pressure on orbit during the first day. Pressures recorded later in the flight were more nearly normal, but the fall during sleep is still present.

Comment

Several general and individual points are illustrated by the 23-hour record. There is great variability in a healthy individual whose usual casual blood pressures are 110/70. Like a large percentage of active males his working pressures are more typically 135/90. In such

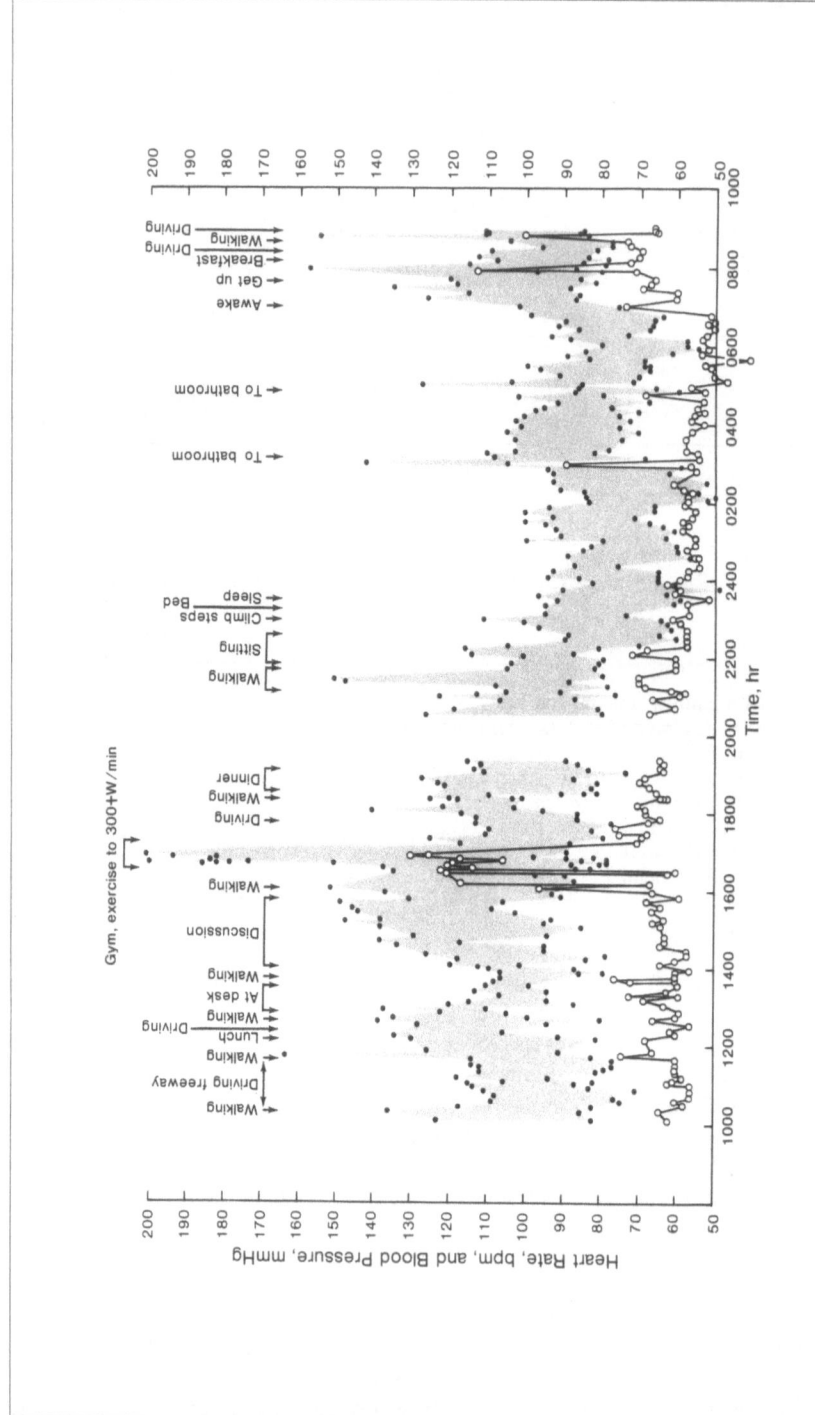

Fig. 2 Twenty-three hour recording of a typical non-flying work day for subject. Exercise was on a bicycle ergometer at levels shown 1640 hrs. Discussion with an emotional content at 1400 hrs.

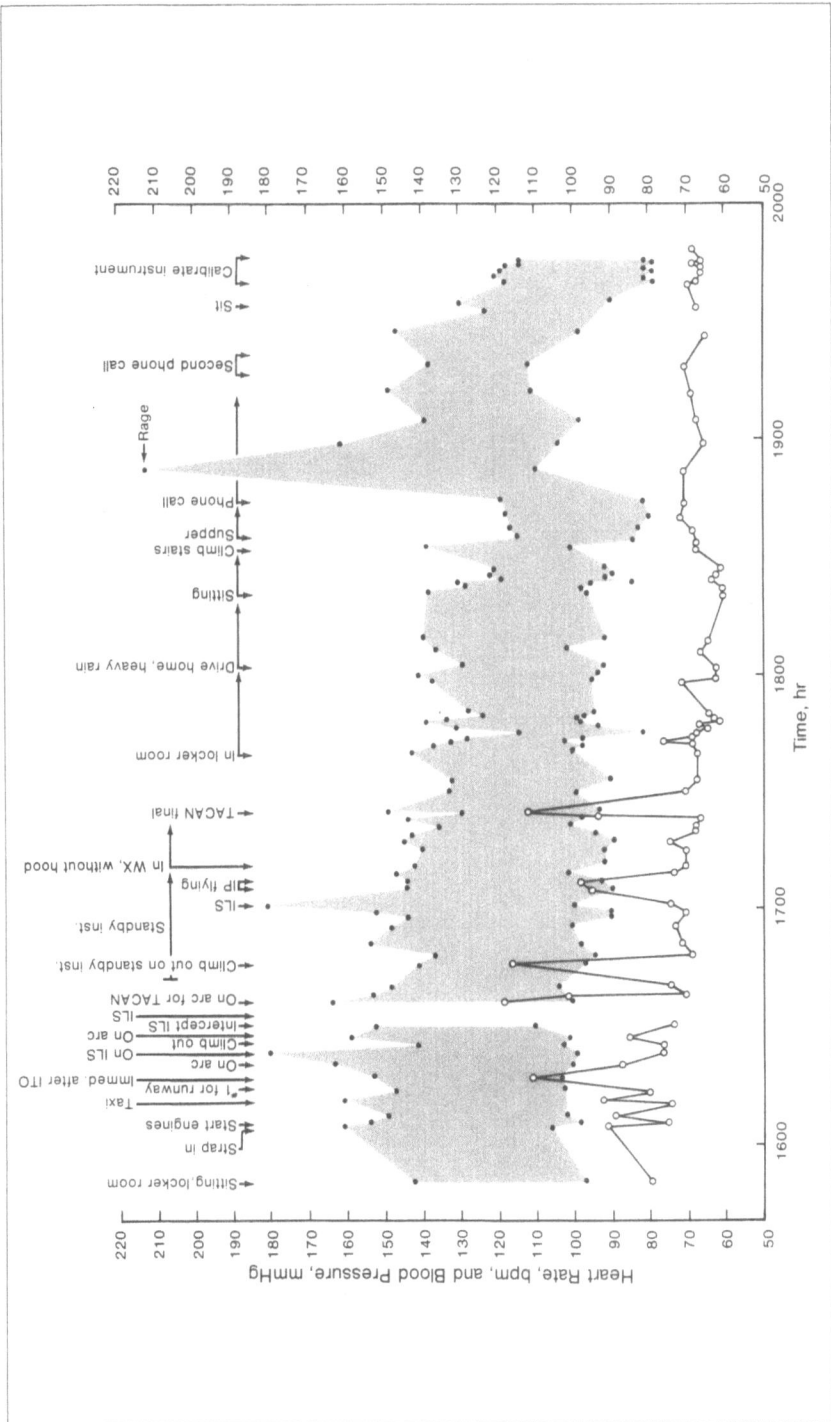

Fig. 3 First flight in T-38 recording blood pressure. Subject was flying on instruments under hood. ILS Instrument Landing System TACAN Tactical Air Navigation System. ITO Instrumental Takeoff.

100

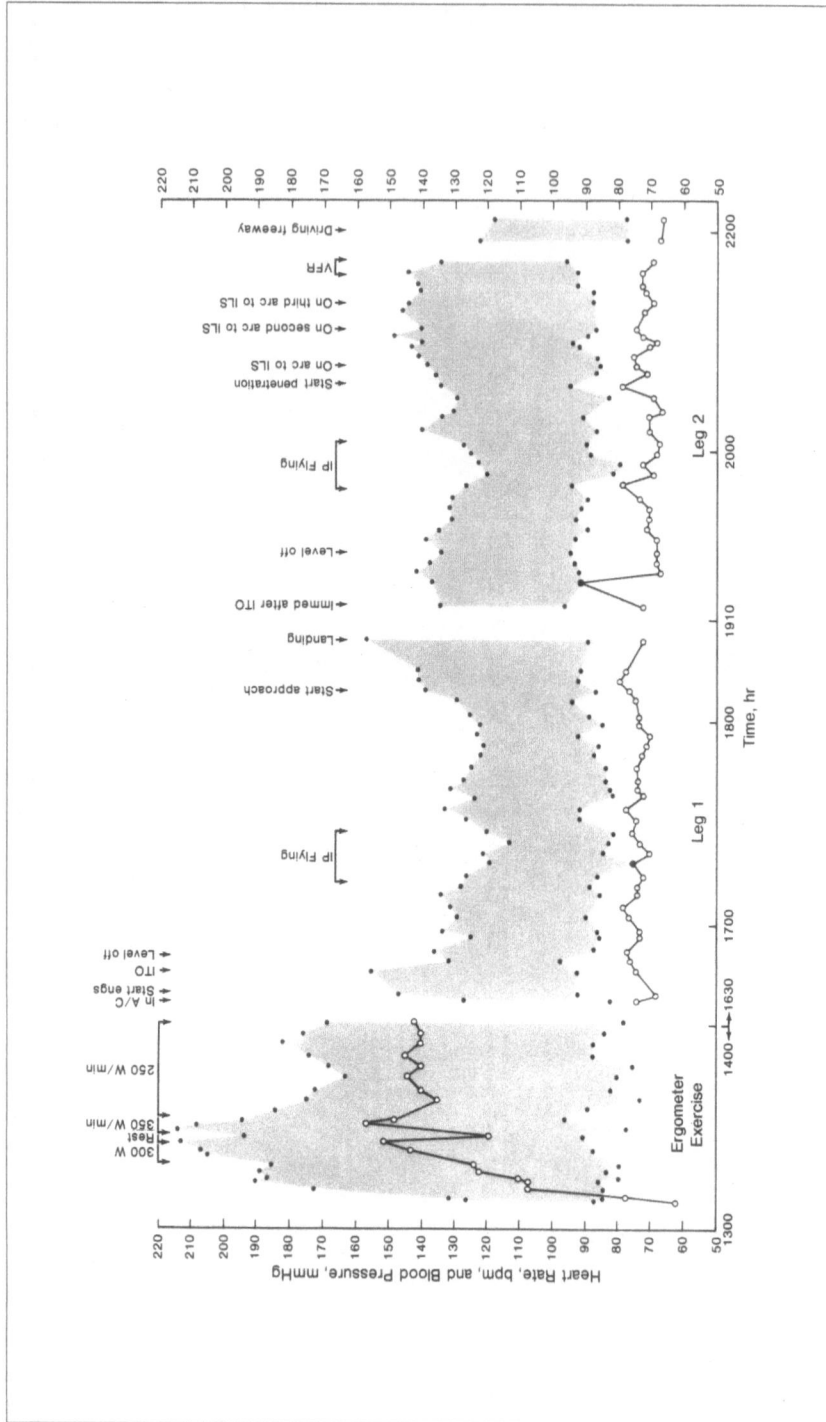

Fig. 4 Second recorded flight in T-38. Subject was again on instruments but flight was 2 legs, cross-country with multiple approaches prior to landing. ILS Instrument Landing System. VFR visual flight rules.

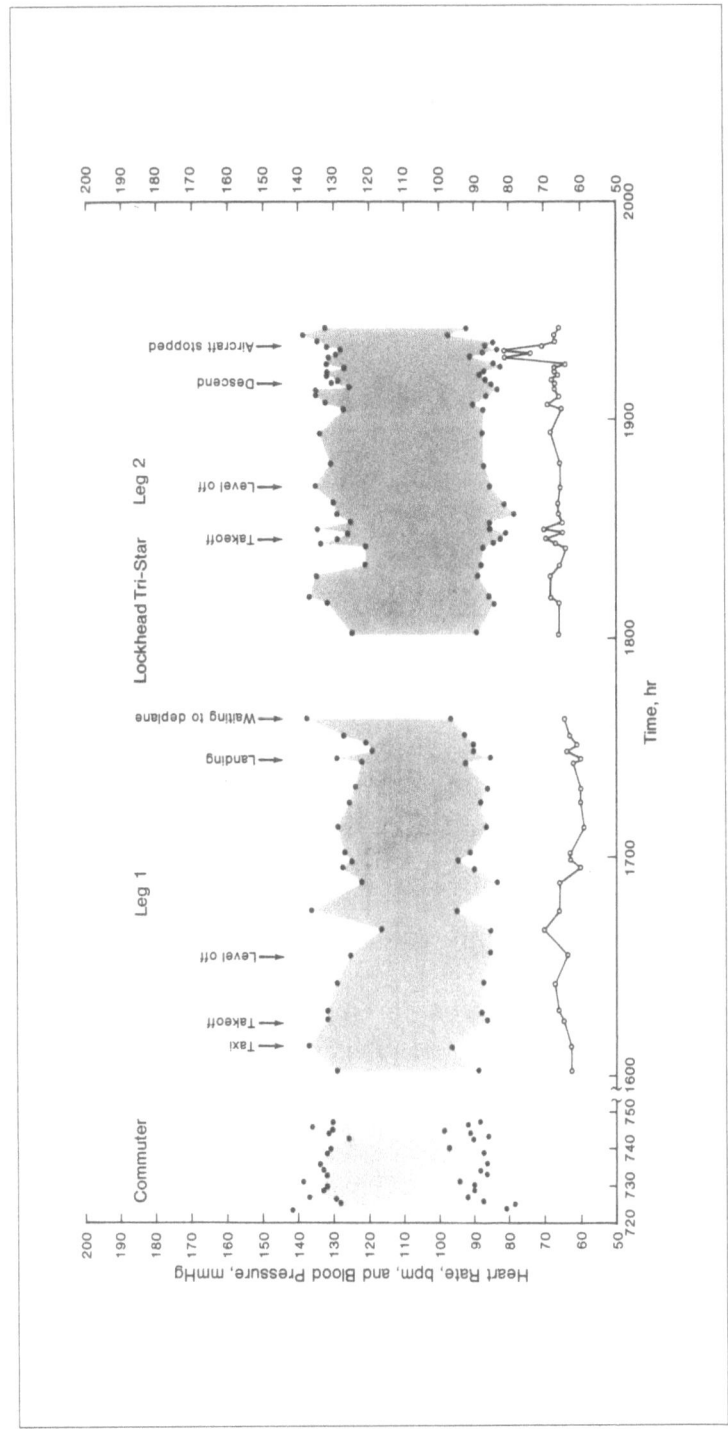

Fig. 5 First recorded flights in civil aircraft (D. H. Otter commuter and lockheed Tri-Star), 3 legs.

101

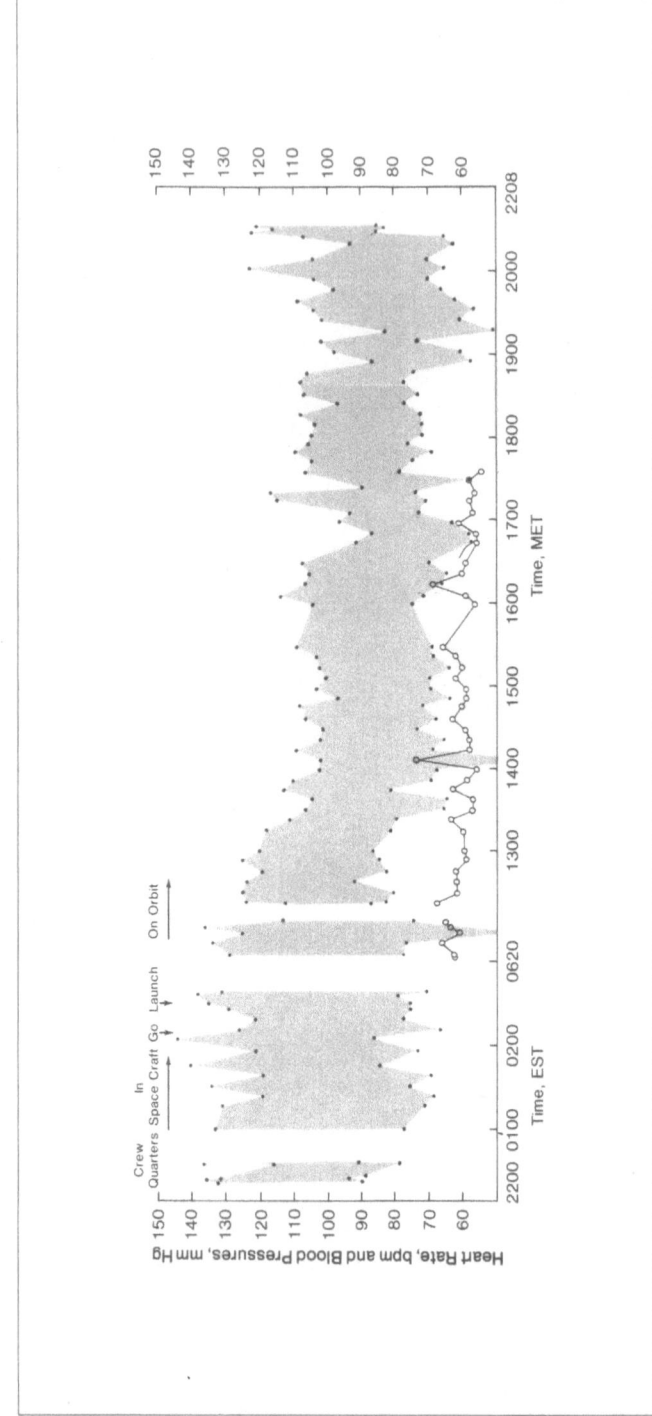

Fig. 6 Launch and first "day" and "night" on-orbit, STS-8. Times are EDT. See text for explanation of various segments.

active individuals, there is a marked fall during sleep. The concept of diagnosis based on some percentage of pressures being above an arbitrary level of pressures, often derived from casual pressure experience, is in our opinion unjustified. A sizeable percentage of normal males show much less increase with work and less decrease in sleep. More recent 24-hour records from the individual are consistent with this one.

The predominant feature of the first inflight record (Fig. 3) is a fall in SBP and DBP during flight. Note that pressures were high before the flight started. While the work load was high during this flight, it was no higher than in a second flight (Fig. 4) made under the same conditions, insofar as possible. The most likely explanation is the effect of the orienting (alerting) (10) reflex, for while the subject was totally familiar with every aspect of the flight, the separate operations, when combined, had a potentially significant impact on both flight operations and other team members. As the impacts were experienced, pressure dropped. This is analogous to the white coat/cuff syndrome that will always plague manual blood pressure measurement, but it also illustrates the danger of a new situation affecting even automatic pressure measurements. The inadvertent measurement made during anger illustrates the potential strength of psychogenic effects. A second T-38 flight illustrates two effects noted by previous investigators e.g., increased BP at the start and end of a flight which is consistent with the increased responsibilities and workload at those times and the "commander's effect", i.e., the pilot responsible for the vehicle always exhibits relatively higher pressures than other equally skilled and knowledgeable pilots present for a given situation (11). This is demonstrated here by decreases in pressure when control was deliberatly relinquished to the I.P. in an undemanding situation.

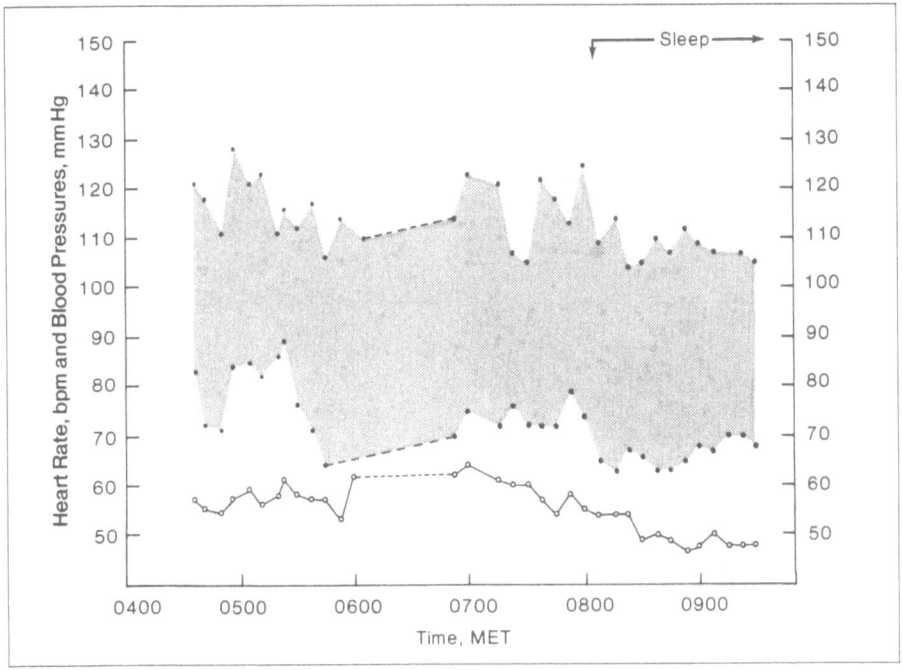

Fig. 7 Portion of "day" and "night" of Mission Day 5, STS-8, MET shown is plus 4 days.

Inflight pressures were considerable (4) lower than those previously recorded (5) and could be attributed to individual physiology, increased flying time in the A/C or differences in physical condition.

The civil flights were remarkable only for the absence of BP effects.

Records from the space flight are complicated by several factors. First is the large fluid shift with probable expansion of central blood volume. The second is neurological effects from weightlessness during the first 36 hours of flight.

Pressure remained normal for the situation during launch (Fig. 6). At 06.00 h the pressure was comparable to ground situations, but from 12.00 h to 17.00 h there was a progressive fall reaching quite low values during the sleep period. However, sleep, if at all present, was brief and episodic. Considerable lability is present. By day 5 onorbit pressure (Fig. 7) had increased to near 1 g values, however, the usual fall with sleep is present. Heart rates had now become quite low by any standards.

In summary, automated Rivi-Rocci techniques can be used to measure blood pressure in a number of aerospace applications including noisy, demanding environments. There are several unique aspects of blood pressure response to aerospace operations, some of which remain to be defined by additional studies, especially in space flight.

References

1. v. Diringshofen H and Belonoschkin B: Experimentelle Untersuchungen über den Einfluß hoher Beschleunigungen auf den Blutdruck des Menschen. Z. Biologie 93: 1 (1932).
2. v. Diringshofen H and Diringshofen B: Elektrokardiographie, Blutdruckschreibung und Pneumotacographie im Motorfluge. Acta Aerophysiologica 6: 48 (1933).
3. McFarland RA and Edwards HT: The Effects of Prolonged Exposures to Altitudes of 8,000 to 12,000 Feet During Trans Pacific Flights. J. of Aviat Med 8: 156 (1938).
4. Kirsch RE: A Physiological Study of Aviators During Combat Flying. J. of Aviat Med 16: 376 (1945).
5. Roman JA: Cardiorespiratory Function Inflight. J. of Aerospace Med 34: 322 (1963).
6. NASA SP-4003: Space Medicine in Project Mercury. U.S.G.P.O. (1965).
7. NASA SP-121: Gemini Mid-Program Conference. U.S.G.P.O. (1966).
8. NASA SP-377: Biomedical Results of Skylab. U.S.G.P.O. (1973).
9. Ramacci CA et al: Esperienze di Sfig Momanometria Automatica su Piloti Militari in Volo. Rivista D Medicina Aeronautica e Spaziale 44: 230 (1980).
10. Pickering GW: High Blood Pressure. J. and A. Churchill (London (1968)).
11. Roman J: Risk and Responsibility as Factors Affecting Heart Rate in Test Pilots. Aerospace Medicine 36: 518 (1965).

Adress for correspondence:
William E. Thornton, M.D.
John M. Wallace, M.D.
Hypertension Service, 5A
University of Texas Medical Branch
Galveston, TX 77550

Understanding hypertension. The contribution of direct ambulatory blood pressure monitoring.

E. B. Raftery

Summary: The description of a fundamental rhythm of circadian variation of blood pressure which is dependant for its expression upon the alpha adrenoreceptor in the peripheral arteriole presents an entirely different way of looking at blood pressure and it is apparent that the effects of drugs which are used to control hypertension upon this rhythm may well be of fundamental importance. The description of this rhythm would not have been possible without the technique of ambulatory intra-arterial blood pressure recording, and there is every possibility that more fundimental discoveries will follow. The abnormality which underlies essential hypertension has yet to be elucidated; these sudies suggest that the abnormality lies in the central nervous system. If it is a primary autonomic defect, then we must look to the hypothalamus rather than the smooth muscle of the peripheral arteriole, the kidney, or genetically – controlled abnormalities of the sodium pump for the "cause" of essential hypertension.

Whatever its mechanism, this rhythm quite clearly presents a much more acceptable method for examining the effects of drugs on blood pressure than taking one-off casual recordings in an out-patient clinic. In particular, the introduction of a time element is bound to provide information missing from conventional clinical trials.

The Concept of Blood Pressure

Physicians have been aware of the arterial pulse for centuries and many diagnostic and therapeutic systems have been built up around it. However it was not until the upsurge of scientific curiosity in the eighteenth and nineteenth centuries that attempts were made to 'measure' blood pressure – i.e. express the sensations of tension and pulsation in the artery in numerical terms (1). Invasive techniques rapidly improved throughout the nineteenth and twentieth centuries in reliability and accuracy, but the non-invasive techniques have lagged sadly behind, and there has been no substantial advance since the full description of the Korotkoff technique at the turn of the century. This presents difficulties because invasive techniques cannot safely be used routinely in man, and yet the non-invasive technique most commonly used is full of known (and unknown) inaccuracies and unexplained discrepancies.

None of this would matter very much but for the fact that blood pressure has been shown to be an accurate predictor of life expectancy (2, 3) and reduction of elevated blood pressure has been shown to reduce the incidence of the cardio-vascular diseases which tend to shorten life expectancy (4). So in recent years attention has focused upon blood pressure as a concept, and methods for accurate clinical measurement have received increasing attention (5).

Northwick Park Hospital & Clinical Research Centre, Harrow, Middlessex, HA1 3UJ, U.K.

However this raises a difficult and complex problem; the blood pressure measurement which is a good predictor for large populations of hundreds of thousands may not be of much value when applied to a single individual from a different, but similar, population. In fact, it is to be hoped that this measurement *is* of no value, because blood pressures which predict a shortening of life expectancy in large populations can be found in as many as 15% of the normal population when surveyed by the same techniques (6).

Most physicians agree that the casual one-off indirect recording of blood pressure which forms the basis of insurance mortality statistics is not good enough to be used as an indicator of the need for treatment in individual patients – whether taken alone or in combination with other factors which are known to increase the risk of cardiovascular disease. The literature abounds with recommendations that the blood pressure should be recorded on three separate occasions under standardised conditions before a decision can be taken. It is not clear why most physicians regard three or more as being better than one, but it is clear that many recordings are thought to be more indicative of the 'truth' than just one.

This is likely to be true. Continuous recordings of intra-arterial blood pressure have shown quite clearly that blood pressure is a continuous variable, and as such is not amenable to simple methods of measurement. Cursory examination of the tracings show that there is considerable beat-to-beat and minute-to-minute variation, and that there may well be considerable inter-action between the measurer and the measured blood pressure. At best, a one-off indirect recording is relevant to the twenty-odd beats which occupy the time taken for the recording. It is inconceivable that it should approximate to any sort of "average" or "representative" measurement of blood pressure in any individual. It may well be that a "better" estimate may be obtained by repeated measurements over a long or short period of time, but nothing is known of this, and nothing can be known until the necessary experiments have been performed.

Intra-Arterial Ambulatory Recordings

The direct methods for measuring blood pressure have the great advantage of well-defined accuracy and precision, but cannot be widely used for the study of blood pressure in the individual because of their invasive nature. However, many of these objections were overcome in the system for continuous recording of intra-arterial blood pressure first desribed by Stott and his co-workers (7) and later refined at Northwick Park Hospital and Clinical Research Centre (8). This system consists of a small cannula which is placed in the brachial artery of the non-dominant arm under local anaesthesia, and is attached to a transducer/perfusion unit which hangs in a bag around the patient's neck. This perfuses the cannula with heparinised saline so that it does not clot, and transforms the pressure wave into an electrical signal which is recorded on a slowly-moving miniaturised tape recorder which hangs on a belt around the patient's waist (Fig. 1). The patient can dress and go about his normal activities, sleeping at home and returning to the hospital at twelve-hourly intervals for calibration and "topping up" of the perfusion reservoir. In this way, an accurate and precise recording of the blood pressure generated by each heart beat can be made while the patient is in his own familiar environment, away from the influence of doctors and nurses and going about his normal daily activities. Each tape cassette will record a full twenty-four hours of data, and heart-rate can be derived from a simultaneous ECG recording. The data can be recalled from the casette at leisure and digitised using a hybrid computer program (9) which stores the information to be used in any way required by the investigator.

While this technique has been shown to be free of serious complications in many hundreds of studies performed at Oxford, Northwick Park and other institutions, nevertheless it must be emphasised that it has all the potential hazards of invasive techniques, and cannot be regarded as anything other than a tool for research, which may shed much-needed light on blood pressure, the way it varies, and the "best" methods of obtaining information about it in individuals.

This technique has been used extensively to describe and enumerate the changes in blood pressure which occur during a wide variety of physical and mental activities (10). While these descriptions are interesting and informative, the wide degree of variation in blood pressure which these recordings clearly reveal emphasises the fundimental problem of characterisation of these records. This is essentially a statistical problem, which is capable of resolution (11) but still requires much work and thought.

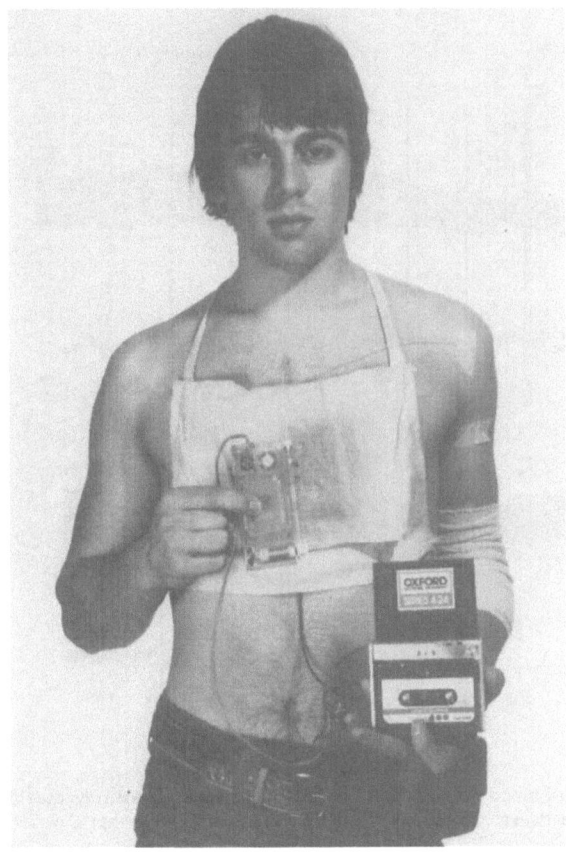

Fig. 1. A subject wearing the Oxford system for continuous intra-arterial blood pressure recording. The cannula is in the left brachial artery, the perfusion unit is worn around the neck, and the tape recorder goes into a pouch on the patient's belt.

Diurnal Variation of Blood Pressure

Complete data on blood pressure throughout each 24 h cycle can readily be obtained from the tape cassettes and printed out using a direct-writing recorder (Fig. 2). This crude presentation is as meaningless as a single one-off recording taken by the indirect technique, since it is full of variability and cannot readily be expressed in a simple numerical fashion. Because of the large number of observations this becomes a statistical problem, but it is readily apparent from the tracings that there is a difference between the blood pressure which is obtained during the day and the blood pressure which is obtained during the night. Simple inspection of the tracings shows the BP falls in the night and so does the amount of variability. This is not a new observation; in fact it can be dated back to 1898 (12), and it has long formed the basis for a suspicion that there is a diurnal rhythm of BP between day and night which may well be intimately related to other circadian rhythms. This information from the tape recordings obtained from hypertensive subjects may well yield important information about blood pressure which is as yet poorly understood. However, ambulatory BP recordings can never be properly standardised because it is quite impossible to establish exactly the same conditions of physical and

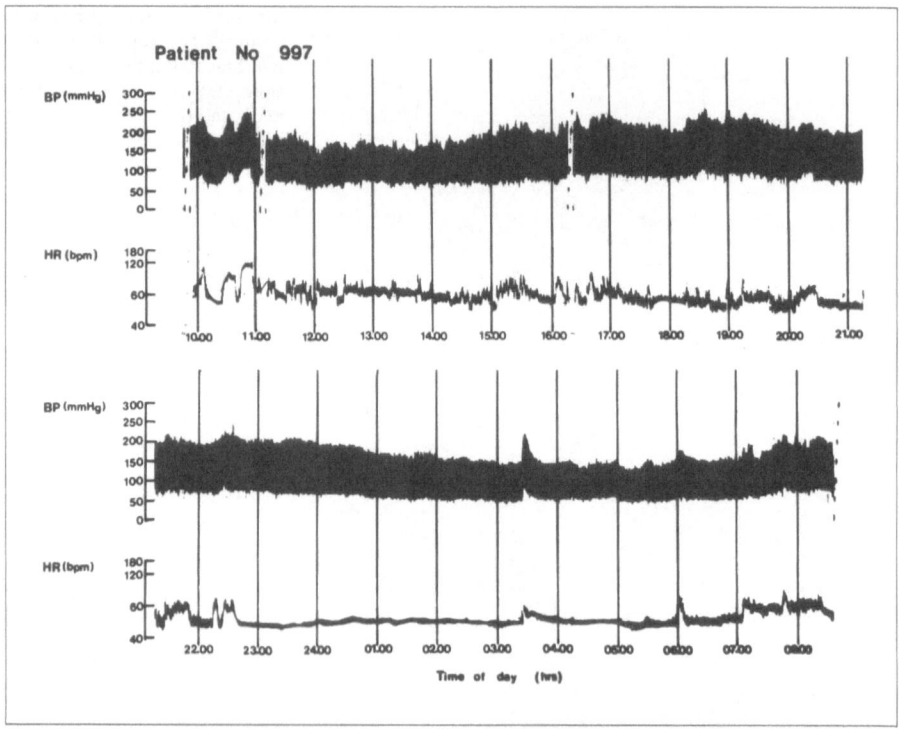

Fig. 2. A complete 24-hour print-out of blood pressure and heart rate. The vertical bars indicate the hours on the time axis. All the data between each bar is meaned by the computer so that a performance curve can be constructed.

emotional activity on any two consecutive days and there must be a considerable amount of random "noise" in any individual tracing. A variety of techniques have been employed to "smooth" these variations and produce a standardised curve for variation over each day and night, but the most successful has been the relatively simple technique of calculating hourly means of systolic and diastolic pressures for each hour during the day and expressing the results on a 24-h axis. This relatively simple description of blood pressure can readily be interpreted by the eye. We have employed this technique in a large number of patients with untreated hypertension and a small group of patients who were completely normotensive, and have revealed a surprisingly simple curve (13) which has many of the characteristics of a true circadian rhythm (Fig. 3). We have found that this curve is not readily apparent in all individual tracings but if the technique is used to describe group performance rather than individual performance then the combination of any three out of any number of recordings will produce a curve which can be very little altered by adding more information to the data base. This is strong evidence that it represents a fundamental rhythm which could be used to describe blood pressure more satisfactorily than a one-off clinic recording.

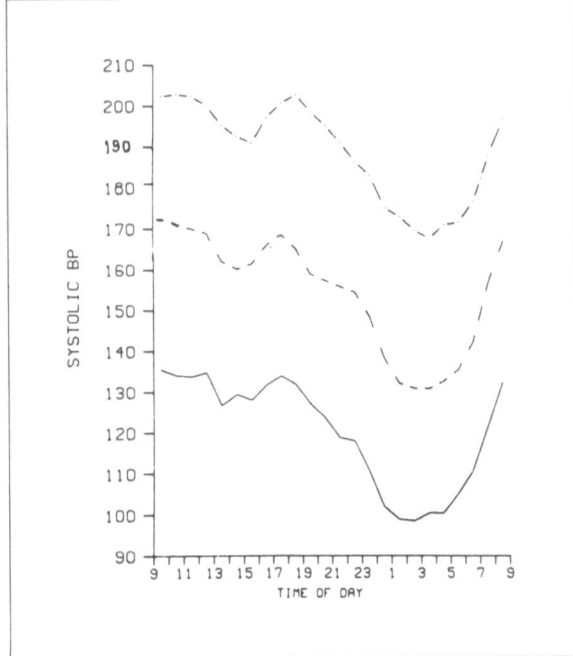

Fig. 3. Systolic blood pressure curves in three groups of subjects. Note the similarity of the curves with peaks at 10.00 h and 17.00 h and a nadir at 03.00 h. Note also the rise in pressure before the hour of awakening. ——— Normotensives' (25), - - - uncomplicated hypertensives (100), ·—·—· hypertensives with LVH (20).

There are two peaks of mean blood pressure: one in the morning around 10.00 h and the second in the afternoon around 11.00 h. From late afternoon onwards the mean BP falls rapidly until about 03.00 h when there is a slow but consistent rise until 07.00 h. This hour in our patients coincided with the time of arousal and rising from bed, and from

109

07.00 until 10.00 h there is a rapid rise in blood pressure to the first peak for the day. The smoothness of this curve and in particular the small rise in pressure between 03.00 and 06.00 h strongly suggests a fundamental rhythm, which is presumably related to activity of the autonomic nervous system.

The curve which can be derived from hourly mean heart rates is superficially similar to that of the blood pressure, but on closer inspection there are a number of differences (Fig. 4). Firstly, the peak for heart rate is to be found at 01.00 h for reasons which are not at all clear. From that point onwards, mean heart rate falls throughout the night, and goes on falling until 07.00 h (which is the hour of arousal) after which it rises rapidly to a peak at 10.00 h. It then falls again until 12.00 h only to rise rapidly to its peak for the day at 01.00 h.

On the basis of these curves, it was proposed that a 24-h tape recording could be represented as a fundamental circadian curve which could be used to describe group behaviour and may also be useful in individuals since the simple statistical technique of hourly means produces a powerful numerical and pictorial expression of blood pressure. However, this is a concept which clearly needs to be firmly established before it can be completely accepted as a method of describing blood pressure.

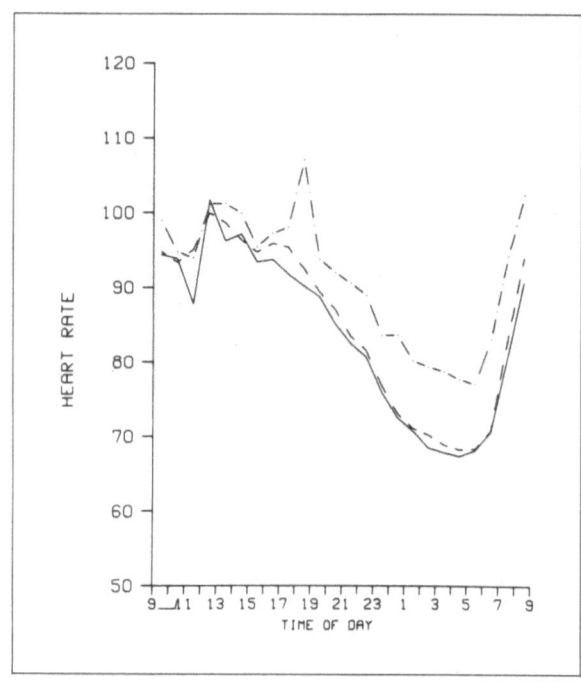

Fig. 4. Heart rate curves from the same groups. The peaks are different, and heat rate continues to fall until the hour of awakening. ——— Normotensives (25), − − − uncomplicated hypertensives (100), ·—··— hypertensives with LVH (20).

Significance of the Preawakening Rise in Pressure

It must be readily apparent that the simple addition of random numbers could easily produce the small rise in pressure before the hour of awakening. Different individuals in the groups described were awakening at different times so that in pooling the data some blood pressures were rising white others were falling. This possible artefact in the curves can be readily corrected by orientating the 24-h axis around the hour of awakening (Fig. 5). This is a very simple task for the computer to perform since the precise time of arousal (i.e. recovery of vision) was clearly identified in all these patients. When this correction was applied, the blood pressure was still seen to rise from 03.00 h in the morning until the hour of awakening and although there was no dramatic change in the pressure until arousal took place, the small but consistent rise in pressure could be shown to be statistically significant ($p < 0.001$) (13). However when the data from the mean heart rate curve was manipulated in the same way it was apparent that heart rate does not rise in conjunction with the blood pressure, but goes on falling until the hour of arousal (Fig. 6). This very simple demonstration of a small but consistent rise in pressure before the hour of arousal is again strong evidence that these curves are representing a true circadian rhythm; furthermore the evidence suggests that this rhythm is dissociated from that shown by mean heart rate when expressed in the same way.

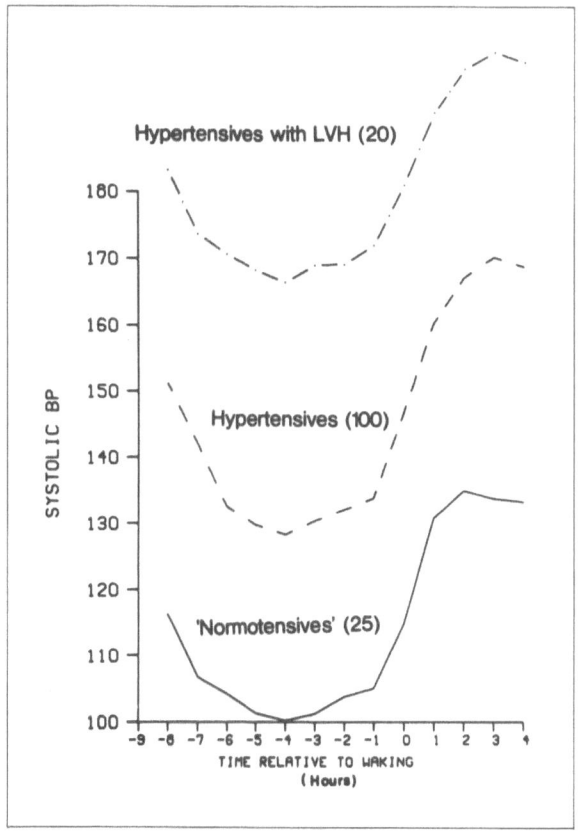

Fig. 5. Blood pressure curves "normalised" around the hour of awakening. The pre-awakening rise of pressure is still present and is strong evidence of a circadian rhythm.

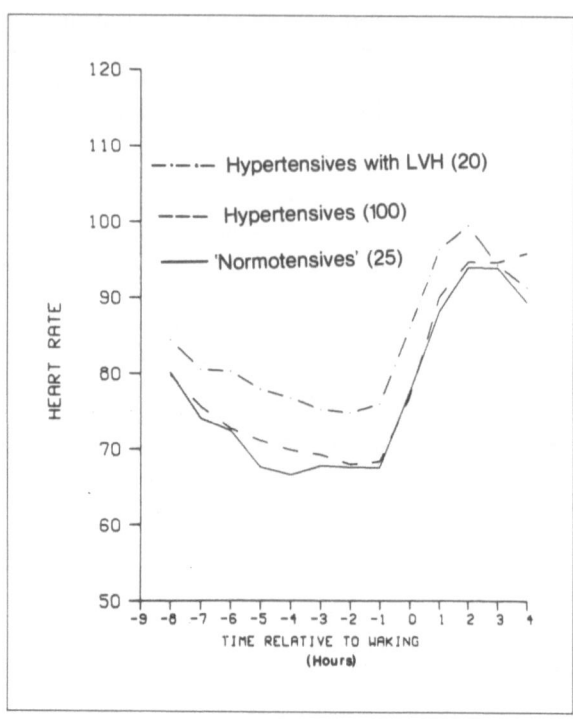

Fig. 6. "Normalised" heart rate curves. Note that heart rate goes on falling until the hour of awakening.

Repeatability of the Curves

If these curves represent a strong circadian rhythm then they should be very repeatable from day to day and even perhaps from week to week. For eight of these patients under study, complete data was available for a full 48-h period and a circadian curve could be constructed for the first and second days (Fig. 7). These plots show that the curves ob-

Fig. 7. Repeating the circadian curves on two consecutive days produces an identical curve, which is evidence of a very strong circadian rhythm.

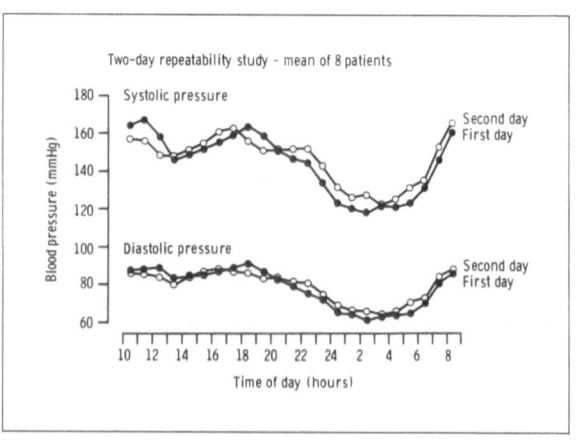

tained are almost identical, with no statistical differences between any pair of hourly mean pressures throughout the whole cycle. Furthermore when these curves were repeated after a six-week interval during which the subjects took placebo tablets (15), the same high degree of repeatability was readily demonstrated. This can only be interpreted as strong evidence of a powerful circadian rhythm which is very little influenced by individual variations in activity, both mental and physical.

Activity Versus Inactivity

It is conceivable that the diurnal variation in blood pressure is simply a reflection of high blood pressures during daytime activities as opposed to low blood pressures during nocturnal inactivity. We tested this hypothesis in ten of our patients by performing a 48-h recording, with the subjects spending one of the 24-h periods completely inactive in bed, and the second period going about their normal everyday activities (16). Comparison of the heart rate curves (Fig. 8) showed (as one might expect) that the high heart rates obtained during the day were almost completely abolished by bedrest, producing a much "flatter" heart rate curve. However direct comparison of the activity/inactivity blood pressure curves showed a very different picture with again no statistical differences between any of the mean hourly points and a remarkable retention of the shape of the curve. This again points to a true circadian rhythm rather than a simple alternation of activity and inactivity.

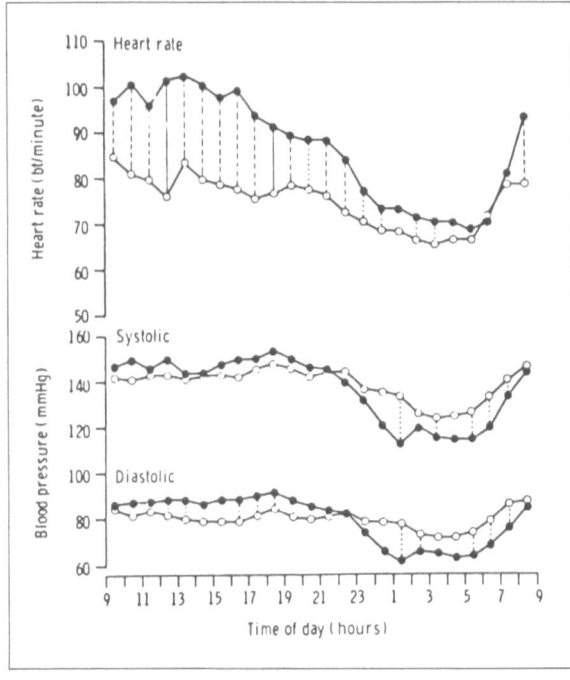

Fig. 8. Bed rest flattens the heart rate curve, but the blood pressure curve remains intact. Circadian variation of blood pressure activity study ● = Ambulant, p ······ < 0.05; ○ = Bedrest, p – – – < 0.01; p ——— < 0.001.

Dissociation Between Heart Rate and Blood Pressure Diurnal Variation

A fundamental part of the observations that have been made so far is the difference in behaviour between mean heart rate and mean blood pressure. It has been generally thought that heart rate and blood pressure are very closely associated and follow similar patterns, so that one might almost be used as an indicator of the relative changes in the other. The findings from our laboratory suggested that there was a dissociation between the behaviour of mean heart and mean blood pressure, and this hypothesis could be tested by performing 24-h curves in patients with fixed-rate pacemakers in whom there could be no variation in the heart rate (17) (Fig. 9). A study performed on eleven patients again quite clearly showed that a general shape of the blood pressure curve was retained, even though the heart rate was absolutely fixed.

Fig. 9. The shape of the blood pressure curve remains intact despite the fact that all the patients had fixed-rate pacemakers and therefore a fixed heart rate.

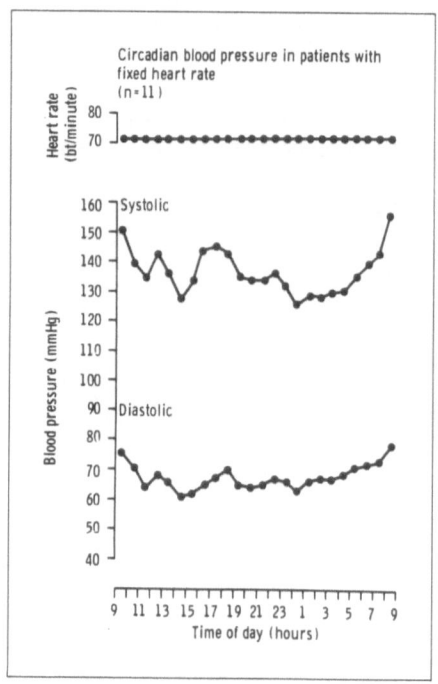

Circadian Variation of Blood Pressure

From these observations it is possible to suggest that there is a very strong circadian rhythm of blood pressure which expresses itself over each 24-h cycle with two peaks occurring at 10.00 h in the morning and 11.00 h in the afternoon, followed by a steady fall in pressure throughout the night until 03.00 h when the mean pressure begins to rise slowly until the hour of arousal. From this point, the blood pressure rapidly rises to its peak for the day once again. Heart rate responses do not follow such a circumscribed curve. But heart rate and blood pressure are under the control of the autonomic nervous sytem and it would appear from these data that while that part of the autonomic nervous system which is responsible for controlling blood pressure follows a circadian rhythm, that part responsible for heart rate is much more sensitive to variations in mental and physical activity and does not follow the same pattern. A simple consideration of the physiological principles underlying blood pressure control would suggest that this is hardly surprising. Heart rate is very largely controlled by variations in vagal tone whereas blood pressure is essentially controlled by variations in sympathetic tone which act on the peripheral arteriole and are mediated there by an alpha adrenoreceptor. The parasympathetic and sympathetic nervous systems are under no obligation to behave in the same way, and a dissociation between the two is well within the bounds of credibility.

This description of a fundamental rhythm of circadian variation of blood pressure which is dependant for its expression upon the alpha adrenoreceptor in the peripheral arteriole presents an entirely different way of looking at blood pressure and it is apparent that the effects of drugs which are used to control hypertension upon this rhythm may well be of fundamental importance. The description of this rhythm would not have been possible without the technique of ambulatory intra-arterial blood pressure recording, and there is every possibility that more fundimental discoveries will follow. The abnormality which underlies essential hypertension has yet to be elucidated; these sudies suggest that the abnormality lies in the central nervous system. If it is a primary autonomic defect, then we must look to the hypothalamus rather than the smooth muscle of the peripheral arteriole, the kidney, or genetically – controlled abnormalities of the sodium pump for the "cause" of essential hypertension.

Whatever its mechanism, this rhythm quite clearly presents a much more acceptable method for examining the effects of drugs on blood pressure than taking one-off casual recordings in an out-patient clinic. In particular, the introduction of a time element is bound to provide information missing from conventional clinical trials.

References

1. Raftery EB: The methodology of blood pressure recording. Brit J Clin Pharm 6: 193 (1978).
2. Actuarial Society of America and the Associations of life insurance medical directors: Supplement to Blood Pressure Study (New York 1941).
3. Metropolitan Life Insurance Co.: Blood pressure: Insurance experience and its implications (New York 1961).
4. Australian national blood pressure study: Lancet, i, 1261 (1980).
5. O'Brien E and O'Malley K: Essentials of blood pressure measurement. Churchill Livingstone (London 1981).
6. Miall WE: Screening for hypertension. Brit J Hosp Med 592 (1982).
7. Bevan AT, Honour AJ, Stott FH: Portable recorder for continuous arterial pressure measurement in man. J Physiol Lond 186, 3P (1966).
8. Millar-Craig, MW, Hawes B, Whittington J: A new system for recording ambulatory blood pressure in man. Med Biol Eng Comp 16: 727 (1978).
9. Cashman PMM, Stott FD, Millar-Craig MW: Hybrid system for fast data reduction of long-term blood pressure recordings. Med Biol Eng Comp 17: 629 (1979).
10. Wertheimer L, Bandu I, Amerasinghe S: Blood pressure in normal subjects. Proceedings of the Second International Symposium on Ambulatory Monitoring. p. 143, Academic Press (London 1977).

11. Sayers BM, Cicchiello LR, Raftery EB, Mann S, Green H: The assessment of continuous ambulatory blood pressure records. Med Inform 7: No. 2, 93–108 (1982).
12. Hill L: On rest, sleep and work and the concomitant changes in the circulation of the blood. Lancet 1, 282–285 (1898).
13. Millar-Craig MW, Raftery EB, Bishop CN: Circadian variation of blood pressure. Lancet i, 795 (1978).
14. Millar-Craig MW, Mann S, Altman DG, Raftery EB: The dissociation between blood pressure and heart rate changes prior to waking. Proceedings Fourth International Symposium on Ambulatory Monitoring. p. 531. Academic Press (London 1982).
15. Gould BA, Mann S, Davies AB, Altman DG, Raftery EB: Can placebo therapy influence arterial blood pressure? Clin Sci, 61, 478s (1981).
16. Mann S, Millar-Craig MW, Melville D, Bala Subramanian V, Raftery EB: Physical activity and the circadian rhythm of blood pressure. Clin Sci 57 Suppl. 5, 291s (1979).
17. Davies AB, Cashman PMM, Bala Subramanian V, Raftery EB: The effect of a ventricular demand pacemaker on blood pressure. Proceedings Fourth International Symposium on Ambulatory Monitoring. p. 582. Academic Press (London 1982).

Address for correspondence:
E. B. Raftery, M.D.
Consultant Cardiologist
Director, Division of Cardiovascular Diseases
Northwick Park Hospital & Clinical Research Centre
Harrow, Middlesex, HA1 3UJ, U.K.

Ambulatory blood pressure in 199 normal subjects, a collaborative study

John M. Wallace, William E. Thornton, Harold L. Kennedy, Thomas G. Pickering, Gregory A. Harshfield, Edward D. Frohlich, Franz H. Messerli, Ray W. Gifford jr., Kennith Bolen.

Summary: The use of ambulatory BP monitoring is increasing, yet few normal data exist. We report a collaborative study (5 Centers) of 199 normal subjects monitored once each for 22.9 h (mean) with the Del Mar Avionics Pressurometer system. There were 149 men age 17–69 yr and 50 women age 18–60 yr; 191 were caucasian and 8 black. All subjects had repeated casual BPs < 140/90 prior to monitoring. Major results were: 1) within the preset normotensive limits of BP there was no difference in SBP with age. During work, DBP was 6.1 mm Hg higher in men > 40 than < 40 yr. 2) In men and women matched for age, SBP was higher in men, DBP slightly higher in women in subjects < 30 yr, and HR was higher in women. 3) With sleep SBP fell ≃ 12%, DBP ≃ 15% and HR ≃ 20% (p < 0.001 vs SBP) in both sexes. 4) BP variability was as great within subjects (mean of individual SDs) as among subjects (SDs of group mean). 5) In all subjects during the work day the mean ambulatory BP, and this mean + 2 SD (all values rounded), were 121/77 and 138/92 for men, and 109/77 and 126/89 for women. Mean ambulatory BPs and the means + 1 SD and + 2 SD are tabulated herein for various age groups. We present these data as tentative yardsticks for the assessment of casual BPs as well as ambulatory BP records.

In individuals with questionable hypertension, a 24 h ambulatory BP recording to establish his or her own mean and SD can be useful in evaluating past and future casual BPs, and in assessing the BP with respect to the present normal data.

Introduction

In May 1981 the authors of this report, their co-workers, and other investigators* having experience with the Del Mar Avionics ambulatory blood pressure monitor, met to share experiences and to discuss early results in normotensive subjects. We agreed to pool these results and now present them in this paper, which analyzes records obtained in five contributing medical centers prior to November 1981.

In the two years following, non-invasive ambulatory BP monitoring has developed rapidly but basic data in normotensive subjects remains insufficient. Kennedy et al. studied

Department of Medicine, University of Texas Medical Branch, Galveston (JMW and WET), The Cardiovascular Division, St. Louis University School of Medicine, St. Louis (HLK), The Cardiovascular Center, The New York Hospital-Cornell University Medical Center, N.Y. (TGP and GAH), The Division of Hypertensive Diseases, Ochsner Clinic and the Division of Research, Alton Ochsner Medical Foundation, New Orleans (EDF and FHM), and The Department of Hypertension and Nephrology, Cleveland Clinic Foundation, Cleveland (RWG Jr and KB). In addition to the above, participants in planning this collaboration included Jan IM. Drayer MD and Michael A. Weber MD, The Hypertension Center and Medical Service, VA Medical Center, Long Beach, and the University of California, Irvine, and Sheldon G. Sheps MD, Division of Cardiovascular Diseases and Internal Medicine, The Mayo Clinic, Rochester.

* Jan Drayer, M.D., Sheldon Sheps, M.D., Michael Weber, M.D.

72 normal men and stressed the similarity of BP over a wide age range (1). Most of their subjects are included in the present analysis. Pickering et al. (2) and Messerli et al. (3), also from centers contributing to this study, reported findings in a total of 38 normal subjects, mostly men. Other studies, stressing hypertension, have presented little detail in normals (4, 5, 6). Pioneer (7) and later work (8) with the Oxford intra-arterial system have contributed basic knowledge of normal ambulatory BP physiology with which non-invasive data have been generally consistent. The latter, however, might be more directly applicable to casual BPs.

Our purpose was to collaborate in building a bank of normal non-invasive ambulatory BP data. In this paper we have sought to analyze these data in a manner we hope will demonstrate their applicability both to everyday casual BPs, and to a major current problem, namely, the uncertainty of the range of normotension.

Methods

Selection of subjects

Two hundred and forty-one normal subjects were studied in 5 centers prior to the decision to pool the data. Upon review, 42 records were rejected as being technically unsatisfactory leaving 199 successful monitorings (Table 1). This number, though small, is at present the largest yet available for a normotensive baseline. Each center employed its own criteria of normotension which, however, uniformly excluded a history of hypertension or hypertensive drug use. Casual BPs were < 140/90. In Centers A and B PEs and extensive laboratory studies were also normal. Most subjects were caucasian and were either students, industrial workers, or medical center personnel.

Monitoring equipment

Approximately half the records were obtained with the Del Mar Avionics Pressurometer II (PII) and half with the newer Pressurometer III (PIII). The brachial transducer common to both is sensitive to infrasonic frequencies from the artery which are coupled to the Korotkov sounds. It is also sensitive to low frequency noise which may accompany movement of the arm, tension of its muscles, and vibrations transmitted from an automobile seat, for example. Therefore, the arm must be relaxed and held away from such noise at the time of a pressure. If so, reliable pressures are usually obtained during normal daily activities. Most incorrect readings are easily recognized when data are edited. Readings with a pulse pressure < 10 mm Hg are automatically rejected and such false ones as diastolic higher than systolic, zero values, or isolated very high or low readings, which are usually due to extraneous vibrations or movement, may be edited out*). Good agreement

---

*) PII tapes were edited by hand after processing by a modified Holter reader. PIII output was initially processed by the Del Mar Avionics 1979 charter which was available to all participants. Further data reduction was performed by the prototype computer for the system (1 center), the Del Mar 1981 analyzer (1 center), a locally developed computer system (1 center), and by hand from 1979 charter records for 2 centers.

between Pressurometer and Hg manometer was obtained in all subjects analyzed. Actual monitoring periods averaged less than a full 24 h (Table 1). Studies were rejected which did not include the normal period of sleep plus at least an equal period of normal awake activity. The shortest study was 16 and the longest 25 hours.

An accurate assessment of the quality of sleep is not available. In one group (n = 77) with determinations every 7.5 minutes day and night, the majority of subjects reported sleeping about as well as usual, a minority about half as well as usual, and only a few slept poorly. Sleeping BP was sampled at 15–30 min in most other subjects. The sleep BPs and HRs reported here are probably higher than in the unmonitored state.

Table 1. Ambulatory BP records of normotensive subjects contributed by five centers (A–E) for pooled analysis.

Center	A	B	C	D	E
Subjects total	78	77	23	17	4
males	64	52	18	9	4
females	12	25	5	8	0
caucasian	78	69	23	17	4
black	0	8	0	0	0
Hours monitored	22.2	23.4	23.0	23.1	21.0
	±2.38	±1.36	±2.15	±0.75	±3.56
Usual frequency of recording (min)					
day	7.5	7.5	15	7.5	7.5 (2), 30 (2)
night	7,5–15	7,5	30	7.5	7.5 (2), 30 (2)
Mean No. BPs recorded per subject	–	167.0	88.4	154.2	98.0
		±21.08	±18.86	±32.23	±51.32
% deletions per subject	–	12.0	16.4	15.7	17.9
		±7.40	±12.58	±12.31	±6.72
Mean No. BPs analyzed per subject	132.2*	148.1	73.9	130.0	80.5

* Center A submitted printouts of valid BPs only (already edited).

Analysis of data

Records were forwarded by Centers A, C, D, and E to Center B for analysis. Each record was divided into three periods, the 9 h of the working day which included work, school, and home-based activity; the actual duration of sleep (Centers B–E) or an 8 h period composed almost entirely of sleep (Center A); and, the entire period of monitoring, the 24 h mean, which was separately analyzed in addition to the periods of work and sleep. Student's t test was used for paired and unpaired data as appropriate.

Results

Blood pressure

In all 149 men the BP (mean ± SD) was 120.6±8.77/76.7±7.65 (working day), 105.5±8.88/65.2±6.15 (sleep), and 115.7±7.81/72.4±6.27 (24 h): in all 50 women it was, respectively, 108.5±8.35/77.3±6.09, 95.3±8.99/64.4±6.40, and 104.2 ± 7.97/73.1 ± 5.50. SBP was always higher in men than women (p < 0.01) but DBP was similar.

In men, SBP was not higher in the older than younger groups during any period. There was a small rise in DBP up to age 40 but not beyond (Fig. 1a). For the working day, DBPs for all ages < 40 and ≥ 40 were, respectively, 74.3±7.89 and 80.4±6.46 (p <0.005). Women of age < 30 and ≥ 30 had similar SBP and DBP (Fig. 1b).

Fig. 1a. Ambulatory BP (means ± SD) in 149 men. See table 3 for numbers in each age group.

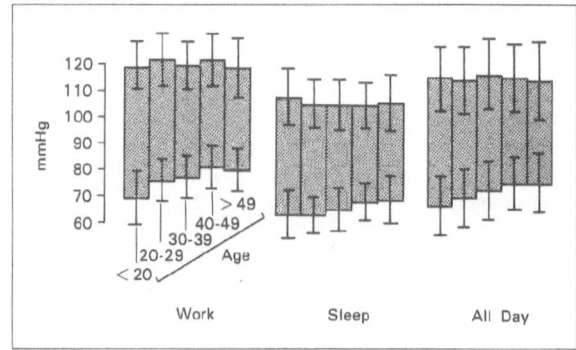

Fig. 1b. Ambulatory BP (means ± SD) in 50 women. Stippled bars, 29 women < 30 yr; cross-hatched, 21 women ≥ 30 yr.

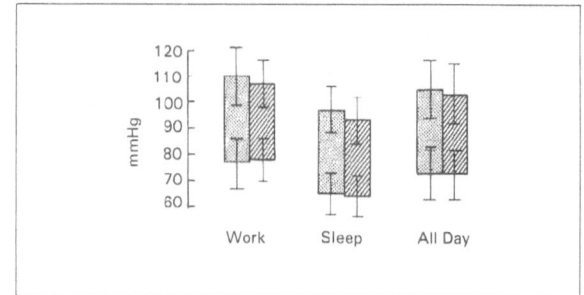

Heart rate

In men the HR (mean ± SD) was 77.7±9.73 (working day), 62.1±7.94 (sleep), and 72.5±8.50 (24 h). Respective HRs in women were 83.3±10.11, 66.6±9.77, and 78.2±8.47. HR was higher in women than men for each period (p < 0.01) but did not differ with age in either sex (Fig. 2 a and b).

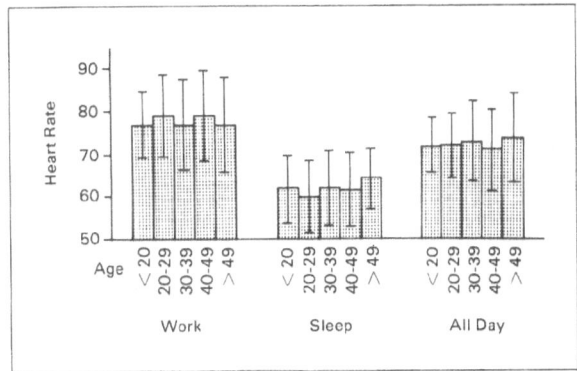

Fig. 2a. Ambulatory HR (means ± SD) in 145 men. HR records were technically unsatisfactory in 4 men with good BP records.

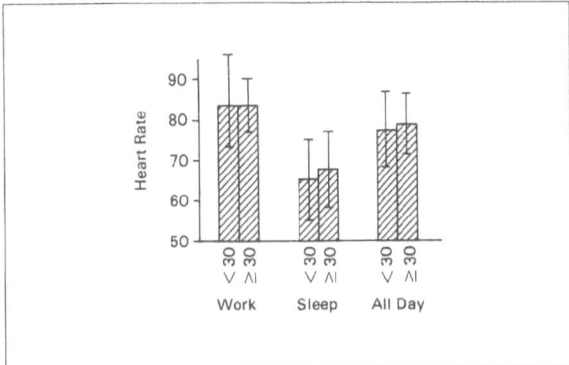

Fig. 2b. Ambulatory HR (means ± SD) in 47 women. HR records were technically unsatisfactory in 3 women with good BP records.

Age-matched men and women

To further assess gender differences, two groups, all caucasian, were created by matching 24 women < 30 and 21 women ≥ 30 with men of similar age (Table 2). When there were more men than women of a given age, the man to be matched was picked at random. In general, SBP was higher in men and HR in women, and DBP was higher in women than men in the younger (p < 0.05 for the 24 h period) but not older pairs. This was due to the lower DBP in younger than older men, a difference not apparent in women. The 14.4 year mean age difference between the groups did not affect SBP or HR in either sex.

Changes with sleep

With sleep, HR fell more than SBP or DBP in both sexes at all ages, Fig. 3. This suggests reduced sensitivity of baroreceptors to the low BP, whereas increased sensitivity to induced rises of BP occurs during sleep (9). Except in males < 20 yr old, DBP fell slightly

121

more than SBP. The data also suggest that sleep BP declined least in the youngest men, yet their HR declined as much. In all men % declines during sleep compared with work were: SBP 12.1 ± 6.44, DBP 14.1 ± 8.28, and HR 19.8 ± 8.72; for all women they were 11.9 ± 7.60, 16.4 ± 8.90, and 19.6 ± 8.65.

Table 2. Comparison of ambulatory BP in normal men and women: two age-matched groups separated by 14.4 years.

	age < 30			age ⩾ 30		
	men	women		men	women	
n	25	25		21	21	
age	24.2 ± 3.11	24.2 ± 3.14		38.6 ± 8.23	38.6 ± 8.11	
	work		p value	work		p value
SBP	120.3 ± 6.54	110.1 ± 8.38	< .001	121.6 ± 6.51	106.7 ± 6.89	< .001
DBP	73.7 ± 5.90	76.7 ± 5.92	NS	78.3 ± 6.89	77.7 ± 5.84	NS
HR	77.8 ± 9.24	84.0 ± 8.92	< .05	78.6 ± 9.36	83.7 ± 6.66	NS
	sleep			sleep		
SBP	105.5 ± 8.90	97.4 ± 9.69	< .01	106.1 ± 7.20	92.0 ± 10.40	< .001
DBP	62.0 ± 6.21	63.7 ± 6.87	NS	65.6 ± 5.91	63.7 ± 5.31	NS
HR	60.8 ± 8.52	65.6 ± 10.36	NS	62.2 ± 8.66	68.0 ± 9.12	< .05
	24 hours			24 hours		
SBP	115.3 ± 5.56	105.7 ± 8.94	< .001	117.1 ± 5.92	102.8 ± 6.39	< .001
DBP	69.7 ± 5.37	72.8 ± 5.57	< .05	73.7 ± 6.61	72.7 ± 4.78	NS
HR	72.1 ± 7.11	78.2 ± 8.25	< .01	73.2 ± 9.38	79.0 ± 7.36	< .05

The SBP, DBP, and HR values are means ± SD for the monitoring periods indicated. Age-matched subjects were treated as pairs for calculation of p values.

Fig. 3. Mean changes (%) in ambulatory SBP, DBP, and HR during sleep compared with work in 145 men and 47 women. In both sexes and all age groups % fall in HR was greater than % fall in SBP by paired analysis, p < 0.05–< 0.001. It was also >% fall in DBP (p < 0.05–< 0.001) in all groups except men > 49 yr and women ⩾ 30 yr.

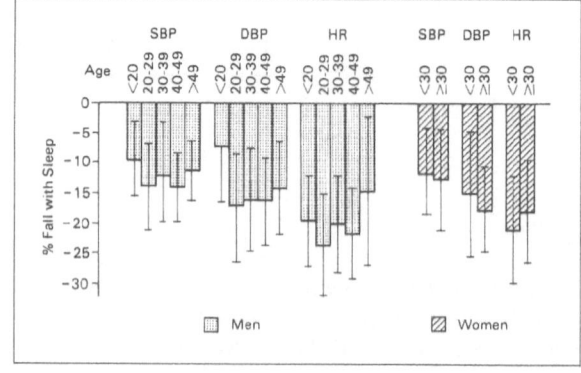

The mean of the SD of each subject's BP (individual SD) as well as the SD of the mean of each group (group SD) were calculated for work and sleep, and the group SD for the entire day (Table 3). Individual SDs for the whole day, a period which includes both work and sleep with widely different BP levels, are less applicable and are not included.

The mean of the individual SDs may be useful in evaluating casual BPs in future patients. For example, from Table 3, a 24 year old man with a screening BP of 127/80 would be within 1 SD of the mean of his ambulating age group, a BP of 137/90 would be between 1 and 2 SD of the mean, and one of 143/95 would be just greater than 2 SD above it. Likewise, the group SDs may be useful in evaluating ambulatory BP records. A 45 year old man with a mean working BP of 126/85 would be within 1 SD of the mean of his age group, a mean BP of 136/95 would be between 1 and 2 SD of it, and one of 142/98 would be just greater than 2 SD above it. Similar assessments may be applied to the period of sleep and the 24 h mean.

Table 3. Mean ambulatory BP and its variability in 199 normotensive individuals arranged for easy application to casual and monitored BP.

Sex	Age	n	Period	Mean	Group SDs		Individual SDs	
					+ 1 SD	+ 2 SD	+ 1 SD	+ 2 SD
F	<30	29	work	110/77	119/83	129/90	121/86	133/95
			sleep	97/65	107/72	117/79	106/73	115/81
			24 hr	105/73	114/79	123/85		
F	≥30	21	work	107/78	114/79	123/85	116/85	125/93
			sleep	93/64	101/69	109/75	102/72	111/80
			24 hr	103/73	109/78	116/83		
M	<20	22	work	119/69	128/78	137/87	129/79	139/89
			sleep	108/63	116/70	125/78	119/72	130/81
			24 hr	116/67	123/75	130/83		
M	20–29	39	work	122/76	130/83	138/91	132/85	142/94
			sleep	105/63	114/69	123/75	114/71	123/79
			24 hr	115/70	122/76	129/82		
M	30–39	39	work	120/77	130/85	140/93	129/85	138/93
			sleep	105/65	114/70	123/76	115/73	125/81
			24 hr	117/73	123/80	134/88		
M	40–49	18	work	122/81	131/89	141/97	132/89	142/97
			sleep	105/68	114/74	123/80	114/75	123/82
			24 hr	116/76	124/82	133/88		
M	>49	31	work	119/80	127/86	136/92	130/88	141/96
			sleep	106/69	116/76	126/83	117/78	128/87
			24 hr	115/76	124/81	133/86		

Mean BPs are group means for the monitoring periods indicated. 1SD and 2SD of these means are added to them in the "Group SDs" columns; means of the individual SDs of all subjects are added to them in the "Individual SDs" columns. All figures were rounded up to the nearest whole number.

Inspection of Table 3 shows that in almost all instances the means of individual SDs are somewhat larger than the SDs of the group means. This suggests that, in these normotensive subjects grouped by age and sex, the variability of BP within an individual is a great as that from individual to individual.

Also of interest in Table 3, is the observation that for most men during the working day, the means + 2 SD are rather close to the traditional BP of 140/90 mmHg, diastolic values diverging (being higher) more than systolic. In the women, systolic values (means + 2 SD) are well below 140 whereas the diastolics are closer to 90.

Discussion

Blood pressure and age

Our study did not show a higher BP in older than younger normotensive subjects over the wide age range represented, which was 17.2 to 56.8 years in the five groups of men. DBP for the work period was 6.1 mmHg higher in men $\geq$ 40 years than in those $<$ 40 (mean of 80.4 vs 74.3, $p < 0.005$). However, not even this small difference was seen in SBP and our oldest group (> 49 yr) included 12 men $>$ age 58 (mean 61.9 yr) with a mean SBP of 116.8 mm Hg during the work period. This was a surprise because atherosclerosis, which frequently accompanies aging, selectively elevates the SBP (10, 11). We did not assess atherosclerosis but it may have been less extensive in our normotensive subjects than in the general population which includes large numbers of hypertensives. In the women, both DBP and SBP were similar in the younger (mean age 22.9 yr) and older (mean age 38.5 yr) groups. Heart rate, as well, did not rise with the years in either sex.

Longitudinal studies performed in presumably normotensive men (12, 13, 14) have generally shown a rise in the average BP with age. We believe there are two major reasons for our different results. Firstly, our study objectives and subject selection were different. By design we excluded BPs $\geq$ 140/90 at all ages to increase the odds that all subjects were normotensive. In contrast, the longitudinal studies were designed to follow BP with time in cohorts initially normotensive, though not exclusively so, all future BPs included.

The results from these different approaches may help to focus the relationship of BP to age. We excluded the possibility of any BPs in the hypertensive range at any age but did not exclude the expression of an age-related increase in SBP as well as DBP within the broad normotensive range. The fact that no such increase was seen in SBP and only a small one in DBP suggests the possibility that the age-related increase in mean BP in longitudinal studies, even though the means themselves remained $< 140/90$, is due to the inclusion of increasing numbers of hypertensive men in each successive age group. Even in the classic "Thousand Aviator Study" (12), in which all men at entry had BPs $< 132/86$, 134 men (of an average of 721 followed) had an SBP > 140 at some point over the 24 years, and the number was much higher in the Royal Canadian Air Force-Manitoba Study in which some men may have been hypertensive at entry (13). Re-analysis of these data minus all entries $\geq$ 140/90 would be of interest; BP in the remainder might rise little or not at all with age. In fact, Oberman et al. specifically indicated this likelihood in their discussion (12). Finally, lingitudinal observation of women through the menopause, controlling for weight gain and other factors, might further clarify the issue. Our two premenopausal groups had similar BPs despite a 15.4 yr age difference. Whether the postmenopausal aging which awaits them will, per se, increase their BP is not yet known.

A second reason our results differ may be our use of the 24 h ambulatory monitor. The other studies were based on casual readings, often only one, and often taken in potentially stressful settings by physicians. Both conditions usually yield higher than average BPs in normotensive and hypertensive subjects (15, 16, 17, 18). For each subject the BP analyzed in our study was the mean of many, thus excluding the likelihood of entering a value 1 or 2 or more SDs above the true average. In studies using casual BP this phenomenon probably accounts for higher than average initial entries and their poor agreement with future BPs within subjects (14). If variability increases with age, the use of casual BPs would be expected to lead to an age related rise in group means. Drayer et al. found variability to be higher in older than younger hypertensives over the whole 24 h period (19), a long interval which includes large differences between work and sleep. However, within the working day when BPs are usually taken for studies, neither we nor Kennedy et al. (1) found higher SDs in older normotensives.

It is common for BP to rise with age but is it normal? Our data and much in the cited longitudinal studies (12, 13, 14) question that it is. In all of these studies a large majority of subjects had little rise in BP. We know now that in our society mild hypertension, especially borderline, is very common, and hypertensive factors such as weight gain, smoking, excessive salt and alcohol, and atherosclerosis are also common. It is likely that these influences, mounting over the years, raise the BP of many into the hypertensive range (no longer included with normal), especially those with a genetic predisposition. When they are averaged in with the normotensives, now defined as individuals who do not become hypertensive in the absence of or despite these factors, BP as a whole goes up. We are hesitant to accept the common assumption that a rise of BP with age is a normal biological progression in our society.

Men and women compared

In our subjects as a whole, without regard to age, SBP was higher in men than women and HR higher in women for each period of the day. There was no difference in overall DBP. These results were confirmed in the two age-matched subgroups except that age-matching revealed a higher DBP in women than men in the younger but not older pairs. Thus, the wider pulse pressure apparent in men was due entirely to their higher SBP. We have found that in young normotensive subjects an unknown 24 h ambulatory BP plot can usually be recognized as female by its narrow pulse pressure (higher DBP and lower SBP) and rapid HR. Our data do not explain the higher male SBP but possible factors include a higher salt intake in men (20). The higher HR in women despite their lower SBP is also unexplained but could be an expression of baroreceptor activity.

BP variability

The main BP data obtained from this study are presented in Table 3, arranged for easy reference to patients. Because our subjects were ambulatory and came from different parts of the country, tha data should be generally applicable to various "walk-in" BPs in caucasian patients. This might include BPs taken in doctors' offices or clinics (when patients do not first sit or lie down for 10 min), in screening booths, with BP machines, or at home. The period mean plus 1 and 2 SDs (mean of the individual SDs for each period), as presented in the last two columns of the table, are offered as tentative yardsticks for such casual BPs. In a subset of the present data (Wallace and Thornton, unpublished) casual and office BPs in some subjects averaged higher than the mean working ambulatory BPs but were almost always within 1 or 2 SDs of it.

Our values for the BP mean and SD for the working day for men < 40 yr are strikingly similar to those for men aged 20–39 published by Rabkin et al (13). Their data were derived from casual BPs in 3580 men (entry examination) and ours from 24 h ambulatory BP recordings in 100 men. For example, for ages 25–29 (n = 1479) their mean BP is $121.1 \pm 10.2/75.2 \pm 7.7$, and for ages 20–29 (n = 39) ours in $122.0 \pm 10.3/75.6 \pm 8.8$ (individual SDs). For ages 35–39 (n = 539) their figure is $121.9 \pm 11.0/77.0 \pm 8.2$, and for ages 30–39 (n = 39) ours in $120.3 \pm 9.2/77.4 \pm 7.9$. Although their mean values result from a single entry in many men and ours from many entries in few men, the close agreement of both the means and SDs in not surprising in view of our Table 3 which shows similar variability within and among subjects.

The SDs may be useful in keeping casual BPs in perspective. In a 25 yr old man a casual BP up to 142/94 would be within 2 SD of his normotensive group mean. Such readings, especially on first examination, should not be greatly unexpected, and even less so readings up to 132/85, within 1 SD. Based upon chance alone repeated readings will regress toward the mean. In addition, repeat visits, and home readings especially, are even more likely to yield BPs close to the mean by minimizing or eliminating the white coat effect. Conversely, neither physician nor patient should be necessarily alarmed if today's reading is 142/94 when at the last visit it was 122/76 (the normotensive mean).

In borderline patients in particular, a 24 h ambulatory BP recording to establish the subject's own mean and SD can be helpful in evaluating past and future casual BPs, and in assessing the BP with respect to the present normal data.

Acknowledgements

We thank Mrs. Carol A. Gullette for her expert help in preparing the manuscript. We thank Mr. Tatsuo Uchida for advice and assistance with all statistical analysis.

References

1. Kennedy HL, Horan MJ, Sprague MK, Padgett NE, Shriver KK: Ambulatory blood pressure in healthy normotensive males. Am Heart J 106: 717–722 (1983).
2. Pickering TG, Harshfield GA, Kleinert HD, Blank S, Laragh JH: Blood pressure during normal daily activities, sleep, and exercise. JAMA 247: 992–996 (1982).
3. Messerli FH, Glande LB, Ventura HO, Dreslinski GR, Suarez DH, MacPhee AA, Aristimuno GG, Cole FE, Frohlich ED: Diurnal variations of cardiac rhythm, arterial pressure, and urinary catecholamines in borderline and established essential hypertension. Am Heart J 104: 109–114 (1982).
4. Sheps SG, Elveback, LR, Close EL, Kleven MK, Bissen C: Evaluation of the Del Mar Avionics automatic ambulatory blood pressure-recording device. May Clin Proc 56: 740–743 (1981).
5. McCall WC, McCall VR: Diagnostic use of ambulatory blood pressure monitoring in medical practice. J Family Practice 13: 25–30 (1981).

6. Corsi V, Germano G, Appoloni A, Ciavarella M, De Zorzi A, Calcagnini G: Fully automated ambulatory blood pressure in the diagnosis and therapy of hypertension. Clin Cardiol 6: 143–150 (1983).
7. Bevan AT, Honour AT, Stott FH: Direct arterial pressure recordings in unrestricted man. Clin Sci 36: 329–344 (1969).
8. Mancia G, Ferrari A, Gregorini L, Parati G, Pomidossi G, Bertinieri G, Grassi G, di Rienzo M, Pedotti A, Zanchetti A: Blood pressure and heart rate variabilities in normotensive and hypertensive human beings. Circ Res 53: 96–104 (1983).
9. Smyth HS, Sleight P, Pickering GW: Reflex regulation of arterial pressure during sleep in man: A quantitative method of assessing baroreflex sensitivity. Circ Res 24: 109–121 (1969).
10. Colandrea MA, Friedman GD, Nichaman MJ, Lund CH: Sytolic hypertension in the elderly: An epidimiologic assessment. Circulation 41: 239–245 (1970).
11. Kannel WB, Wolf PA, McGee DL, Dawber TR, McNamara P, Castelli WP: Systolic blood pressure, arterial rigidity, and risk of stroke. The Framingham Study. JAMA 245: 1225–1229 (1981).
12. Oberman A, Lane NE, Harlan WR, Graybiel A, Mitchell RE: Trends in systolic blood pressure in the thousand aviator cohort over a twenty-four year period. Circulation 36: 812–822 (1967).
13. Rabkin SW, Mathewson MB, Tate RB: Relationship of blood pressure in 20–39-year old men to subsequent blood pressure and incidence of hypertension over a 30-year observation period. Circulation 65: 291–299 (1982).
14. Froom P, Bar-David M, Ribak J, Van Dyk D, Kallner B, Benbassat J: Predictive value of systolic blood pressure in young men for elevated systolic blood pressure 12–15 years later. Circulation 68: 467–469 (1983).
15. Hypertension Detection and Follow-up Program Cooperative Group: Blood pressure studies in 14 communities, a two-stage screen for hypertension. JAMA 237: 2385–2391 (1977).
16. Kain HK, Hinman AT, Sokolow M: Arterial blood pressure measurements with a portable recorder in hypertensive patients. I. Variability and correlation with "casual" pressures. Circulation 30: 882–892 (1964).
17. Floras JS, Hassan MO, Sever PS, Jones JV, Osikowska B, Sleight P. Cuff and ambulatory blood pressure in subjects with essential hypertension. Lancet 2: 107–109 (1981).
18. Mancia G, Grassi G, Pomidossi G, Gregorini L, Bertinieri G, Porati G, Ferrari A, Zanchetti A: Effects of blood pressure measurement by the doctor on patient's blood pressure and heart rate. Lancet 2: 695–697 (1983).
19. Drayer JIM, Weber MA, DeYoung JL, Wyle FA: Circadian blood pressure patterns in ambulatory hypertensive patients. Effects of age. Am J Med 73: 493–499 (1982).
20. Stoltz PK, Wallace JM, Thorton WE, Wang C-H, Himi K: Gender differences in blood pressure effects of salt revealed by 24 hour ambulatory monitor (abstr.). Clin Res 27: 417A (1979).

Address for correspondence:
John M. Wallace, M.D.
Hypertension Service, 5A
University of Texas Medical Branch
Galveston, TX 77550

Non-invasive automated blood pressure monitoring in ambulatory normotensive men

Jan I. M. Drayer, Michael A. Weber, Eleanor R. Chard

Summary: In this study non-invasive automated ambulatory blood pressure monitoring techniques have been used to evaluate patterns of blood pressure in 34 healthy normotensive men. The results of the monitoring reveal that, as in hypertensive patients, blood pressure is highest during daytime and lowest at night in these volunteers. The average of daytime blood pressures ($128 \pm 12/80 \pm 7$ mmHg) were significantly higher (p <0.01) and nighttime blood pressure averages ($109 \pm 11/67 \pm 9$ mmHg) were significantly lower (p <0.01) than the conventionally measured casual blood pressure ($119 \pm 13/76 \pm 9$ mmHg). On average, 15.6% of systolic blood pressure readings in each tracing were greater than 140 mmHg. More than 25% of these elevated readings were found in 6 of the 34 subjects. The percentage of diastolic blood pressures greater than 90 mmHg in each tracing was 14.4%. Again, six subjects accounted for more than 25% of elevated diastolic blood pressures during the 24hour monitoring period. The incidence of these elevated blood pressure readings was not age-dependent. However, subjects with a positive family history for hypertension had, on average, more elevated systolic blood pressures than patients with a negative family history (24 vs. 9%, p <0.05), even though casual blood pressures were not different between these groups. The correlation coefficient between casual and whole-day average systolic blood pressures was highly significant (r = 0.60, p < 0.001) as was the correlation coefficient between casual and whole-day average diastolic blood pressure (r = 0.72, p < 0.001). However, both correlation coefficients were stronger after substitution of casual blood pressures by the averages of blood pressure recorded between 8.00 and 10.00 a.m.
The data presented in this paper helps define blood pressure in healthy normotensive volunteers. Ultimately, these data may be used as an aid in the diagnosis of patients with high blood pressure.

Introduction

Ambulatory blood pressure monitoring has frequently been used in the evaluation of hypertensive patients. Non-invasive automated blood pressure monitoring systems provide a convenient and safe method in the evaluation of daytime and nighttime blood pressures in hypertensive patients and normotensive control subjects. Recently, research projects have focused on the use of such systems in the diagnosis of patients with borderline hypertension (1) and essential hypertension (2), the effects of aging on blood pressure patterns (3), the relationship between blood pressure and the presence of cardiac hypertrophy (4, 5) and the effectiveness of antihypertensive therapy (6). However, the monitoring systems have rarely been used in normotensive control subjects (7).

In this study we report our findings using a non-invasive atuomated ambulatory blood pressure monitoring system (Pressurometer III, Del Mar Avionics, Irvine, California) in 34 healthy normotensive men.

Section of Clinical Pharmacology and Hypertension Veterans Administration Medical Center Long Beach, California and the University of California Irvine, California

Methods

Healthy normotensive men were chosen to participate in the study. The volunteers denied a history of hyperension and all had casual seated blood pressures less than 150/95 mmHg. In fact, only 3 of the 34 volunteers had a casual seated systolic blood pressure greater than 130 mmHg. (136, 139 and 145 mmHg, respectively) and 2 other subjects had diastolic blood pressures which were greater than 90 mmHg; 95 and 91 mmHg, respectively.

On the day of the study, the patient's height and body weight were obtained. Ideal body weight was estimated using the Metropolitan Life Tables and actual weight then was expressed as a percentage of ideal body weight. The average time of the hook-up was 11 ± 1 hours in the morning. The subjects were requested to perform their normal daily activities on the day of the study. Automated ambulatory blood pressure monitoring was then performed during 24 h using the Pressurometer III (Del Mar Avionics, Irvine, California). With this instrument, readings of systolic and diastolic blood pressure and heart rate were obtained at 7.5 min intervals throughout the 24-h day. After completion of the monitoring, the data were printed using a 1979 Pressurometer Charter (Del Mar Avionics).

Readings which showed an inconsistent increase or decrease in systolic or diastolic blood pressure of greater than 20 mmHg, and readings with a calculated pulse pressure of less than 5 mmHg were deleted prior to further analysis of the data. Analysis of the tracings was only performed if at least 75% of the maximal number of 192 readings per 24 h passed the deletion criteria provided that no data were lost for a period greater than one hour. The following analyses of systolic and diastolic blood pressure were performed using an Apple II Plus microcomputer; average of all readings obtained during the 24-h monitoring, average of the readings obtained during 12 consecutive 2-h periods starting at midnight and the averages of daytime (06.00 to 22.00 h) and nighttime (22.00 to 06.00 h) blood pressures. In addition, a histogram of the blood pressure data from each 24-h tracing was obtained.

Blood pressures measured in the seated position just prior to the start of the monitoring using a standard sphygmomanometer were used as causal seated blood pressures. The

Table 1. Clinical Characteristics of 34 Normotensive Male Subjects.

	Mean ± SD	Range
Age (yrs)	37.9 ± 9.7	23–60
Height (cm)	181 ± 7	166–193
Weight (kg)	82.5 ± 12.1	65.6–112.6
Ideal Weight* (%)	111 ± 15	83–145
Casual Systolic Blood Pressure (mmHg)	119 ± 13	76–145
Casual Diastolic Blood Pressure (mmHg)	76 ± 9	58–95

* Actual weight as a percentage of ideal weight according to Metropolitan Life Tables.
SD = Standard deviation

performance of the monitoring equipment was checked immediately after the hook-up of the patient and upon return of the patient 24 h later. Blood pressures recorded by the Pressurometer were compared to those measured simultaneously with a standard mercury sphygmomanometer. The average of two readings were used in the comparison of both techniques. The correlation coefficient between the two systolic blood pressures obtained in this way at the start of the monitoring was highly significant ($r = 0.98$, $p < 0.001$) as was the correlation coefficient obtained at the completion of the monitoring period ($r = 0.90$, $p < 0.001$). The correlation coefficients between the diastolic blood pressure obtained with the Pressurometer and those measured simultaneously with the sphygmomanometer also were significant; $r = 0.92$, $p < 0.001$ at the beginning and $r = 0.83$, $p < 0.001$ at the end of the monitoring period. These data confirm earlier studies on the validation of the Pressurometer (8).

The subjects were requested to return to the office approximately 7 weeks later (32 ± 13 days), for another measurement of their causal blood pressure. Standard statistical tests, paired and unpaired Student t-tests, and Pearson correlation coefficients were used in the analysis of the data. All data are expressed as mean $\pm$ standard deviation. Two-tailed p values are used to express significance of the results of the statistical tests.

Results

In this study, ambulatory blood pressure monitoring was performed in 34 healthy normotensive men. The clinical characteristics of the subjects are given in Table 1. The volunteers were 23 to 60 years old. The ideal weight of 6 volunteers exceeded 125%. Casual systolic blood pressure was greater than 140 mmHg in one 57 year old man. Diastolic blood pressure was 78 mmHg in this subject. Casual diastolic blood pressure exceeded 90 mmHg in 2 men, but these men had no history of hypertension and both systolic and diastolic blood pressure were normal on repeated examination; 115/78 and 137/85 mmHg, respectively.

The comparison of casual blood pressures and averages of blood pressures obtained during ambulatory monitoring is presented in Table 2. The whole-day average blood pressure was not different from the casual blood pressure. The average of the daytime blood pressures, and the average of the blood pressures measured between 8.00 and 10.00 a.m.

Table 2. Comparison of Casual Blood Pressures and Averages of Blood Pressures Obtained During Various Time Periods of the Day in 34 Normotensive Male Subjects.

	Casual Blood Pressure	Whole-Day Average	Daytime Average	Nighttime Average	2-Hr Morning Average
Systolic Blood Pressure (mmHg)	119 ± 13	122 ± 11	$128 \pm 12^*$	$109 \pm 11^*$	$129 \pm 12^*$
Diastolic Blood Pressure (mmHg)	76 ± 9	76 ± 7	$80 \pm 7^*$	$67 \pm 9^*$	$82 \pm 7^*$

* $p < 0.01$ when compared to casual blood pressure

were significantly higher, and the average nighttime blood pressures were significantly lower than casual blood pressures. These differences were slightly more pronounced for systolic than for diastolic blood pressure.

The histogram of the blood pressures recorded in all volunteers is given in Fig. 1. Overall, 15.6% of systolic blood pressures were greater than 140 mmHg and 14.4 percent of readings of diastolic blood pressures were greater than 90 mmHg. More than 25% abnormal systolic blood pressures (> 140 mmHg) were found in 6 subjects and more than 25% of abnormal diastolic blood pressures (> 90 mmHg) were found in another 6 subjects. Only one subject had both more than 25% abnormal systolic and more than 25% abnormal diastolic blood pressures.

A family history of hypertension, defined as the known presence of hypertension in at least one of the parents, brothers or sisters of the participant in this study, was present in 14, absent in 19 and unknown in one subject. It is of interest to note that the incidence of abnormal systolic blood pressures (> 150 mmHg) was higher in normotensive subjects with a positive family history of hypertension than in those with a negative family history of hypertension (24 ± 26 and 9 ± 11 percent, respectively, $p < 0.025$). However, the incidence of abnormal diastolic blood pressures (> 90 mmHg) was similar for both groups of subjects (18 ± 15 and 12 ± 16 percent, respectively, not significant). Casual blood pressures were not different between the two groups ($122 \pm 11/77 \pm 8$ and $116 \pm 14/75 \pm 10$ mmHg, respectively, not significant).

The correlation coefficients between casual systolic and diastolic blood pressure and whole-day blood pressure averages are given in Fig. 2. Highly significant correlation coefficients were obtained for both systolic and diastolic blood pressure. However, the correlation coefficients between the average of 16 blood pressures obtained between 8.00 and 10.00 a.m. and the whole-day average blood pressure were higher than those between casual and whole-day average blood pressures.

The volunteers returned for a repeated measurement of their casual blood pressure 32 days after the day of the blood pressure monitoring. The average casual blood pressure

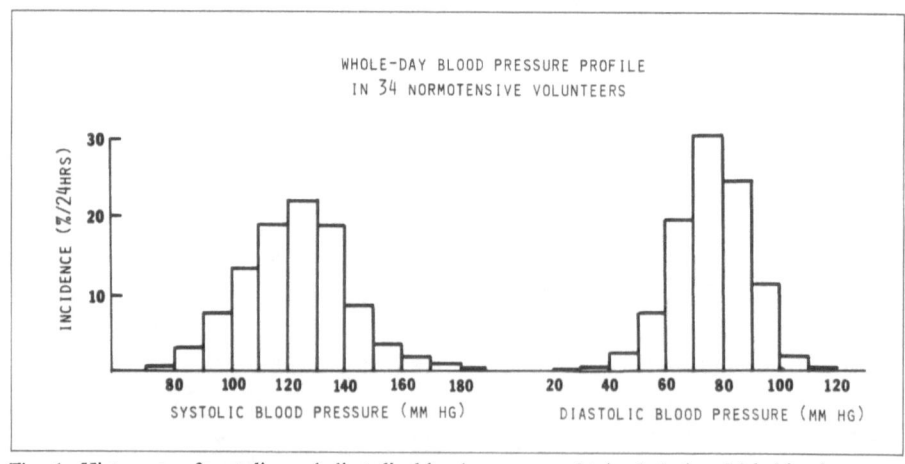

Fig. 1. Histogram of systolic and diastolic blood pressures obtained during 24-h blood pressure monitoring in 34 healthy normotensive volunteers.

132

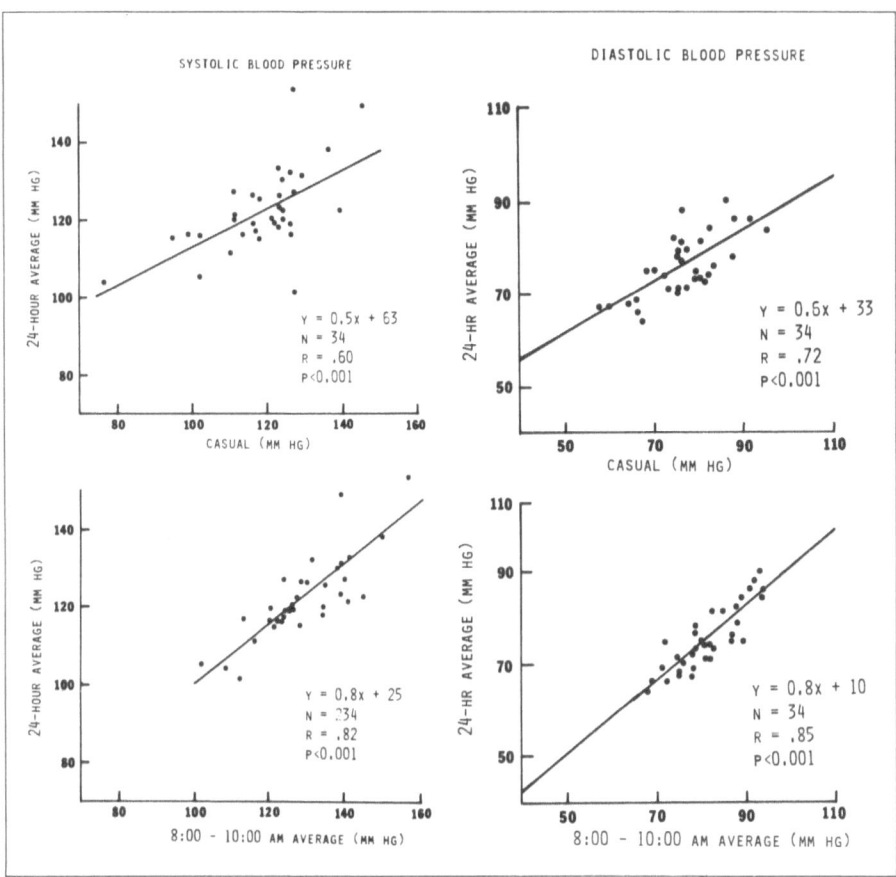

Fig. 2. Relationship between casual blood pressure (top) and average morning blood pressures (bottom) and whole-day averages of blood pressure in normotensive volunteers. The left panel depicts data for systolic blood pressure and the right panel shows the relationships for diastolic blood pressure.

Table 3. Correlation Coefficients Between Repeated Casual Blood Pressures and Various Measures of Blood Pressure Obtained During Ambulatory Blood Pressure Monitoring.

	Repeated Casual Systolic Blood Pressure	Repeated Casual Diastolic Blood Pressure
Initial Casual Blood Pressure	r = 0.75**	r = 0.60**
Whole-Day Average Blood Pressure	r = 0.67**	r = 0.51**
Daytime Average Blood Pressure	r = 0.71**	r = 0.47**
Nighttime Average Blood Pressure	r = 0.42*	r = 0.47**
8.00 to 10.00 a.m. Average Blood Pressure	r = 0.62**	r = 0.51**

* p < 0.05; ** p < 0.01

133

obtained on the day of the monitoring was not different from the casual blood pressure obtained 32 days later; $119 \pm 13/76 \pm 9$ and $119 \pm 12/73 \pm 9$ mmHg, respectively. The correlation coefficients between the various measures of blood pressure obtained on the day of the monitoring and the repeated casual blood pressure are given in Table 3. The correlation coefficients between blood pressure averages and repeated casual blood pressures were not better than the correlation coefficients between initial and repeated casual blood pressures.

Discussion

In this study, an average of 184 blood pressures were obtained during a 24-h period in 34 healthy normotensive men using a non-invasive automated ambulatory blood pressure monitor. The results confirm data obtained previously in normotensive volunteers (7, 9). Higher blood pressures were most often found during daytime and blood pressure decreased significantly at night.

The incidence of abnormally high systolic and diastolic blood pressures was higher in this study than that recently reported by Kennedy et al. (7). More than 25% abnormal systolic or diastolic blood pressures were found in 11 of the 34 men. We found a significant relationship between the incidence of abnormally high systolic blood pressures and the presence of a positive family history of hypertension. The effect of the positive family history on the prevalence of elevated systolic blood pressure was independent of the age of the subjects studied or the height of their casual systolic blood pressure. However, the age of subjects has been shown to play a role in the incidence of abnormal readings in a study of a larger number of normotensive men (7). It seems obvious that a careful analysis of the prevalence of abnormal blood pressures in normotensive and hypertensive patients is needed for the definition of normalcy of results of whole-day ambulatory blood pressure monitorings. Fewer than 25% of abnormal readings have been found in many patients with borderline hypertension as well as in patients with established essential hypertension (1).

It has been shown that, in patients with hypertension, casual blood pressures do not reliably predict the whole-day average blood pressures (3, 10). Averages of multiple blood pressures recorded during a 2-h period in the morning significantly better predict the whole-day average blood pressure than single casual blood pressure readings. In this study, the correlation coefficient between average morning blood pressures and the whole-day average blood pressures also were higher than the correlation coefficients between casual blood pressures and whole-day average blood pressures. However, the correlation coefficients did not increase as markedly in healthy normotensive men as was found in hypertensive men. This difference in the results of both studies might be related to the smaller range of blood pressures found in normotensive control subjects.

Finally, we have evaluated whether a careful analysis of the blood pressure of normotensive control subjects during a 24-h period might help to better predict blood pressure levels found during repeated examination. The data presented in this study reveal, however, that casual blood pressures measured on the day of the monitoring equally well predict the whole-day average blood pressure as the latter predict future casual blood pressures. The comparison between the reproducibility of casual blood pressures and the reproducibility of whole-day averages of blood pressures obtained in normotensive control subjects using non-invasive automated ambulatory blood pressure monitoring techniques is presented elsewhere (11).

References

1. Horan MJ, Kennedy HL, Padgett NE: Do borderline hypertensive patients have labile blood pressure? Ann Intern Med 94: 466–468 (1981).
2. Pickering TG, Harshfield GA, Kleinert HD, Blank S, Laragh JH: Blood pressure during normal daily activities, sleep and exercise. JAMA 247: 992–996 (1982).
3. Drayer JIM, Weber MA, DeYoung JL, Wyle FA: Circadian blood pressure patterns in ambulatory hypertensive patients. Effects of age. Am J Med 73: 493–499 (1982).
4. Devereux RB, Pickering TG, Harshfield GA, Sachs I, Jason J, Hollis DK, Laragh JH: Left ventricular hypertrophy in patients with hypertension: importance of blood pressure response to regularly occurring stress. Circulation 68: 470–476 (1983).
5. Drayer JIM, Weber MA, DeYoung JL: Blood Pressure as a determinant of cardiac left ventricular muscle mass. Arch Intern Med 143: 90–99 (1983).
6. Garrett BN, Kaplan NM: Lofexidine in the treatment of hypertension: A twice-daily vs. once-daily dose comparison with 24-hour blood pressure monitoring. J Clin Pharmacol 21: 173–180 (1981).
7. Kennedy HL, Horan MJ, Sprague MK, Padgett NE, Shriver, KK: Ambulatory blood pressure in healthy normotensive males. Am Heart J 106: 717–722 (1983).
8. Harshfield GA, Pickering TG, Laragh JH: A validation study of the Del Mar Avionics ambulatory blood pressure system. Ambulatory Electrocardiogr 4: 7–12 (1979).
9. Raftery EB, Millar-Craig MW: Information derived from direct 24-hour recordings. In: Blood Pressure Variability DL Clement (ed.) University Park Press (Baltimore, USA, 1979).
10. Weber MA, Drayer JIM, Wyle FA: A representative value for whole-day blood pressure monitoring. JAMA 248: 1626–1628 (1982).
11. Weber MA, Drayer JIM, Nakamura D: Blood pressure fluctuation and amplitude in normal human subjects. In: Ambulatory Blood Pressure Monitoring. MA Weber, JIM Drayer (eds.) Steinkopff-Verlag (Darmstadt, West Germany (in press) 1983).

Address for correspondence:
Jan I. M. Drayer, M. D.
Hypetension Center (W 130)
VA Medical Center
5901 East Seventh Street
Long Beach, CA 90822

Chronobiologic assessment of human blood pressure variation in health and disease

Franz Halberg*, Erna Halberg*, Julie Halberg**, Francine Halberg***

Summary: Once long and dense measurement series are available, biologic rhythm characteristics are readily computed. To assess such characteristics, we present suitable methods for blood pressure data collection and analysis. Since intra- and inter-individual differences are greater for blood pressure than for many other physiologic variables, any rhythm should and can be assessed for the individual subject by an inferential statistical approach. Circadian rhythms are thus mapped in human blood pressure in health and disease, under ordinary conditions and in social isolation, and can be shifted in their timing by changes in work schedule. Under all of the foregoing conditions, these rhythms account for a large part of the variability in blood pressure measurements. Their assessment renders changes in blood pressure predictable to a substantial degree, whereas their neglect can lead to false positive and false negative diagnoses of "hypertension". Changes in a measure of the extent of reproducible change, such as the circadian amplitude, can lead to amplitude-hypertension occurring before the 24-h mean becomes elevated: mesor-hypertension. When changes in biologic rhythm characteristics precede an elevation of the 24-h mean of systolic blood pressure, they are harbingers of cardiovascular disease. Once automatic and/or self-measurement covers at least 48 hours with proper density, rhythmometry yields stable characteristics. High school students and adults alike can handle inferential statistical tests whereby rhythm characteristics a) are determined in actual or presumed health and b) may be found to be altered, the alteration (indicating, e.g., amplitude and/or mesor-hypertension) prompting intervention. Statistical tests also gauge the effect of intervention, motivate compliance and thus contribute toward the success of preventive or curative measures. A system of education and software for rhythm analysis, wedded to hardware for self- and automatic blood pressure measurement, is particularly suitable for screening, diagnosis and the optimization by timing of non-drug and drug treatments to enhance the desired effect and to reduce side effects. Rhythmometry of data from room-restricted automatic monitoring demonstrates the effect of a shift from a beta-blocker to a placebo within 24 hours and corroborates it within 48 hours.

Introduction

Automatic monitoring can lead to the recognition of odd-hour blood pressure elevation ("evening" or "morning" hypertension) as an initial diagnosis or under treatment that may seem to be satisfactory on the basis of a conventional check at the "wrong" time. A

* University of Minnesota, Minneapolis, Minnesota
** University of Connecticut, Farmington, Connecticut
*** Stanford University, Stanford, California

Support: National Institute of General Medical Sciences (GM-13981); National Cancer Institute (CA-14445); Hoechst Italia Foundation

glance at a 24-h record, however, may not allow one to make objective statements as to a change in pattern, e.g., after a given intervention. This paper illustrates how by objective rhythmometry, some ot the uncertainties of a subjective interpretation of a record may be removed by practitioners of medicine, as well as basic scientists interested in mechanisms of blood pressure variability (Fig 1 and 2).

Rhythm characteristics and their uses

Rhythms can be defined as algorithmically-formulatable recurring biologic changes with a waveform validated by inferential statistical means. The point and (confidence) interval estimates of their characteristics include a midline-estimating statistic of rhythm, the mesor, a rhythm-adjusted mean (which differs from the arithmetic mean when measurement series do not cover an integral number of cycles and/or vary in density, when the mesor is more representative of the average pressure upon the vessels' walls than the mean). Another characteristic, the amplitude (one-half the total predictable rhythmic change defined by a mathematical function fitted to the data), objectively estimates the condition of amplitude-hypertension. Mesor- and/or amplitude-hypertension are transient or lasting elevations of the circadian mesor and/or amplitude, validated to lie outside the upper 90% prediction limit established earlier for the given individual and/or an age- and sex-matched peer group. Human amplitude-hypertension characterizes 1) the mesor-hypertensive's first response to therapy, a stage in which the return toward normally from abnormality mirrors the development toward abnormality from normalcy; or 2) an early stage of blood pressure rhythm alteration. The handled SHR-SP rat shows a systolic amplitude-hypertension prior to a genetically-determined mesor-hypertension (11).

A third characteristic is the acrophase, the lag from zero-time of the peak in the fitted function, one of the measures of timing. After shifts of the sleep-wake routine, which is a dominant synchronizer of circadian rhythms, different variables can show differences in rate and even in direction (delay vs. advance) of adjustment; comparison of the shift-behavior of blood pressure itself and of functions possibly underlying the coordination of changes in blood pressure can yield differential diagnostic clues. Such clues may point to the factors (such as aldosteronism) underlying circadian mesor- and/or amplitude-hypertension.

The period, another measure of timing, is fixed for the analysis of short time series collected under conditions likely to be associated with a given rhythm, such as a prominent circadian rhythm in blood pressure, usually but not invariably synchronized with the (e.g., 24 h) living routine. The period is allowed to vary for the analysis of long series and then becomes an estimated characteristic. In disease, the systolic blood pressure may desynchronize, at least transiently, from the diastolic one and from the core temperature rhythm, as well as from the 24-h clock. The same can occur in health and in mesor-hypertension during social isolation. During social isolation, circadian circulatory rhythms can exhibit average periods differing in length from precisely 24 h (e.g., of 24.32 and 24.30 h, with 95% confidence limits that do not cover 24 h and have no exact environmental match). Such findings suggest the contribution to rhythmicity of an intrinsic mechanism, yet the desynchronized periods are transiently synchronizable by (presumably geophysical) 24-h cyclic factors. (Unpublished data of E. Lucas, L. E. Scheving, R. B. Sothern et al.)

138

Blood pressure and endocrine rhythm alteration can signal cardiovascular disease risk (21, 24). Once rhythmometry by cosinor and chronobiologic serial section validates the diagnosis of amplitude-hypertension and/or mesor-hypertension, it provides a reference for and quantifies the effects of drug or non-drug therapy of blood pressure-related isease,e.g., the effect of interventions such as salt and/or dietary caloric restriction, assessed on an individualized basis by the comparison of characteristics in tests of parameters from cosinors. Instruction in chronobiology and the self- (or if need be automatic) measurement and analysis of blood pressure rhythms in the context of secondary education, initiated in several geographic areas as an initial step toward self-help in health care, can eventually become part of every citizen's scientific literacy (15, 18).

Variability

Limited variability by only a few mmHg in human systolic or diastolic blood pressure is implied by publications such as that of the National Center for Health Statistics (1964). It is often the misinterpreted result of averaging across values obtained at arbitrary times for a population, or of averaging consecutive values along the scale of minutes or even hours for the individual (cf. 8, 15). The actual range of variation, even under conditions when a

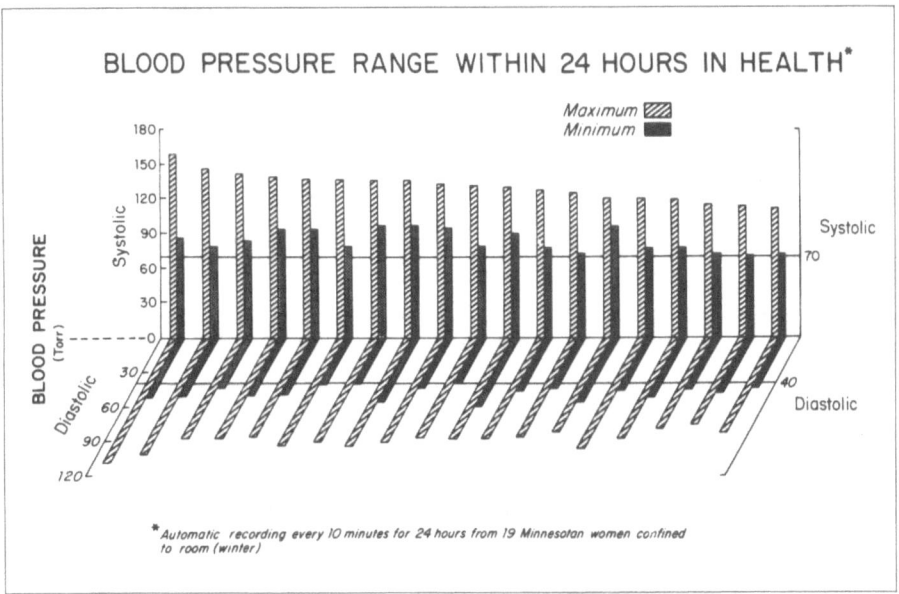

Fig. 1. Within 24 hrs, the highest diastolic pressure can be higher than the lowest systolic one of the same individual. In view of such variability, the practice of indicating that the systolic and diastolic blood pressure is a certain number of mmHg (or Torr) is hardly warranted. This is recognized when single values are complemented by the use of means. One need not refer to time-unqualified means only, however, when some components of variability can be resolved as characteristics of a basic rhythm (see Fig. 3), and also as gauges of health, risk or disease.

person is restricted to a room, is properly revealed by the automatically-monitored direct or indirect blood pressure. Figure 1 shows within-day differences for individuals restricted to a room (12). Figure 2 shows them for several age groups of clinically healthy subjects (cf. Drayer et al. (9) for patients with an elevated blood pressure). The task then arises to extract information on any predictable components of such variability.

Fig. 2. The statements in the legend of Figure 1 apply to different age groups. Average differences in systolic and diastolic pressure of at least 40 mmHg are apparent in most automatically monitored records. Variability is artificially reduced by averaging, e.g., for a given individual, data for consecutive hours or, for a population, data irrespective of time.

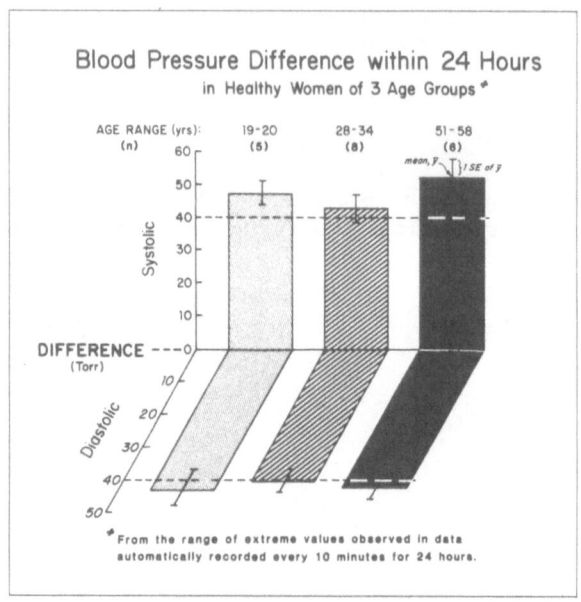

Background

This task was undertaken against the background of information from around-the-clock self-measurements by some of the authors on most days, with few interruptions, for spans of over 5 or even 15 years (20). Beyond the detection of ultradian variation (with a frequency higher than 1 cycle in 20 hrs), the occurrence of about-24-hour (circadian), about-7-day (circaseptan), about-monthly (circatrigintan) and about-yearly (circannual) rhythms in blood pressure, in conjunction with age trends, has thus been documented (11, 12, 15, 20, 21, 37).

Given appropriately dense and long data series, part of the variability can be resolved as a predictable one insofar as it is rhythmic with several frequencies. The characteristics of each rhythm can be assessed by a special set of inferential statistical computer methods. The method of plexo-serial linear-nonlinear rhythmometry (12, 14) and others are particularly applicable to automatic ambulatory measurements. Their output, intended for the clinician and the researcher, has already been used by school children (33), leading to normative data. If instrumentation could be made available on a proper scale, the combined hardware-software package should eventually serve each citizen interested in self-help for health maintenance. An individualized mesor and other rhythm characteristics and their prediction intervals serve as personal reference standards (16, 12).

It has become routine to follow the action potentials of the heart with electrocardiograms for at least 24 hours and in some chronobiologic research for much longer (26). Comparable studies of human blood pressure are under way. Whether one's interest is in basic science, e.g., genetics or actual day-to-day practice, one should realize that the parameters of predictable blood pressure rhythmicity (Fig. 3) are readily obtained by computer and even by pocket calculator (5). These parameters can be exploited by all those who practice ambulatory or other repeated blood pressure monitoring, preferably for spans of at least 48 (rather than 24) hours (23).

Standardized room-restricted data collection

Results of automatic blood pressure monitoring while the subject is confined in activity to a room, e.g., at home or at the workplace, must be considered separately from an entirely ambulatory profile. For automatic room-restricted monitoring, at 10- to 60-min intervals, usually for 24 or 48 hours, and occasionally for longer spans (12), we used mostly equipment manufactured by Nippon Colin (Komaki, Japan, model BP203X), hereinafter called Nipco. The Nipco uses the oscillometric method and provides a printout with calendar date and clock-hour of systolic and diastolic blood pressure, heart rate and some approximation of ventricular ectopy. It is equipped with a conventional pressure cuff without microphone or transducer. The Nipco weighs 9.1 kg; it cannot be worn, but is provided with a handle so that it can be carried, e.g., back and forth from workplace to home. Recording may be carried out whenever the subject intends to stay for a while, mostly in the same room, be it at home, awake or asleep, or at work, while sitting or standing. For short departures from the room, the cuff can be slid off without unfastening it. The Nipco can be connected through an RS232 port to a personal microcomputer (Apple II or other) to allow for automatic data transfer and subsequent analysis, e.g., by single cosinor (14, 19, 4). After data transfer to a mini-computer (such as a PDP11/34), additional analyses and graphs are prepared (12). The restriction to a room has the disadvantage that one is unable to monitor the subject while walking or running. That the record does constitute a standardized profile descriptive of sedentary activity as well as rest may be an advantage, however.

Data evaluation

A 48-h test of blood pressure, measured mostly at 10-min intervals (with interruptions when the cuff is removed for departures from the machine, for up to 1 h) provides the individual with a personalized set of reference standards for the interpretation of the characteristics of circadian and any ultradian rhythms. Figure 4 shows data monitored automatically for 7 days, but stacked ("folded" in a plexogram) along the scale of a single idealized day. Thus, each datum is plotted as a dot at the corresponding clock-hour. Superimposed upon the data is the best-fitting 24-hour cosine curve, computed by the single cosinor method (12). Note from Figure 4 that the peak detected (macroscopically) by the naked eye differs in its location from the acrophase, and that the amplitude covers

DEFINITION OF RHYTHM PARAMETERS

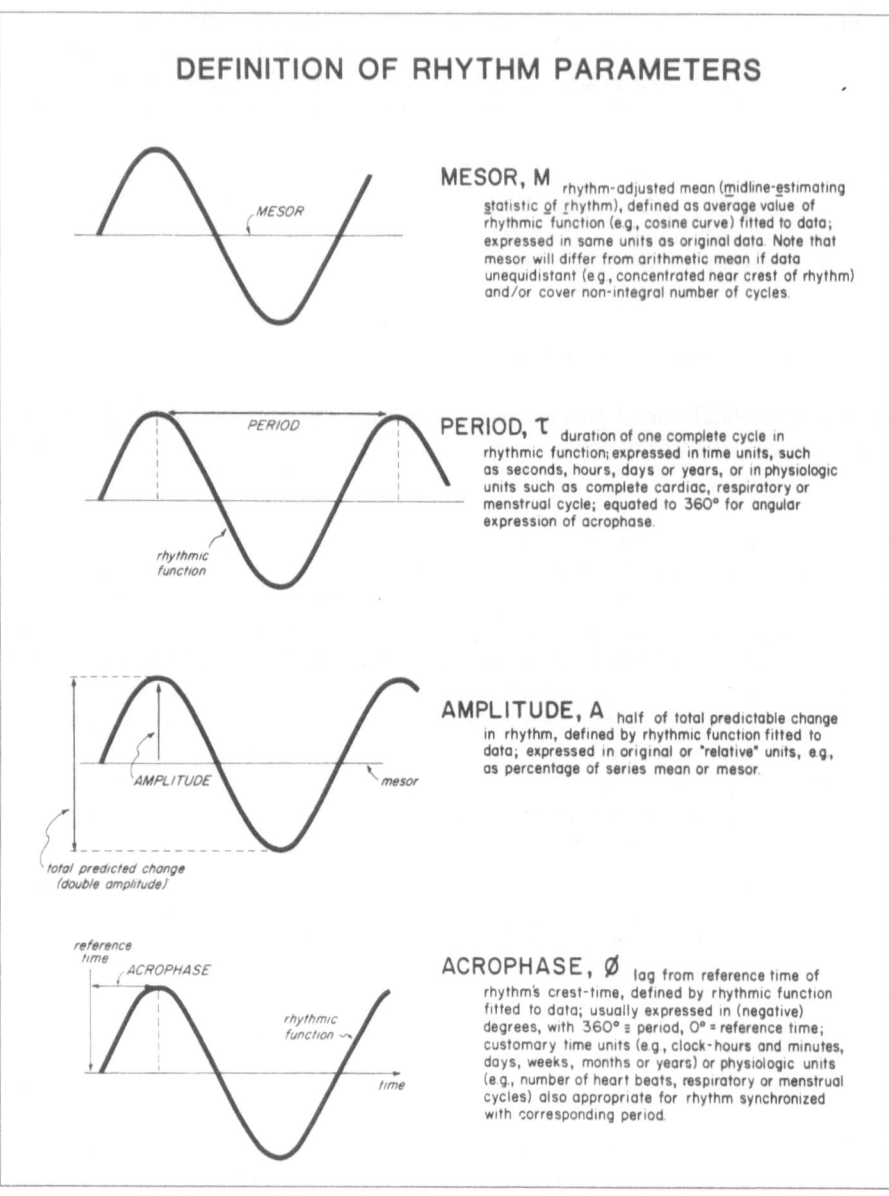

MESOR, M rhythm-adjusted mean (midline-estimating statistic of rhythm), defined as average value of rhythmic function (e.g., cosine curve) fitted to data; expressed in same units as original data. Note that mesor will differ from arithmetic mean if data unequidistant (e.g., concentrated near crest of rhythm) and/or cover non-integral number of cycles.

PERIOD, τ duration of one complete cycle in rhythmic function; expressed in time units, such as seconds, hours, days or years, or in physiologic units such as complete cardiac, respiratory or menstrual cycle; equated to 360° for angular expression of acrophase.

AMPLITUDE, A half of total predictable change in rhythm, defined by rhythmic function fitted to data; expressed in original or "relative" units, e.g., as percentage of series mean or mesor.

ACROPHASE, Ø lag from reference time of rhythm's crest-time, defined by rhythmic function fitted to data; usually expressed in (negative) degrees, with 360° ≡ period, 0° ≡ reference time; customary time units (e.g., clock-hours and minutes, days, weeks, months or years) or physiologic units (e.g., number of heart beats, respiratory or menstrual cycles) also appropriate for rhythm synchronized with corresponding period.

Fig. 3. Abstract characteristics of a rhythm, valuable endpoints of physiology and pathology that can be exploited for the assessment of health and risk as well as for diagnosis and treatment. One of these characteristics is the rhythm-adjusted mean or mesor (more reliable than a time-unspecified mean); another is the amplitude, which allows objective quantification of amplitude-hypertension (in lieu of reference to labile or borderline hypertension) and yields insights that focus upon the mesor (only) does not provide. The acrophase and period, measures of timing, gain in interest from the viewpoint of differential diagnosis (see schedule shifts) and under extraordinary conditions (e.g. social isolation).

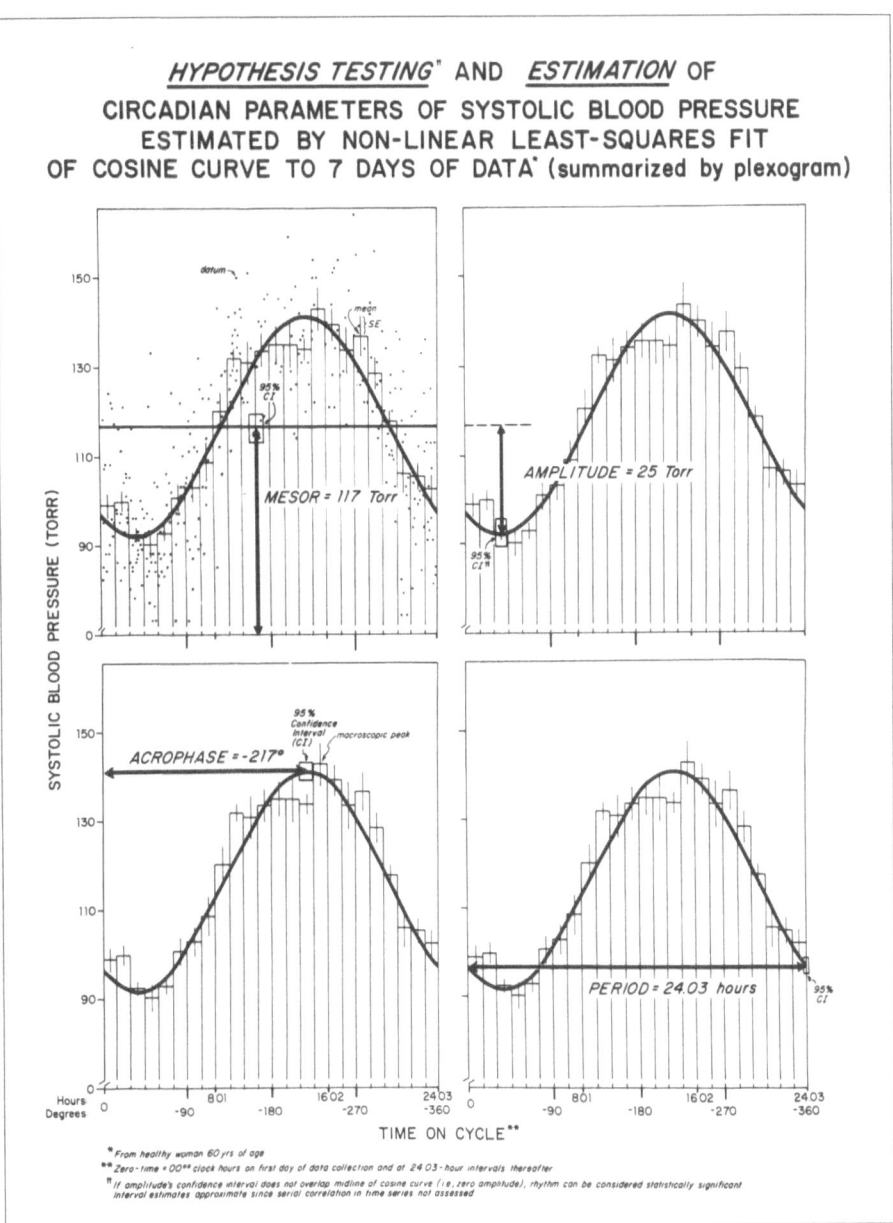

Fig. 4. Rhythm characteristics derived by the single cosinor method from original data; useful first approximations of blood pressure "dynamics". (For a qualification of the interval estimates in this figure, see text.)

one-half of the predictable portion of the variability accounted for by the fit of a cosine curve. The mesor, as a location index for a data set, is usually much more reliable than an arbitrary mean whenever the data are obtained at unequal intervals and/or do not cover an integral number of circadian or other rhythms characterizing the data.

The parameters in Figure 4 have all-too-tight confidence intervals, because correlation in the data has not been assessed. The confidence intervals are not considered when a personal or peer-group chronobiologic reference interval, a paradesm (one of the so-called chronodesms), is used for the interpretation of a parameter (7a, 32). When the confidence interval of a parameter is considered in its own right on the basis of dense data, several solutions are available (7, 29). The simplest, though not necessarily a rigorous approach, consists of circadian cosinor analyses on data averaged for appropriate, perhaps 1.5 h intervals.

Chronodesms

In any quality control, the acceptability of measurements depends on whether a given value lies within certain limits; such limits indicate whether particular observations (or sets of observations) are from the same population as a previous sample used to determine the limits. Chronodesms are such intervals constructed at points along a time scale (e.g., of 24 hours for circadian chronodesms). They are time-qualified reference intervals, e.g., tolerance intervals (17, 22) or prediction intervals (31, 32). Chronodesms may be built around means from observations obtained at a single sampling time (monodesm) or may be separately computed at each of several sampling times (merodesm), or may be built around a model, such as a curve with one or several cosinusoidal components (e.g., but not necessarily, harmonics) describing the entire time series (cosinordesm or rhythmodesm (1, 13, 22)). In the latter case, the computed reference limits at any number of timepoints may be connected to form a chronodesmic band about the fitted model.

A chronodesm can be built for an individual (Figs. 5–9). A tolerance chronodesm built for a peer group contains, with a specified probability, a certain proportion of the individuals in the population. For the case of blood pressure, however, individualized interpretation is highly desirable, if not indispensable. For the individual, a tolerance chronodesm contains, with specified probability (confidence), at least a certain proportion of a distribution of values. For example, Figures 6 and 7 are built to contain (on the basis of a profile measured in 1976), with 90% confidence, 90% of the distribution of future values. The systolic and diastolic blood pressures obtained in 1980, four years after the data used for constructing the time-specified reference interval (in 1976) fall mostly into that interval (Figs. 8 + 9).

Acrophase-shifts

A differential diagnosis may be aided by a comparison of the direction and rate of adjustment of the acrophases for blood pressure and other variables, including some that may be implicated in the coordination of blood pressure. Figure 10 illustrates this possibility. A physician changed his routine by staying up at night and retiring for sleep by day. A so-called chronobiologic serial section in Fig. 10 shows for several variables that, after an abrupt change in routine, the circadian acrophases adjust to the new schedule grad-

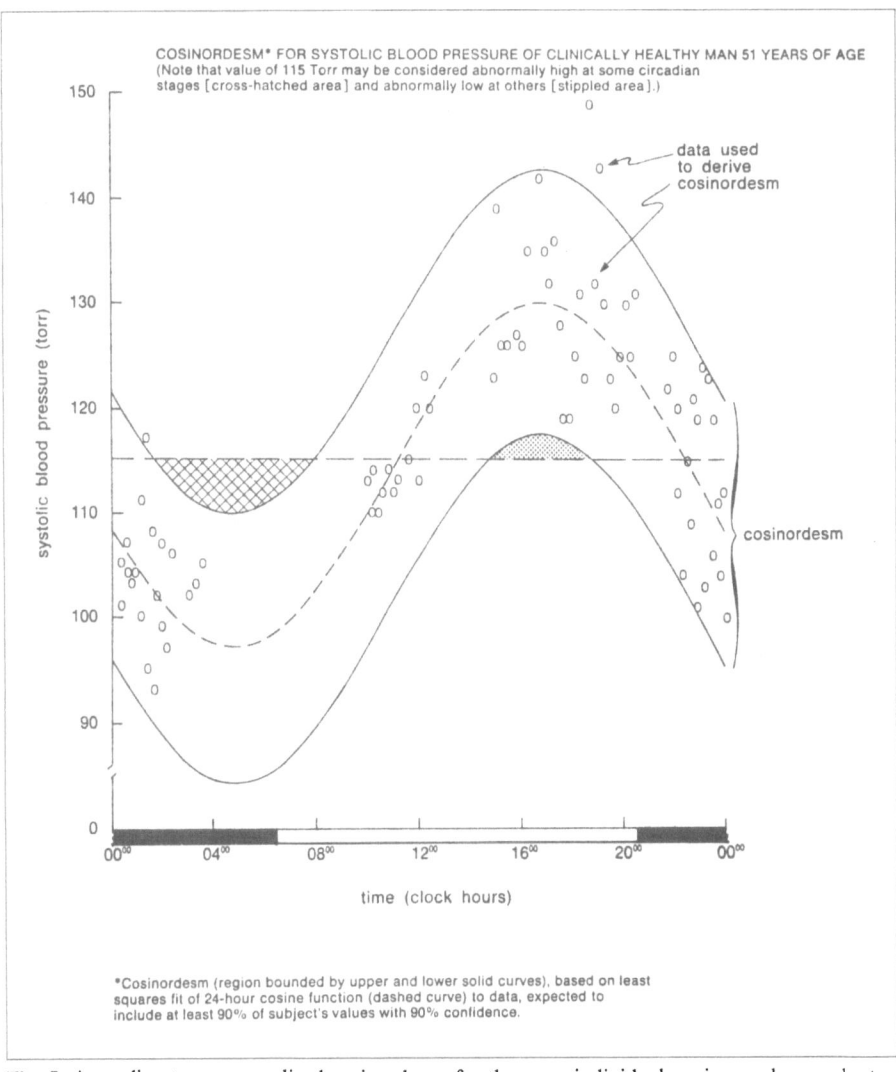

Fig. 5. According to a personalized cosinordesm, for the same individual, a given value can be too high at one time, perfectly acceptable at another and too low at a third.

ually (rather than abruptly). Moreover, systolic and diastolic blood pressure adjust with a delay; a few days after the shift in routine, their acrophases occur at a later time than at the outset (the acrophase at the outset being equated to 0 °). A few days after the shift in routine, the acrophases of other variables that may not be directly pertinent to the coordination of blood pressure rhythms occur earlier than at the outset. It can also be seen in Fig. 10 that in this case systolic and diastolic blood pressure move in the same direction as does the ratio of sodium to potassium. A correlation between the rhythm char-

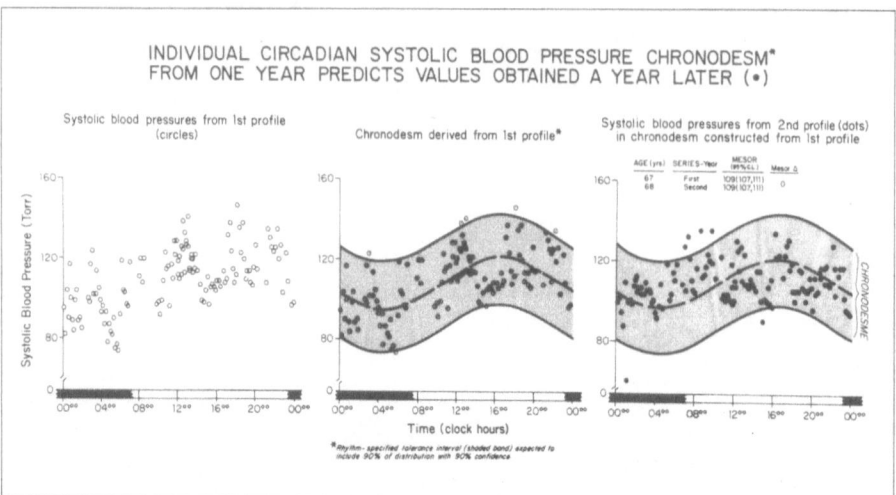

Fig. 6. Chronodesm in the middle is built as cosinordesm on the basis of data on the left. New data obtained a year later (dots on right) fit as well as anticipated.

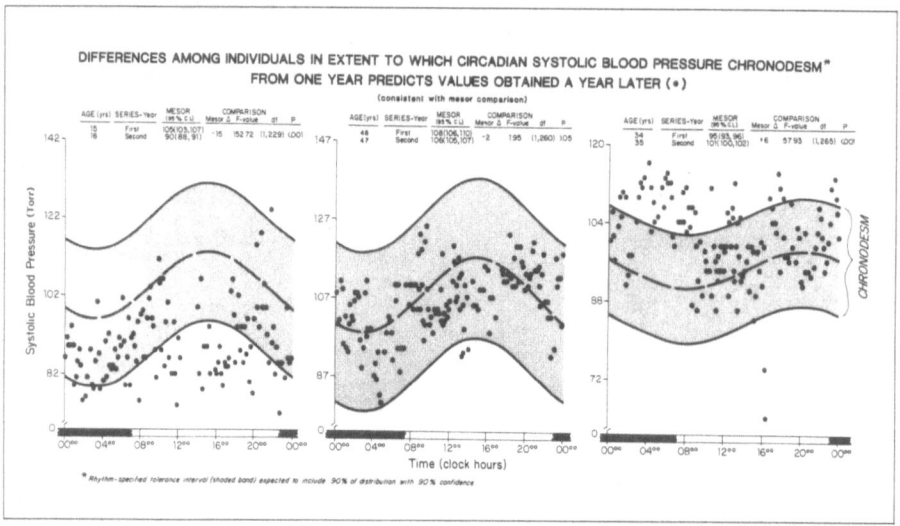

Fig. 7. A new data set (dots) is interpreted for 3 clinically healthy subjects in the light of a personalized cosinordesm built on the basis of data obtained one year earlier. The new profile in the middle is acceptable; the new one on the left, on the average, is low, yet it is likely that the subject had been anxious on the occasion of the first profile, in keeping with a novelty effect; hence, these values are also acceptable. The profile on the right is clearly higher tnan anticipated. Inquiry reveals that just prior to the recording of the second profile, the subject had been asked for a divorce.

acteristics of this ratio in urine and the human urinary excretion of aldosterone has been established by Lee et al. (28). In the case summarized in Fig. 10, aldosteronism was subsequently documented by conventional means, including adrenal vein cannulation.

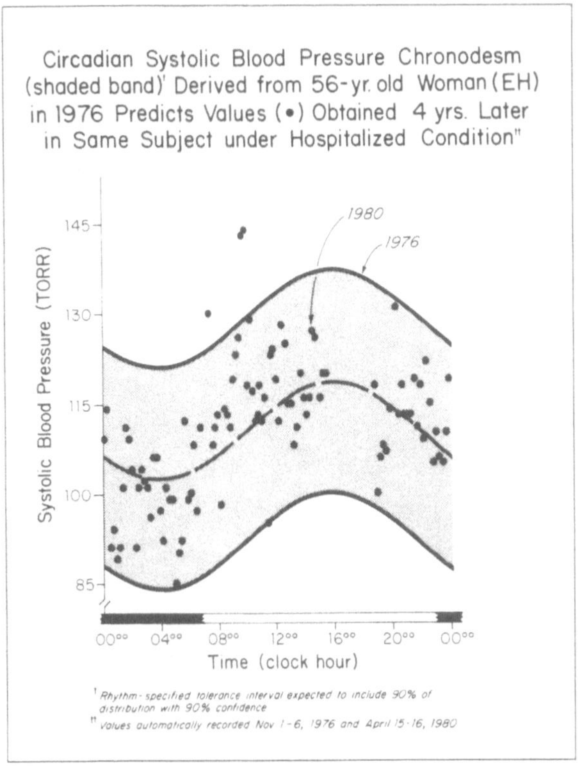
Circadian Systolic Blood Pressure Chronodesm (shaded band)' Derived from 56-yr. old Woman (EH) in 1976 Predicts Values (•) Obtained 4 yrs. Later in Same Subject under Hospitalized Condition"
Systolic Blood Pressure (TORR)
145
130
115
100
85
1980
1976
00⁰⁰
04⁰⁰
08⁰⁰
12⁰⁰
16⁰⁰
20⁰⁰
00⁰⁰
Time (clock hour)
' Rhythm-specified tolerance interval expected to include 90% of distribution with 90% confidence
" Values automatically recorded Nov 1-6, 1976 and April 15-16, 1980

Fig. 8. Most of the systolic blood pressures (dots) obtained 4 years after construction of a cosinordesm fit within the anticipated limits.

Acrophase-drifts and jumps

Figure 11 shows an acrophase-drift of the circadian rhythm in blood pressure (but not of that in core temperature) in a child hospitalized for intermittent fever but studied during an afebrile span on a 24-h hospital routine (by 3 shifts of special nurses around the clock for nearly a month) (16). Other variables of the same child, including diastolic blood pressure, pulse, core temperature and motor activity, were 24-h synchronized. The mechanisms of this internal circadian desynchronization are not known. The phenomenon points to separate periodic internal mechanisms for systolic as compared to diastolic blood pressure, among other variables.

Drug treatment – individualized inferential statistical assessment of effect

Figure 12 shows blood pressure behaviour in a patient receiving a beta-blocker and on the two days following a switch (unknown to the subject) to a placebo. As noted by Romano et al. (34) and Scarpelli et al. (35, 36) and by Güllner with us (10), an increase in the circadian amplitude of blood pressure may occur in response to cessation of treat-

Fig. 9. Most of the diastolic blood pressures (dots) obtained 4 years after construction of a cosinordesm fit within the anticipated limits.

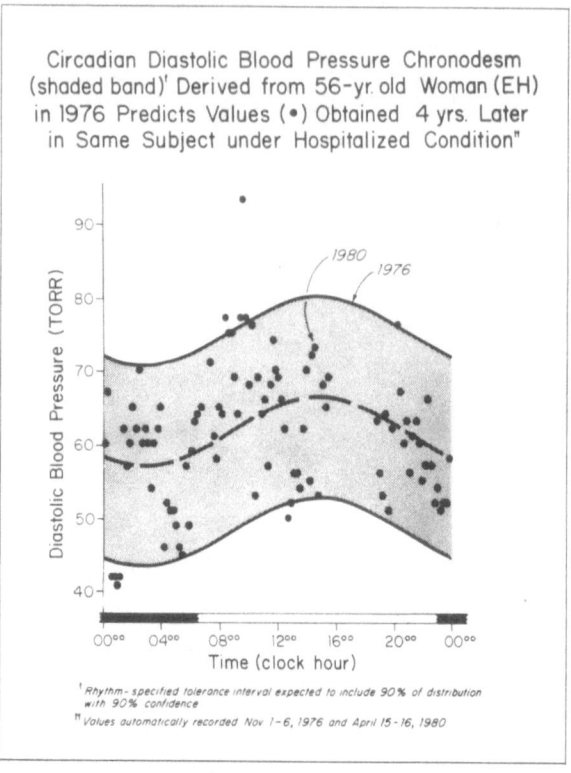

Circadian Diastolic Blood Pressure Chronodesm (shaded band)' Derived from 56-yr. old Woman (EH) in 1976 Predicts Values (•) Obtained 4 yrs. Later in Same Subject under Hospitalized Condition"

' Rhythm-specified tolerance interval expected to include 90% of distribution with 90% confidence

" Values automatically recorded Nov 1–6, 1976 and April 15–16, 1980

ment. The methods here illustrated objectively show the statistical significance (for the given individual!) of the gradual fading of a beta-blocker effect, within the first 2 days of its discontinuance.

Non-drug treatment – individualized inferential statistical assessment of effect

Figure 13 shows that an increase in circadian amplitude of systolic blood pressure can also occur as the result of salt restriction in a mesor-hypertensive individual. As a result of the relatively large amplitude in the stage associated with salt reduction, the highest systolic pressures reached as a function of circadian stage are almost as high as the highest values observed during the reference stage. A mesor reduction occurs with statistical significance in Stages II and III as compared to Stage I ($P < 0.005$). The mesor drop associated with salt restriction is relatively small, that associated with weight reduction much larger. Moreover, the circadian amplitude of systolic blood pressure is reduced only by the weight reduction ($P < 0.005$). The decrease in blood pressure to 120 mmHg after body weight reduction is clearly significant, not only in statistical but also in biologic terms. A reduction by 16.4 mmHg from an average pressure of 136 mmHg can indeed add to longevity in the light of work reviewed elsewhere (27). Thus, the methods here il-

148

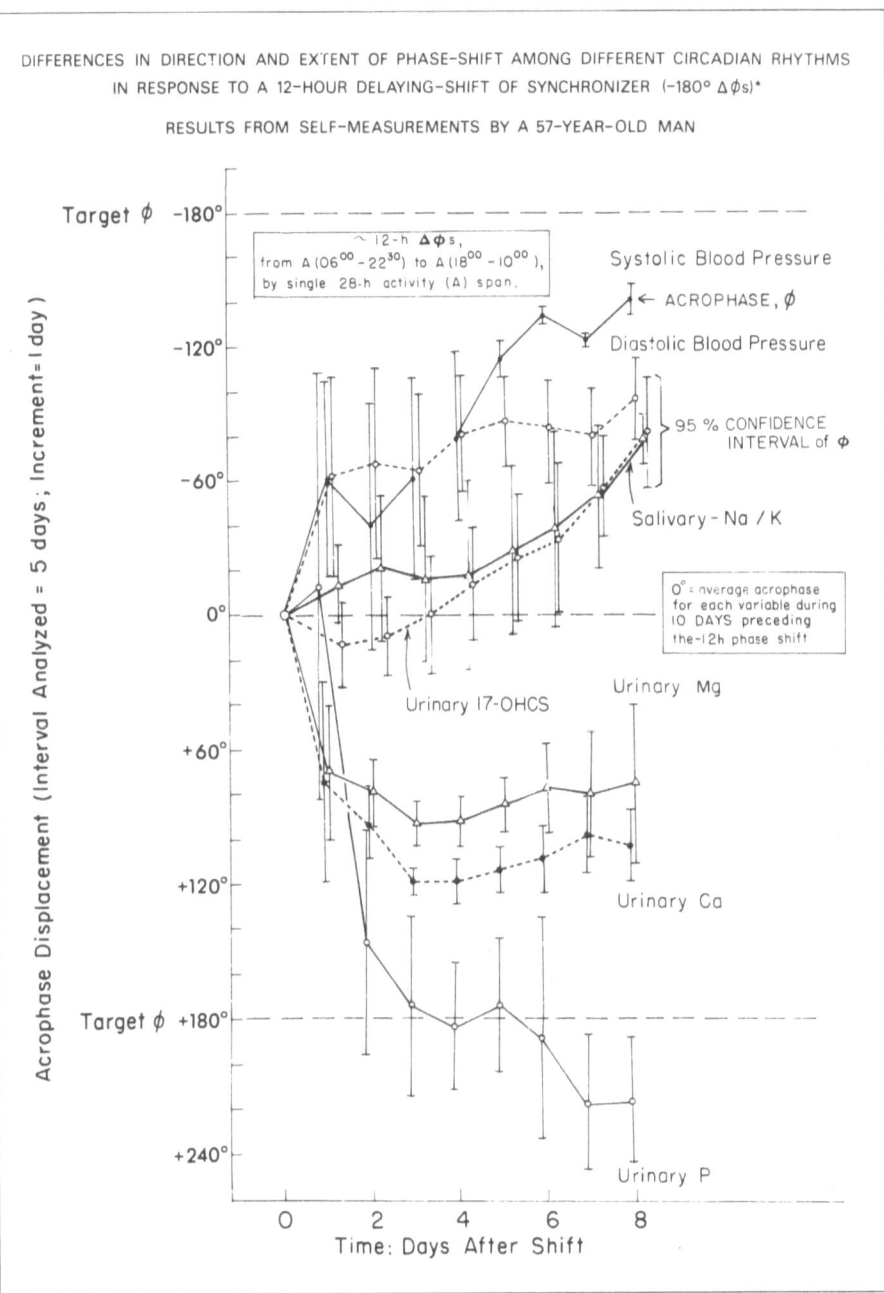

Fig. 10. Part of a so-called multiple chronobiologic serial section showing changes in timing following a change in routine from work by day to work by night. The acrophases for the variables investigated prior to the shift in routine are equated to 0 °. Their time course is then followed by the fit of a 24-h cosine curve, and the plot of the acrophase is thus obtained. It can be seen that the salivary sodium/potassium ratio shows the acrophase behavior closest to that of systolic and diastolic blood pressure. The sodium/potassium behaviour in urine has been correlated with that of aldosterone (28). (For a differential diagnostic value of this shift analysis, see text).

Fig. 11. Part of chronobiologic serial section describing reasonably steady course of rectal temperature acrophase occurring slightly after noon during most days (with noon equated to − 180 °). By contrast, the blood pressure acrophase is found early in the record during the morning hours; eventually, it occurs at noon, and at the end of the recording span, it occurs at night. Systolic blood pressure in this case desynchronized from the diastolic one and other variables, for reasons not known.

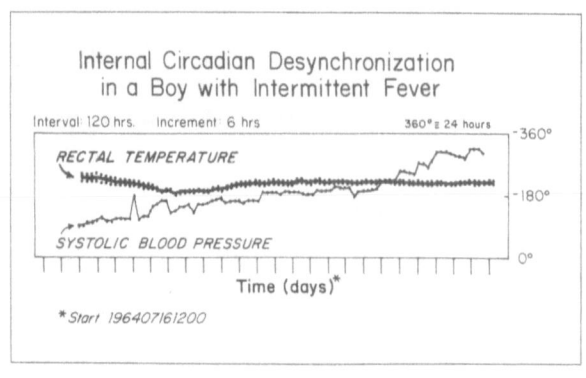

lustrated allow one to consider salt-sensitivity separately for the systolic vs. diastolic blood pressure, separately for the circadian amplitude vs. the mesor and with a view of statistical, as well as medical significance in each case.

Many studies on human subjects show that a substantial salt reduction alone can lower a previously high blood pressure in a sizeable fraction of patients and thus reduce cardiovascular complications (27). It has also been shown that many individuals may not be salt-sensitive, including subjects studied by us on an individualized basis (27). Genetically salt-susceptible individuals, however, are not a negligible minority; in the estimation of Jacobson and Liebman (25) or Berglund (3), salt restriction is effective in achieving "normotension" in 20 or 50% of "hypertensive" patients, respectively. Differences in estimates may stem from many factors but these need no longer include the failure to use individualized statistical tests on dense and long data, as advocated herein.

Since salt sensitivity, overweight and mesor- or amplitude-hypertension are mass phenomena in many geographic areas, and since mesor-hypertension and perhaps amplitude-hypertension, if not treated, can lead to cardiovascular complications, an appropriate reduction in salt and/or caloric intake may favorably affect millions of people. It does not suffice to emphasize the preventive value of salt restriction and weight reduction on a population basis; in implementing the intervention, it is essential to gauge its effects on an individualized basis.

Problem areas

It is tempting to separate individuals who are salt-sensitive from those who are not, and thus to describe types both in the clinic and in the experimental laboratory. The classification into types requires a full assessment of the several frequencies that characterize blood pressure in health and disease. In data from around-the-clock monitoring obtained after changes in salt intake, mesor tests (2, 4, 14) document that the transition from the "usual" to a low-salt intake can be associated with an increase rather than a decrease in systolic or diastolic blood pressure (e.g., from a mesor of 144 to one of 150

150

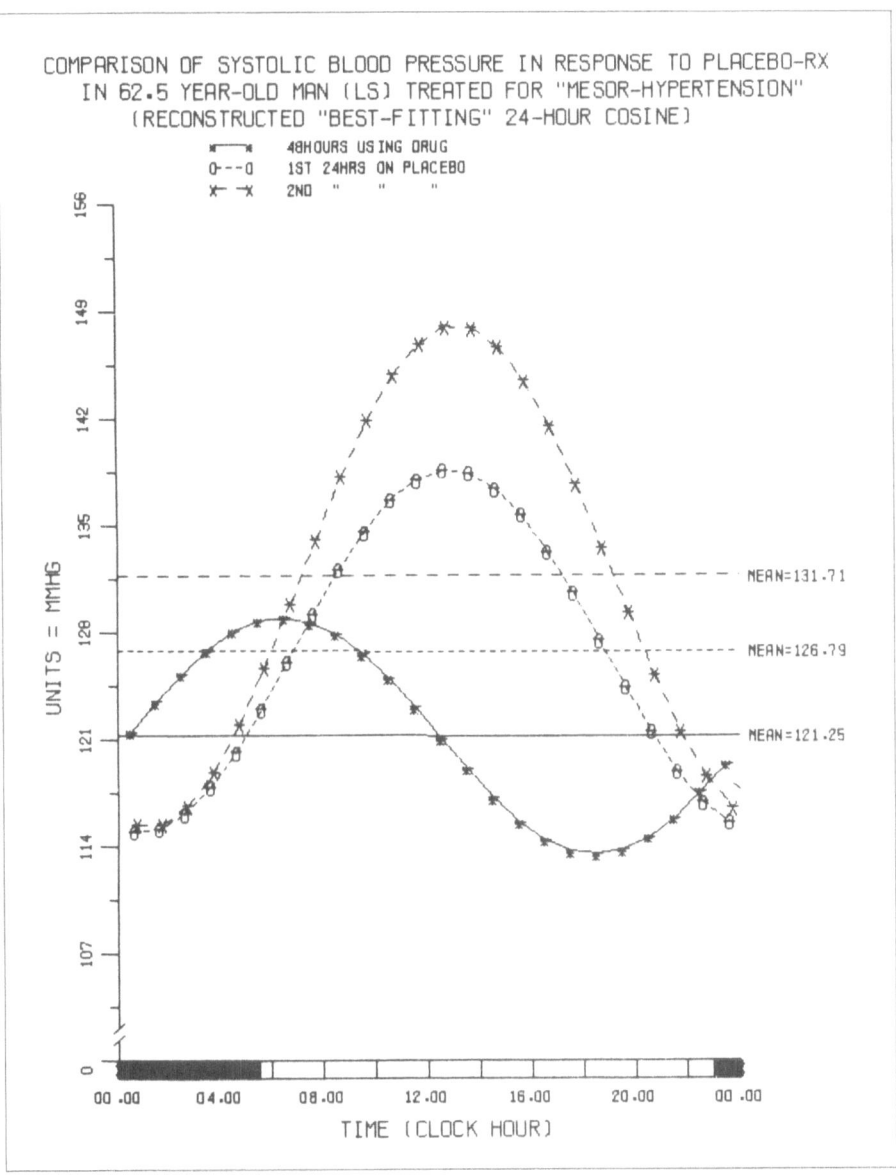

Fig. 12. Changes in blood pressure mesor during the 2 days immediately following a change (unknown to the subject) from a β-blocker to a placebo. Parameter tests show high statistical significance for a change in the combination of three rhythm parameters, namely of a mesor change of 5.5 mmHg, an amplitude increase of 4.1 mmHg, and an acrophase delay by 95°. Even the change in amplitude-acrophase pair, without taking the mesor change into account, is significant below the 1% level, as is the mesor change on the second day; each parameter is statistically significantly altered as compared to the 48 hours before the switch from drug to placebo. Corresponding prompt changes are not seen on day 1 in diastolic pressure, but are seen for the 3 rhythm parametres combined in a comparison of the second day on placebo with the result on the drug. For the pulse, the changes are the most dramatic, and are statistically significant within 1 day for each parameter separately as well as for combinations of parameters. Courtesy of Prof. L. E. Schering.

151

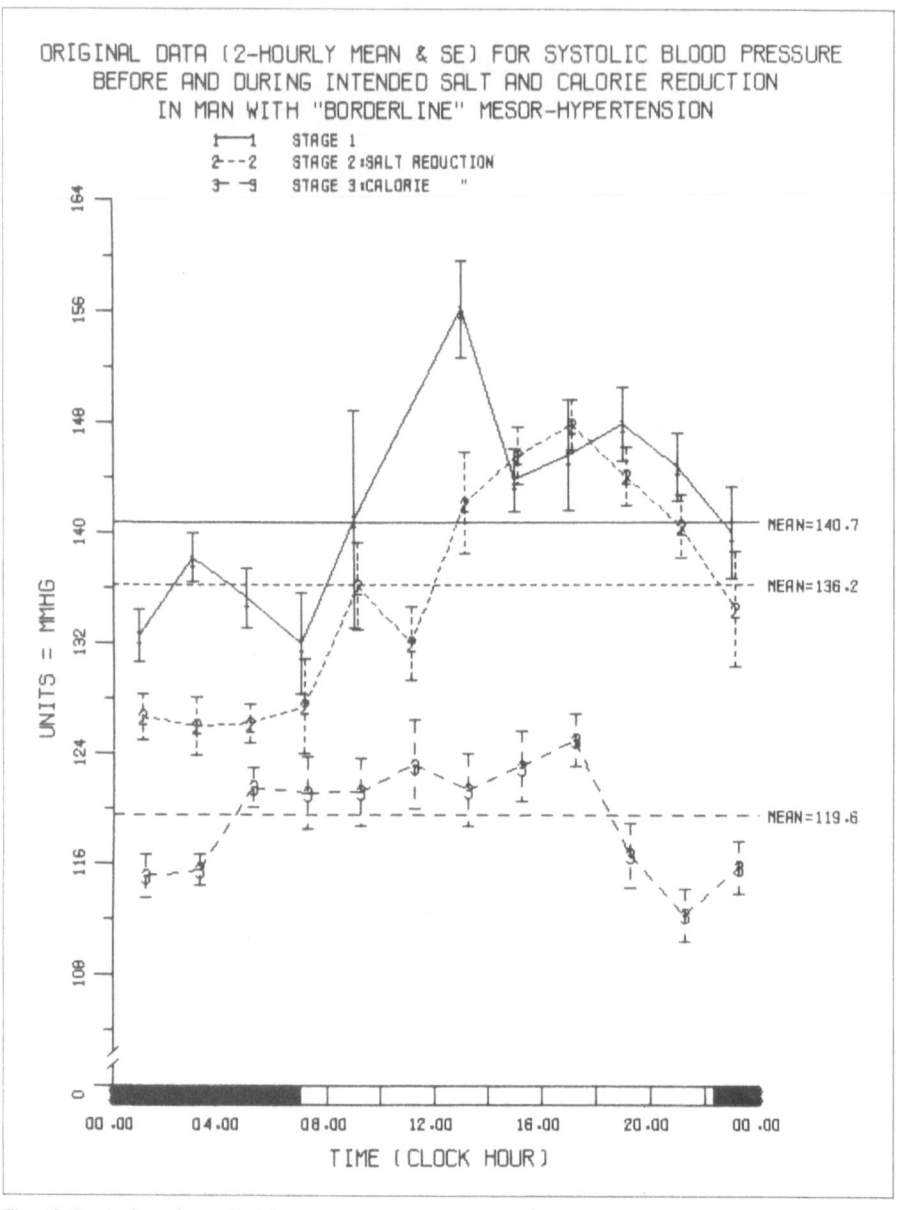

Fig. 13. Lowering of systolic blood pressure by reduction of salt intake and dietary calories (see text).

mmHg, P < 0.05). By the same token, the transition from a "usual" to a high salt intake can be associated with a decrease in both systolic or diastolic blood pressure (e.g., from 161 to 150 or from 110 to 103 mmHg, respectively) (P < 0.05). These results of our analyses of data obtained with Catherine S. Delea and the late Frederic C. Bartter by Prof. Terukazu Kawasaki, now at Kyushu University in Fukuoka, Japan, have led us to postulate three types of responses to changes in salt intake, namely no response or a statistically significant change in either direction. Whether the change in either direction is biologically significant, however, remains an open question amenable to rigorous study with the hardware and software now available. Certainly, more than a single day's even dense monitoring is required to obtain a reasonably stable mesor of human blood pressure (23).

Systolic mesor and/or amplitude-hypertension in 15- to 18-year old Minnesotan students

Several earlier publications have emphasized the educative merits of chronobiologic literacy at all ages and the particular role of chronobiology in secondary education for self-help in health maintenance (15, 18). Chronobiologic self-measurement for this purpose has been documented in technical detail (17) and remains the first practical step in school screening, complemented when need be by automatic measurement series and by endocrine spotchecks. Rhythms with multiple frequencies indeed gauge cardiovascular and other disease risk (21). International endocrine studies completed with a view of the prevention of the major diseases of our civilization have led to the specification of blood tests of neuroendocrine function for cost-effective risk assessment (based on only one or two samples of blood) (24). A thorough test of chronobiologic approaches to the assessment of individualized human variability, that of blood pressure in particular, is pertinent and cost-effective in schools (18, 33). When based upon self-measurement, this test requires sampling for 48 hours at hourly intervals during waking, with at least one added measurement near midsleep (38). It is much more densely and cost-effectively done by automatic monitoring, e.g., with the Nipco (23).

Against this background, students at a suburban high school were introduced to the elements of chronobiology in lectures. They learned and implemented the automatic and/or self-measurement of blood pressure around the clock and the interpretation of such measurements. The biology teacher thereafter assembled some of the students for a 24-hour autorhythmometry session in the high school library. 24 students participated on this occasion and a few had 24-h follow-ups at home; a total of 19 self-measured and 9 automatic series were obtained. 8 of the students in this study had been pre-diagnosed as "hypertensive" in prior screening of more than 1200 students by the school nurse according to conventional criteria.

According to as-yet tentative chronobiologic criteria, a population (rhytm-adjusted) mean (mesor) of 128 mmHg represents the intersect of two distributions found earlier for the systolic blood pressure of a few hundred adults. According to this mesor criterion, which refers to a mean including values during sleep and/or rest as well as wakefulness, three students previously classified as "normotensive" were found in this study to be potentially mesor-hypertensive, and two others to be potentially amplitude-hypertensive. A mesor for systolic blood pressure equal to or larger than 128 mmHg was found in 11 subjects, with 2 additional subjects reaching that value when the amplitude was added to the mesor. 6 of these subjects actually had a systolic blood pressure mesor equal to or higher than 135 mmHg, whereas in 3 others, the mesor and amplitude reached that value. Diastolic blood pressure mesors above 85 or even above 80 mmHg were not observed; only in two cases did the sum of the mesor and amplitude exceed 80 and it one in exceeded 85 mmHg.

153

All of the students were provided with rhythm-adjusted reference intervals for the interpretation of any follow-up single measurements and with rhythmometric summaries provided parameters to be interpreted in the light of population paradesms (31, 32). The diagnosis of mesor- and amplitude-hypertension, however, must be established on the basis of at least 48-hour (rather than 24-hour) profiles (23). Once the diagnosis of mesor- or amplitude-hypertension is established, timely and time-specified intervention is indicated, e.g., by diet or drugs. The effects of such intervention are also best assessed in an individualized fashion on the basis of chronobiologic criteria (27), preferably with automatic monitoring of the blood pressure, rhythmometric analysis and interpretation in the light of time-specified reference intervals from appropriate data bases. Whether one's aim is prevention, screening or treatment, a proper chronobiologic hardware-software system will require a cost-effective wedding of self- and automatic measurements stored in appropriate, readily accessible and updatable data bases.

Acknowledgements

The authors are indebted to Chronobiologia for permission to reproduce the materials, including graphs and tables, originally prepared for that journal. Germaine Cornelissen Guillaume, Research Associate, Chronobiology Laboratories, University of Minnesota, programmed several tests and gave helpful advice. Instrumentation for chronobiologic assessment of human blood pressure has been generously provided for follow-up research by Mr. Masayuki Shinoda of Nippon Colin Ltd. (Komaki, Japan) and Dr. Roger Adams of Minnesota Mining and Manufacturing Co. (St. Paul, MN).

References

1. Arbogast B, Lubanovic W, Halberg F, Cornelissen G, Bingham C: Chronobiologic serial sections of several orders. Chronobiologia 10: 59–68 (1983).
2. Bartter FC, Delea CS, Baker W, Halberg F, Lee JK: Chronobiology in the diagnosis and treatment of mesor-hypertension. Chronobiologia 3: 199–213 (1976).
3. Berglund GB: Should salt intake be cut down to prevent primary hypertension? Acta med Scand 204: 241–244 (1980).
4. Bingham C, Arbogast B, Cornelissen Guillaume G, Lee JK, Halberg F: Inferential statistical methods for estimating and comparing cosinor parameters. Chronobiologia 9: 397–439 (1982).
5. Cornelissen G, Halberg F, Stebbings J, Halberg E, Carandente F, Hsi B: Data acquisition and analysis by computers and pocket calculators. La Ric Clin Lab 10: 333–385 (1980).
6. Cornelissen G, Nelson W, Halberg E, Halberg F: Individualized reference region for circadian rhythm paremeters of systolic (S) and diastolic (D) blood pressure and heart rate (HR). Minn Acad Sci 51: 9–10 (1983a).
7. Cornelissen Guillaume G, Halberg F, Fanning R, Kanabrocki EL, Scheving LE, Pauly JE, Redmond DP, Carandente F: Analysis of circadian rhythms in human rectal temperature and motor activity in dense and short series with correlated residuals. In: Biomedical Thermology, M Gautherie, E Albert eds, pp. 167–184, Alan R Liss (New York 1982).
7a. Cornelissen G, Nelson W, Halberg F, Montalbetti N, Cagnoni M: Reference region for parameters – parameterdesms – of circadian cortisol rhythm. Chronobiologia 10: 117 (1983).
8. Delea CS: Chronobiology of blood pressure. Nephron 23: 91–97 (1979).
9. Drayer JIM, Weber MA, De Young JL, Wyle FA: Circadian blood pressure patterns in ambulatory hypertensive patients: effects of age. Am J Med 73: 493–499 (1982).

10. Güllner, HG, Bartter FC, Halberg F: Timing antihypertensive medication. p. 527, The Lancet September 8 (1979).

11. Halberg E, Halberg J, Halberg Francine, Halberg Franz: Infradian rhythms in oral temperature before human menarche. In: Menstrual Cycle: A Synthesis of Interdisciplinary Research, A Dan, E Graham, C Beecher, eds., Springer pp. 99–106, Publishing Co. (New York 1980).

12. Halberg E, Halberg F, Shankaraiah K: Plexo-serial linear-nonlinear rhythmometry of blood pressure, pulse and motor activity by a couple in their sixties. Chronobiologia 8: 351–366 (1981).

13. Halberg F: Quo vadis basic and clinical chronobiology: The promise for health maintenance of a temporal anatomy. Am J Anat 68: 543–594 (1983).

14. Halberg F, Carandente F, Cornelissen G, Katinas GS: Glossary of chronobiology. Chronobiologia 4 (Suppl. 1): pp. 189 (1977).

15. Halberg F, Fink H: Juvenile human blood pressure: need for a chronobiologic approach. In: Hypertension in Children and Adolescents, G Giovanelli, M New, S Gorini, eds, pp 45–73, Raven Press (New York 1981).

16. Halberg F, Good RA, Levine H: Some aspects of the cardiovascular and renal circadian system. Circulation 34: 715–717 (1966).

17. Halberg F, Halberg E, Nelson W, Teslow T, Montalbetti N: Chronobiology and laboratory medicine in developing areas. In Proc. 1st African and Mediterranean Congress of Clinical Chemistry, N Montalbetti ed, pp 113–156 (1982).

18. Halberg F, Haus E, Ahlgren A, Halberg E, Strobel H, Angellar A, Kühl JFW, Lucas R, Gedgaudas E, Leong J: Blood pressure self-measurement for computer-monitored health assessment and the teaching of chronobiology in high schools. In: Chronobiology, Proc Int Soc for the Study of Biological Rhythms, Little Rock, Ark, LE Scheving, F Halberg and JE Pauly, eds, Georg Thieme Publishers, Stuttgart; pp 372–378, Igaku Shoin Ltd (Tokyo 1974).

19. Halberg F, Johnson EA, Nelson W, Runge W, Sothern R: Autorhythmometry procedures for physiologic self-measurements and their analysis. Physiol Tchr 1: 1–11 (1972).

20. Halberg F, Lagoguey JM, Reinberg A: Human circannual rhythms in a broad spectral structure. Int J Chronobiol 8: 225–268 (1983).

21. Halberg F, Cornelissen G, Sothern RB, Wallach LA, Halberg E, Ahlgren A, Kuzel M, Radke A, Barbosa J, Goetz F, Buckley J, Mandel J, Schuman L, Haus E, Lakatua D, Sackett L, Berg H, Kawasaki T, Ueno M, Uezono K, Matsuoka M, Omae T, Tarquini B, Cagnoni M, Garcia Sainz M, Griffiths K, Wilson D, Wetterberg L, Donati L, Tatti P, Vasta M, Locatelli I, Camagna A, Lauro R, Tritsch G, Wendt H: International geographic studies of oncological interest on chronobiological variables. In: Neoplasms – Comparative Pathology of Growth in Animals, Plants and Man. H Kaiser ed. pp 553–596, Williams & Wilkins Co. (Baltimore 1981).

22. Halberg F, Lee JK, Nelson WL: Time-qualified reference intervals – chronodesms Experientia (Basel) 34: 713–716 (1978).

23. Halberg J, Halberg E, Hayes DK, Smith RD, Halberg F, Delea CS, Danielson RS, Bartter FC: Schedule shifts, life quality & quantity – modeled by murine blood pressure elevation & arthropod lifespan. Int J Chronobiol 7: 17–64 (1980).

23a. Hanson BR, Halberg F, Tuna N, Bouchard TJ Jr, Lykken DT, Cornelissen G, Heston LL: Rhythmometry reveals heritability of circadian characteristics of heart rate of human twins reared apart. Cardiologia, in press.

24. Hermida Dominguez R, Halberg F, Halberg E, Del Pozo F: Toward a psychoneuroendocrine hemopsy. Clin Chem Newsletter 2: 191–198 (1982).

25. Jacobson M, Liebman B: Dietary sodium and the risk of hypertension. N Eng J Med 303: 817–818 (1980).

26. Leach C, Halberg F, Sothern RB: Infradian variability in total (TE) and longest runs (LE) of cardiac ectopies, heart rate (H), blood pressure and temperature (T) of a comatose man. Chronobiologia 10: 138 (1983).

27. Lee JY, Gillum RF, Cornelissen G, Koga Y, Halberg F: Individualized assessment of circadian rhythm characteristics of human blood pressure and pulse after moderate salt and weight restriction. In: Toward Chronopharmacology, Proc 8th IUPHAR Cong and Sat Symp, Nagasaki, July 27–28, 1981, R Takahashi, F Halberg and C Walker, eds, pp 19–28, Pergamon Press (Oxford/ New York 1982).

155

28. Lee JY, Cugini P, Halberg F, Cornelissen G, Uezono K, Gillum RF, Scavo D: Rhythmometry on "borderline hypertensives" documents "false positives" and statistically significant (SS) correlation of urinary Na/K with aldosterone (Aldo). Chronobiologia 9: 347 (1982).

29. Malbecq W, De Prins J: Application of maximum entropy methods to cosinor analysis, J Interdiscipl Cycle Res 12: 97 (1981).

30. National Center for Health Statistics/Division of Health Examination Statistics: Blood presure of adults by race and area, United States, 1960–1962. U.S. Department of Health, Education and Welfare (U.S. Government Printing Office) (Washington, DC 1964).

31. Nelson W, Cornelissen G, Halberg F, Haus E: Time-specified reference intervals for plasma prolactin and cortisol, based on hybrid sampling design. Chronobiologia 10: 143 (1983a).

32. Nelson W, Cornelissen G, Hinkley D, Bingham C, Halberg F: Construction of rhythm-specified reference intervals and regions, with emphasis on 'hybrid' data, illustrated for plasma cortisol. Chronobiologia 10: 179–193 (1983b).

33. Rabatin JS, Sothern RB, Brunning RD, Goetz FC, Halberg F: Circadian rhythms in blood and self-measured variables of ten children, 9 to 14 years of age. In: Chronobiology, Proc. XIII Int Conf Int Soc Chronobiol, Pavia, Italy, Sept. 4–7, 1977, F Halberg, LE Scheving, EW Powell DK Hayes, eds, pp 373–385, Il Ponte (Milan 1981).

34. Romano S, Buricchi L, Gizdulich P, Scarpelli PT, Corti C: An experimental design for individualized adjustment of treatment in hypertensive patients based on autorhythmometry. Internal Medicine, Proc. XIV Int Cong Internal Medicine ISIM, Rome, Oct 15–19 pp 1482–1484 (1978).

35. Scarpelli PT, Romano S, Buricchi L, Corti C, Menniti P, Gizdulich P: Controllo dell'effetto antiipertensivo del prazosin mediante autoritmometria della pressione arteriosa. In: Problemi e prospettive dell'ipertensione arteriosa, C Bartorelli, A Bertelli, A Giotti, U Teodori eds, ESAM, pp 173–190 (Rome 1978a).

36. Scarpelli PT, Romano S, Lamanna S, Buricchi L, Cai MG: Autorhythmometry in hypertension: some methodological aspects and clinical implications. Chronobiologia 5: 407–424 (1978b).

37. Scheving LA, Scheving LE, Halberg F: Establishing reference standards by autorhythmometry in high school for subsequent evaluation of health status. In: Chronobiology, Proc Int Soc for the Study of Biological Rhythms, Little Rock, Ark, LE Scheving, F Halberg, JE Pauly, eds, pp 386–393, Georg Thieme Publishers Stuttgart/Igaku Shoin Ltd, Tokyo (1974).

38. Sothern RB, Halberg F: Sampling requirements for description of circadian blood pressure (BP) amplitude (A) Minn Acad Sci 51: 11 (1983).

39. Tarquini B, Benvenuti B, Moretti R, Neri B, Cagnoni M, Halberg F: Atherosclerotic chronorisk – recognized by autorhythmometry combined with hemopsies as a step toward chronophylaxis. Chronobiologia 6: 162–163 (1979).

Address for correspondence:
Franz Halberg
Professor of Laboratory Medicine & Pathology
Director, Chronobiology Laboratories
5-187 Lyon Laboratories
University of Minnesota
420 Washington Avenue, S.E.
Minneapolis, MN 55455 USA

The effect of age on circadian rhythm of blood pressure, catecholamines, plasma renin activity, prolactin and corticosteroids in essential hypertension

N. Stern*, E. Beahm**, J. Sowers, D. McGinty*, P. Eggena**, M. Littner, M. Nyby*, and R. Catania

Summary: With aging, blood pressure and norepinephrine (NE) levels gradually increase, and the duration and quality of sleep decrease. This raises the possibility that nighttime enhanced sympathetic nervous sytem activity may affect blood pressure and sleep patterns in aging men. We studied 12 normotensive aging men and 13 age and weight matched essential hypertensives (ages 55–70), as well as 9 young normotensive and 7 hypertensive subjects (ages 22–46 yrs) on a 100 mEq Na/80 mEq K diet. Supine blood pressure and hormone levels were determined at bi-hourly intervals between 09.00–21.00 h and every 30 min between 21.00–09.00 h. Elderly hypertensives and normotensives exhibited circadian rhythms of blood pressure, with the highest levels recorded in the late morning hours and the lowest between 01.00–04.00 h. Contrary to the findings in early essential hypertension, older hypertensives had lower mean 24 h levels of NE (377 ± 9 vs 455 ± 9 pg/ml; $p < 0.001$) than normotensives. The nighttime decrease in NE levels encountered in young individuals was not observed in aging subjects. Elderly hypertensives had lower mean 24 h PRA (0.92 ± 0.03 vs. 1.41 ± 0.06 ng/ml/h; $p < 0.01$). Circadian rhythm for PRA was barely detectable in older hypertensives. The circadian patterns of aldosterone, prolactin (PRL), and cortisol in older hypertensive and older normotensives were similar to those observed in younger hypertensives and normotensives.
Since the secretory pattern of both sleep-independent hormones (cortisol, aldosterone) and sleep responsive hormones (PRL) is unchanged, the disrupted circadian rhythm of NE and PRA in aging hypertensives represent specific abnormalities.

Introduction

Essential hypertension is more prevalent in older males, particulary in obese individuals. Hypertension may be caused in part by increased peripheral vascular resistance that could be related in turn to release of norepinephrine at sympathetic nerve endings in smooth muscles of peripheral arterioles. An age-related gradual increase in plasma catecholamines, probably reflecting both enhanced sympathetic nerve impulse traffic and decrease in clearance of norepinephrine, is well established (1, 2). Sympathetic nervous system activity as reflected by plasma ans urinary catecholamines has been shown to decline during sleep (3, 4). However, older age is associated not only with a decreased duration of sleep and impaired sleep quality (3) but also with an increased prevalence of distinct sleep-related breathing disorders such as central and occlusive sleep apnea (5). The etio-

Departments of Endocrinology*, Hypertension**, Pulmonology and Neuropsychology**, UCLA-San Fernando Valley Program, Sepulveda, California and Department of Endocrine-Hypertension, VA Medical Center, Richmond, Virginia

logy for enhanced sympathetic nervous system activity in older subjects remains poorly understood and the possibility that it is related to an age-dependent increment in sleep disturbances has not been thoroughly explored. Hormones implicated in the regulation of blood pressure such as catecholamines and corticosteroids could serve as mediators of both sleep disturbances and alterations in blood pressure in aging men. Other hormones with sleep related or inherent circadian rhythm such as prolacthin and renin could be also affected, thus potentially constribution to the altered control of blood pressure. This study investigates the circadian rhythm of catecholamines, plasma renin activity corticosteroids and prolactin in elderly normotensive and essential hypertensive subjects as related to blood pressure. Data are assessed in comparison to younger essential hypertensive and normotensive individuals previously studied in this laboratory.

Materials and Methods

Subjects

A total of 25 males, 12 essential hypertensives (blood pressure 140/90–170/115 and 13 normotensives (blood pressure < 135/85) older than 55 years of age were studied. Nine young hypertensives and seven young normotensives (ages 22–46) previously sudied in this laboratory served as controls. Absence of history or physical or laboratory evidence of heart disease, neurological, renal or endocrine deficiency or chronic lung disease (defined FEV_1 < 80%, using age corrected norms) were prerequisites for participation in this study. Participants had no history or evidence of regular alcohol use or use of hypnotic drugs. All medications were withheld for at least three weeks preceding the study.

Study protocol

Subjects were admitted to the geriatric metabolic ward and placed on a diet containing 100 mEq Na^+ and 80 mEq K^+/24 h for 5 days. They underwent three nights (nights 3–5) of adaptation and graded familiarization with the sleep lab. and monitoring equipment subsequently used on night 5 [continuous EEG, EOG, chin and anterior tibialis, EMG, EKG, ear oximeter, nasal and muchal thermister signals, chest and abdominal strain gauges for respiratory related movements, simulated blood sampling and blood pressure measurements (Arteriosonde, Hoffman-La Roche, Nutely, New Jersey)]. Studies were conducted in a sound-proofed room. Simulated and real blood sampling was carried out via a venous catheter connected to a sampling line passing through a port in the wall. 24 h of circadian studies were conducted on day and night 5. Between 09.00–21.00 h blood samples were obtained at bi-hourly intervals, after the patient had been in the supine position for at least 30 min. Between 21.00–09.00 h samples and blood pressure measurements were obtained every 30 min.

Assays

Plasma norepinephrine and epinephrine were analyzed by a modification of the single isotope radioenzymatic assay of DePrada and Zurcher (6). Plasma renin activity, aldosterone, cortisol and prolactin were measured by RIA according to previously described methods (7–10). Assessment of chronobiological characteristics of the various parameters was done by cosinor analysis using a computerized program obtained from the Institute of Work Physiology, Oslo, Norway.

Results

The two groups of elderly subjects did not significantly differ from each other in age (63.8 $\pm$ 1.2 years-normotensives; 64.8 $\pm$ 1.3-hypertensives) and percent. Ideal body weight (115.8 $\pm$ 3.2% for the normotensive or 120.1 $\pm$ 4.0% for the hypertensive group). 60% of the participants displayed distinct sleep related breathing disorders, i.e. central or occlusive sleep apnea, defined by the occurance of more than eight episodes of hemoglobin desaturation (of at least 4%) per hour of sleep. These were evenly distribution between the two groups (7 hypertensives, 8 normotensives). Total sleep time and the distribution of the various sleep stages was also similar in the older hypertensives and normotensive in the study.

Mean arterial blood pressure (MAP) and heart rate (HR) showed a clear diurnal rhythm and the nocturnal decreases were similar magnitude in both groups. Maximal nocturnal decreases in MAP were 27.2 $\pm$ 3.2 mmHg and 24.8 $\pm$ 4.4 mmHg and the maximal decrements in HR were 11.6 $\pm$ 1.9 and 9.2 $\pm$ 1.7 beats per min for hypertensives and normotensive subjects respectively (p = n.s. for both comparisons). The onset of the nocturnal reduction in MAP was usually related to the onset of sleep. MAP rose abruptly in both groups upon awakening. These patterns were essentially indistinguishable from those observed in the reference younger hypertensives and normotensives.

Significant circadian rhythm of norephinephrine secretion as determined by cosinor analysis was detected only in 3 normotensives and 4 hypertensives. Even in these subjects the correlation between actual hormone levels and the calculated best fitting cosine curve was weak (r = 0.206–0.404). This mainly reflected the absence of consistent and continuous nocturnal decrease of norepinephrine levels in elderly subjects. (Figs. 1, 2). A nocturnal decline in plasma noreprinephrine took place in younger subjects, whether hypertensive or not. Consequently in sharp contrast to the reference younger groups where the circadian changes in MAP were strongly related to plasma norepinephrine (r = 0.67, 0.63 in hypertensive and normotensive subjects respectively; p < 0.01 for both), MAP could not be correlated with plasma norepinephrine in older subjects.

Contrary to findings in early essential hypertension, mean 24 h levels of norepinephrine were lower in elderly hypertensive subjects than in age matched controls (377 $\pm$ 9 vs. 455 $\pm$ 9 pg/ml respectively; p < 0.001).

Both hypertensive and normotensive elderly subjects displayed, however, a nocturnal descrease in plasma epinephrine. Individual examples of the relationship between plasma cetecholamines, heart rate and mean arterial blood pressure during sleep are given in Figs. 1 and 2.

Mean 24 h PRA was lower in elderly hypertensives than in age matched normotensives (0.92 $\pm$ 0.03 vs. 1.41 $\pm$ 0.06 ng/ml/h; P < 0.01). The circadian rhythm of PRA in elderly normotensives followed the pattern previously observed in younger subjects: an overall markedly lower mean nighttime (21.00–09.00 h) PRA (1.28 $\pm$ 0.04 vs. 1.86 $\pm$ 0.07 ng/ml/h during the day – 09.00–21.00 h) with secretion surges taking place in the morn-

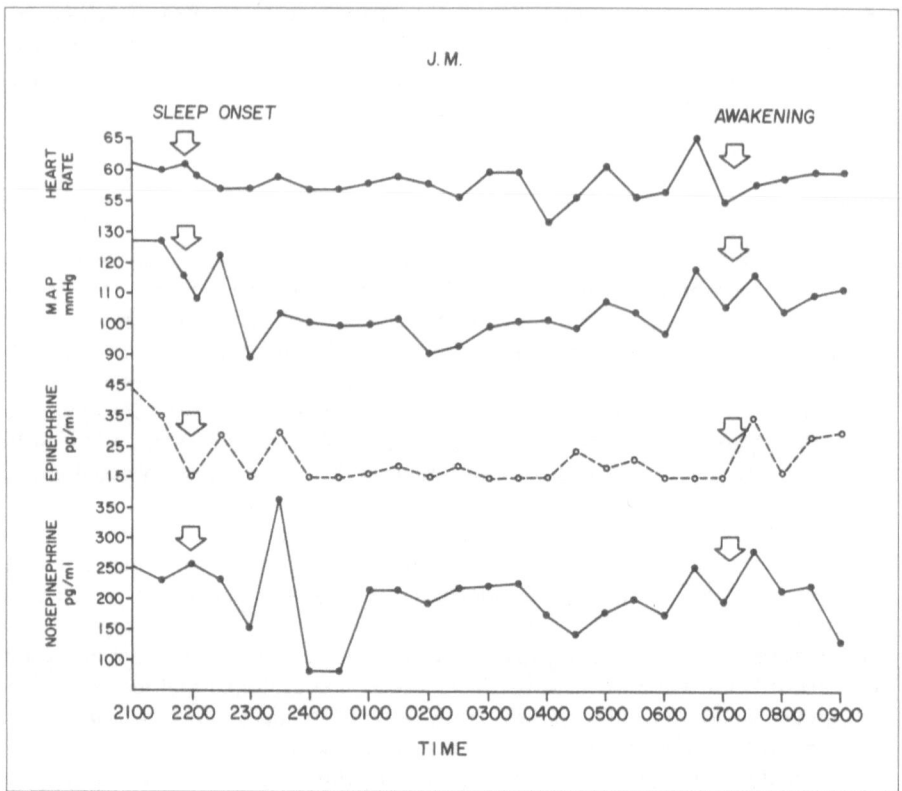

Figs. 1 and 2. Relation of sleep to heart rate, mean arterial pressure, plasma norepinephrine and plasma epinephrine in two older hypertensive subjects. Norepinephrine could not be correlated with MAP. In both patients MAP was positively correlated with plasma epinephrine; (r = 0.54 for J.M. [Fig. 1]; r = 0.45 for H.H. [Fig. 2]; p < 0.01 for both correlations.

ing (08.00–10.00 h), between 19.00–21.00 h (p < 0.05) and again between 01.00–05.00 h (p < 0.05). The circadian rhythm of PRA in elderly hypertensives appeared to be blunted with only small mean day to night variation (1.12 ± 0.03 vs. 0.86 ± 0.02 ng/ml/h respectively, an absence of evening surges and a much smaller rise in the early pre-awakening morning hours.

Despite these differences in the 24 h secretion pattern of PRA the diurnal rhythm of plasma aldosterone in elderly hypertensives and normotensives was indistinguishable and resembled that observed in younger subjects. Moreover, whereas mean 24 h PRA was lower in the hypertensive group, mean plasma aldosterone was not different (7.81 ± 0.54 ng/dl in elderly hypertensives and 8.42 ± 0.55 ng/dl in elderly normotensives). Similarly the diurnal rhythms of cortisol and mean 24 h cortisol levels (7.9 ± 0.6 and 8.4 ± 0.6 μg/dl in hypertensives and normotensives respectively of the two groups were indistinguishable. Diurnal changes in plasma aldosterone were highly correlated (r = 0.91, p < 0.001) with plasma cortisol, but not with PRA, in both groups.

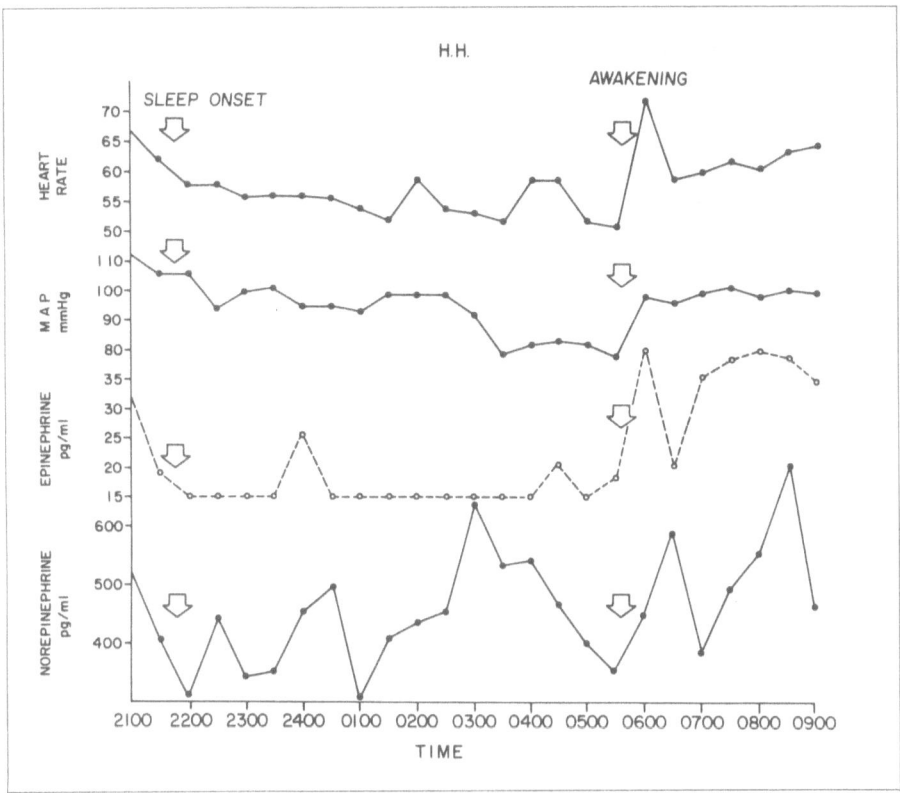

Fig. 2

Despite decreased sleep efficiency the well known nocturnal surge of prolactin release was observed in the elderly individuals, peaking between 01.00–06.00 h at 145 ± 26% of mean 24 h prolactin in the older hypertensive subjects, and at 139 ± 11% in the normotensive subjects.

Discussion

Results of this study suggest that the hypothesis that high blood pressure in the elderly is related to enhanced sympathetic nervous system activity secondary to impaired sleep quality or specific sleep related breathing disorders is inapplicable. First, subjects with sleep apnea were evenly distributed between the two groups and overall sleep quality was not different. Moreover, norepinephrine levels encountered in the group of elderly hypertensives were lower than in age matched normotensive controls indicating that a relatively enhanced sympathetic nervous sytem activity in hypertension of the elderly is unlikely. Further, older subjects, both hypertensives and normotensives, enjoyed a nighttime, sleep related decrease in MAP of the same magnitude observed in young individuals. This occurred in the absence of a circadian rhythm of plasma norepinephrine, reflecting the lack of consistent nocturnal in circulating norepinephrine in both elderly groups. Thus, in sharp contrast to younger subjects where plasma norepinephrine is higher in hypertensive patients than in normotensive controls and is strongly related to concomitant hour to hour MAP, elderly subjects display no correlation between MAP and circulating norepinephrine. The relatively blunted circadian secretion of PRA may be related to the disrupted secretion of norepinephrine.

Sleep sensitive hormones such as prolactin and stress-ACTH responsive hormones such as cortisol and aldosterone exhibit no differential circardian pattern in elderly hypertensives. Thus if disordered sleep is to be implicated in the hypertension of the elderly, mechanisms other than an altered secretion of the classical blood pressure modulating hormones need to be explored.

References

1. Ziegler MG, Lake CR, Kopin IJ: Plasma noradrenaline increases with age. Nature 261: 333–335 (1976).
2. Henry DP, Luft FC, Weinberger MH, Finebert NS, Grim CE: Norepinephrine in urine and plasma following provocative maneuvers in normal and hypertensive subjects. Hypertension 2: 20–28 (1980).
3. Prinz PH, Halter J, Benedetti C, Raskind M: Circadian variation of plasma catecholamines in young and old men: relation to rapid eye movement and slow wave sleep. J Clin Endocrinol Metab 49: 300–304 (1979).
4. Messerli FH, Glade LB, Ventura HD, Dreslinski GR, Suarez DH, MacPhee AA, Aristimuno GG, Cole FE, Frohlich ED: Diurnal variations of cardiac rhythm, aterial pressure and urinary catecholamines in borderline and established essential hypertension. Am Heart J 104: 109–114 (1982).
5. Carskadon NA, Demment WC: Respiration during sleep in the aged human. J Geront 36: 420–423 (1981).
6. Deprada M, Zurcher G: Simultaneous radioenzymatic determination of plasma and tissue adrenaline, noradrenaline and dopamine within the fentomole range. Life Sci 19: 1161–1174 (1976).
7. Eggena P, Barret JD, Sambhi MP, Weidman CE: The validity of compairing measurements of angiotensin I generated in human plasma by radioimmunoassay and bioassay. J Clin Endocrinol Metab 39: 865–870 (1977).
8. Mayes DM, Furuyama S, Kem DC, Nugent Ca: A radioimmunoassay for plasma aldosterone. J Clin Endocrinol Metab 30: 682–685 (1970).
9. Sowers JR, Berg G, Tuck ML, Martin VI, Chandler DW, Mayes DM: Dopaminergic modulation of 18-hydroxycorticosterone secretion in man. J Clin Endocrinol Metab 54: 523–527 (1982).
10. Sowers JR, Hershman JM, Skowsky WR, Carlson HE, Park J: Osmotic control of the release of prolactin and thyrotropin in euthyroid subjects and patients with pituitary tumors. Metabolism 27: 187–193 (1977).

Address for correspondence:
James R. Sowers, M.D.
VA Medical Center
Endocrinology Section
Richmond, Virginia 23249

Blood pressure monitors in studies of cardiovascular response

Bonita Falkner, David T. Lowenthal, and Harvey Kushner

Summary: We have used indirect blood pressure monitors including the Arteriosonde and Vita-Stat (900-D) instruments to measure cardiovascular response to the central stressor of forced mental arithmetic in adolescents. With the use of these instruments we have identified characteristic response patterns in normotensives, young hypertensives and a group at genetic risk for hypertension. Within-subject reproducibility of the response pattern has been proven statistically (cluster analysis). This investigation technique has also been used to study the effect of other factors such as dietary sodium and pharmacologic agents on the stress response. The indirect blood pressure monitors are useful in situations involving limited movement by the subject. Reliable measurements are obtained at frequency intervals of one minute.

Introduction

Investigations of blood pressure in the young have described a progressive increase in blood pressure with age (1). Reports of dynamic testing have also demonstrated marked variation in blood pressure under different conditions of stress. Studies are currently under way to evaluate the correlation of these response patterns to other risk factors for cardiovascular disease. The development of non-invasive instruments has enabled expansion of those studies to larger and younger populations.

This report will describe our findings on the use of two indirect blood pressure monitors, the Arteriosonde (Roche) and the Vita-Stat (900-D). We have used these instruments to measure the cardiovascular response to the stressor of forced mental arithmetic in the young.

Methods

In the first phase of our studies the Arteriosonde (Roche) was used. This instrument utilizes ultrasonics, transmitting the brachial artery pulsations. Parallel mercury columns provide the pressure readings. When the systolic pressure is obtained the left column remains fixed at the level of systolic pressure while the right mercury column drops until the diastolic pressure (4th phase) is obtained. An amplifier transmits the pulse as an auditory signal between systolic pressure and diastolic pressure. In our studies this auditory

Departments of Pediatrics, Medicine, and Physiology Hahnemann University Philadelphia, Pennsylvania signal was timed to obtain the heart rate. Measurements were obtained at one min intervals by a timed automatic cuff inflation pump. The later studies were performed with a Vita-Stat indirect blood pressure monitor. This instrument similarly utilizes ultrasonic techniques. Measurements of systolic pressure, diastolic pressure and heart rate are displayed digitally. Variable timing of blood pressure measurements can be adjusted with the shortest interval being that of one min.

The mental stress testing methodology has been described previously (2). In brief, each subject rested supine for 30 min. Monitoring of blood pressure and heart rate was then begun with measurements obtained in the right arm by one of the above indirect blood pressure monitors. After 10 min of recordings at one min intervals the baseline blood pressure and heart rate were determined from the mean of the last five recordings. Each subject was then challenged to perform difficult serial subtraction for a period of 10 min during which time the blood pressure and heart rate continued to be monitored at one min intervals. Upon completion of the stress, blood pressure and heart rate measurements continued for another five min in the recovery phase.

Results

To examine the reproducibility of the mental stress testing, including the reliability of the instruments, data were examined from 58 stress tests of 20 individual subjects. The time intervals between tests ranged from two weeks to several years. The analysis was based on the time series data measured at one min intervals and included systolic pressure, diastolic pressure and heart rate (3). For analysis of reproducibility within subjects a cluster analysis (4) for each cardiovascular parameter was performed using the 10 equally spaced measurements obtained during the stress test. Cases were a priori allocated to five clusters. It was expected that if the test were reproducible, the outcome of the clustering would be such that the hypertensive subjects would all cluster in the same group and a similar pattern would occur for the normotensives, those at genetic risk, borderline hypertensives and hypertensives. A small group of nonreactors was also expected. For all cardiovascular parameters there was a statistically significant clustering among repeated testing from the same individual. For example, with systolic pressure, 85% had two or more tests in the same cluster ($x = 8.73$, $p < 0.01$). Similar results were observed with the other cardiovascular paramters. These results then indicate that the mental stress testing methodology within subjects is reproducible and also that these instruments used in this manner are reliable.

Discussion

Further mental stress testing studies have been performed which involve a pretest, intervention, posttest design. An investigation of sodium sensitivity in the young demonstrated that offspring of normotensive parents were resistant to sodium loading in that their baseline blood pressure and stress response were unchanged following two weeks of salt loading. Young offspring of hypertensives were sensitive to sodium in that the sodium loading augmented both the baseline and stress response (5). The effect of pharmacologic intervention on stress response has also been investigated in hypertensive adolescents. A centrally acting drug (clonidine) dampened the stress response while diuretics (hydrochlorothiazide) imposed no significant change (6). Thus, the methodology with these monitoring instruments provides a useful means to evaluate the impact of various interventions on the cardiovascular response to central stress.

The monitors described have proven effective in studies to investigate cardiovascular response patterns in the young. Advantages of the instruments are that they are reliable, and non-invasive. Occasional problems were encountered with spontaneous movement by the subject. Distorted recordings occurred when the subject exhibited upper arm movement. Difficulty also occasionally occurred when the subject had a relative bradycardia. In the latter case an accurate diastolic pressure was difficult to obtain. However, this occurred rarely.

In summary, examination of our data on repeated studies demonstrates significant within-subject reliability. The reproducibility of the stress response pattern indicates the validity of the stress testing method and also the reliability of these monitors.

References

1. Task Force on Blood pressure Control in Children. Report of the Task Force. Pediatrics 59 (suppl): 797–820 (1977).
2. Falkner B, Onesti G, Angelakos ET, Fernandez M, Langman C: Cardiovascular response to mental stress in normal adolescents with hypertensive parents. Hypertension 1: 23–30 (1979).
3. Kushner H, Falkner B: A harmonic analysis of cardiac response of normotensive and hypertensive adolescents during stress. J Human Stress 7: 21–27 (1981).
4. Cooley WW, Lohnes PR: Multivariate data analysis. N. Wiley (1971).
5. Falkner B, Onesti G, Angelakos ET: The effect of salt loading on the cardiovascular response to stress in adolescents. Hypertension 3 (suppl II): 195–199 (1981).
6. Falkner B, Onesti G, Affrime MB, Lowenthal DT: The effect of a centrally acting agent versus diuretics on the cardiovascular response to mental stress in adolescent hypertension. Clin Sci 68: 455s–458s (1982).

Address for correspondence:
B. Falkner, M.D.
Hahnemann University
Department of Pediatrics
Broad and Vine Streets
Philadelphia, Pennsylvania 19102

Familial influences on ambulatory blood pressure: studies of normotensive twins

Richard J. Rose

Summary: As a follow-up to a twin study of cardiovascular reactivity to laboratory stress, we are evaluating familial influences on the lability of blood pressure measured in naturalistic environments. Adolescent and young adult twins, differentiated by zygosity and familial history of essential hypertension, are trained to monitor their casual pressures 6 times daily for 3–4 weeks. In addition, co-twins concurrently wear ambulatory monitors for one 18–24 hour period. Preliminary data analyses indicate that lability, as well as level, of blood pressure is a stable characteristic of individuals, and that it exhibits significant familial aggregation due, in part, to genetic factors. Initial analyses suggest that increased lability may be associated with a parental history of hypertensive disease.

Twin-family studies establish that the level of casual blood pressure exhibits familial aggregation attributable, in large part, to genetic influences. To document that fact in a novel way, we exploited the multiple genetic and social relationships found within kinships of monozygotic (MZ) twin parents (1). Children of MZ twins are genetic half-siblings who are reared as cousins in separate households, and a nested analysis of variance of the offspring data permits an incisive partitioning of shared genes from shared experiences. Using maximum likelihood procedures to estimate sources of variance in the systolic pressures of 76 adult MZ twins and their 341 children, we obtained a heritability estimate of 0.63 with no evidence of common environmental effects or maternal influences (2).

In subsequent research, we have assessed familial sources of variance in blood pressure responses to laboratory stress in 478 normotensive adolescents and young adults. That sample included 111 pairs of MZ twins, 66 dizygotic (DZ) twin pairs, and 54 pairs of unrelated individuals recruited from high school and college student populations in Indiana and representing an age range from 14–33 years. The laboratory protocol included five stressors, each of exactly two minutes duration interspersed with a relaxation/recovery period of three minutes, 40 seconds. The first three stressors required active, coping responses to psychological challenge, while the last two were passive, physical stress experiences. Co-twins were concurrently tested in adjacent, but separate rooms. Blood pressures were measured at 40-second intervals during stress with two Arteriosonde 1216 monitors simultaneously triggered by a laboratory computer. Preliminary analyses of these data (3, 4) reveal that the pressor responses exhibit genetic variance: the profiles of

Departments of Psychology and Medical Genetics Indiana University cardiovascular reactivity of MZ twins are significantly more concordant than those of DZ twins, which in turns are significantly more similar than those of the unrelated pairs. In addition, initial analyses suggest that familial risk, indexed by a documented parental history of essential hypertension (EH), is associated with an exaggerated pressor response, as shown in the work of others (5).

In follow-up research with these twins (and newly ascertained twin pairs drawn from the same resources) we are now studying the level and lability of blood pressure observed in the home environment. Pressures are taken at least six times daily in the home environment with digital monitors. Twin pairs are trained to monitor their own blood pressures at two sittings, once in the morning before arising, the other in the afternoon or evening while seated. Whenever possible, the pairs are also evaluated for the level and lability of ambulatory blood pressure as measured with Del-Mar P-III monitors throughout an 18–24 hour period. The major interest in the Del-Mar records is the degree to which the level and lability of ambulatory blood pressure is predictive of the level and lability of pressure self-monitored in the home environment and the degree to which both of these naturalistic records are predictive of the stress reactivity patterns previously observed in the laboratory protocol. A major question addressed in this research is whether a standardized stress protocol is predictive of the level and lability of blood pressure observed in the naturalistic environment.

Results from this research will address the familial nature of labile blood pressure, evaluate its genetic determinants, and assess its association with parental history of hypertensive disease.

Ambulatory blood pressures are observed concurrently for each twin pair. Typically, the subjects report to the laboratory in mid-afternoon and return 20–24 hours later. Before leaving the laboratory, pressures are observed in response to an abbreviated stress protocol in which each subject engages in isometric hand-grip for 160 seconds at 1/4 maximum voluntary contraction. Subsequently, the subjects' monitors are set to obtain pressures at 7 1/2 minute intervals throughout waking periods and at 30-minute intervals during sleep. In addition, subjects are encouraged to manually take their pressures at all other convenient times. Typically, a sample of 80–140 artifact-free measures of systolic and diastolic blood pressure is obtained for each subject. The Del-Mar monitors are routinely checked against a standard mercury column, recharged battery packs are alternated every five days, and voltage checks of internal batteries are periodically made by our electronics technician. Memory from the monitors is dumped into a custom Z-80 laboratory computer programmed to decode the stored blood pressure data. Subsequently, the data are edited, artifactual data points identified according to criteria based on pulse pressure (6) are eliminated, and the edited profiles are plotted using routines of Indiana University computer facilities.

Results from this on-going study can be illustrated with profiles of systolic pressures observed in representative twin pairs differentiated by genetic similarity and familial medical history. Ambulatory systolic blood pressure profiles for a pair of male monozygotic twins, age 22, are shown in Figure 1. The twins are at risk for essential hypertension (EH) by virtue of a documented history of the disease in their mother, who experienced angina and was diagnosed as hypertensive at age 47, a decade prior to our study of her twin sons. She has been under continuous treatment since then.

The figure plots the twins' successive systolic blood pressure (SBPs) recorded over a 22-hour period. As is typically true for MZ twins, levels of SBP are highly concordant:

168

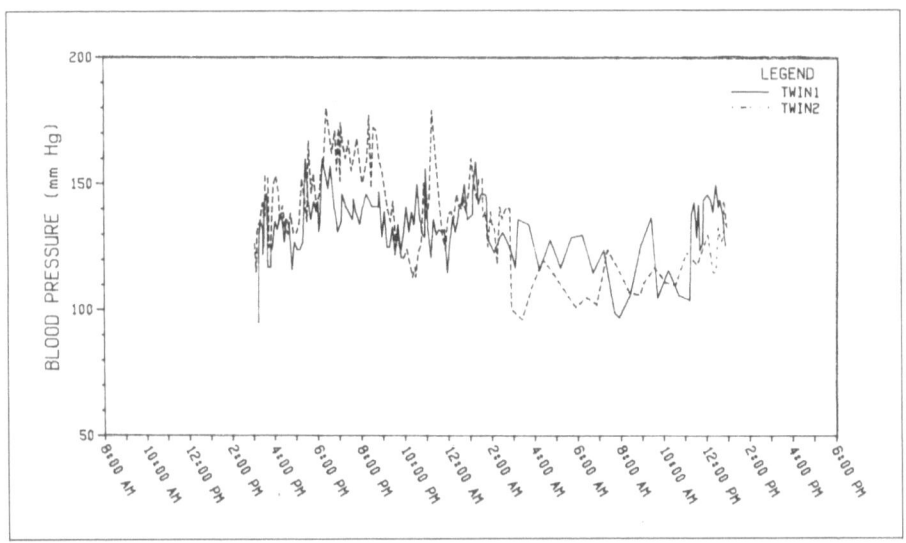

Fig. 1. Ambulatory systolic blood pressures, male, MZ cotwins, age 22, hypertensive parent(s)

systolic pressures of these identical twin brothers, averaged over > 130 observations for each co-twin, are 132.9 and 137.8, differing by < 5 mm. Again as typically found for normotensive young adults with a parental history of EH, the individual pressures are quite labile: the standard deviations of the SBPs for these at-risk twins are 18.2 and 12.0. In contrast, Figure 2 plots 22-hour records of a pair of twins with a negative parental history of EH. Lability of the SBPs is modest; the standard deviations are < 11 mm for each of these 21 year-old women. These are DZ twin sisters, and their systolic pressures are strikingly discordant in average level (93.8 vs. 110.2).

Figure 3 illustrates the very labile SBPs observed in a pair of 28 year-old DZ brothers at elevated risk for EH by virtue of parental history. Standard deviations of the SBP profiles for these at-risk males are 14.7 and 16.5; the means, averaged across 126 observations for one twin and 132 for his co-twin, are 117.8 and 126.6, an average difference of 8.8 mm.

The initial question asked of these data was whether lability of casual blood pressure is a stable characteristic of individuals. Level of blood pressure is established as a reliable characteristic: a group of individuals, whose pressures are monitored on two occasions or concurrently measured by two observers, maintain their rank order. Is lability also a trait-like characteristic of blood pressure? Our preliminary data provide an affirmative answer. Table 1 presents evidence that the standard deviations of SBP data are stable over time and across procedure. Individuals with more labile SBPs in the morning are also more labile in the evenings, and lability of self-monitored casual pressures signif-icantly correlates with lability of ambulatory profiles. In short, while less stable than the level of blood pressure, the lability of SBP is a reliable characteristic of individual varia-tion.

What are its determinants? We have performed conventional twin analyses of the pres-sures recorded over 14–30 days of at-home monitoring (7). Results indicate significant

169

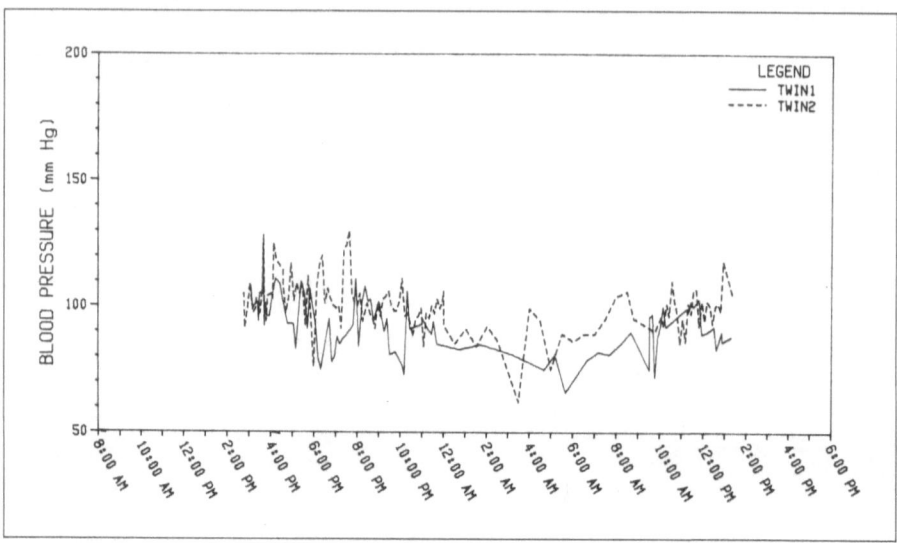

Fig. 2. Ambulatory systolic blood pressures, female, DZ cotwins, age 21, normotensive parents

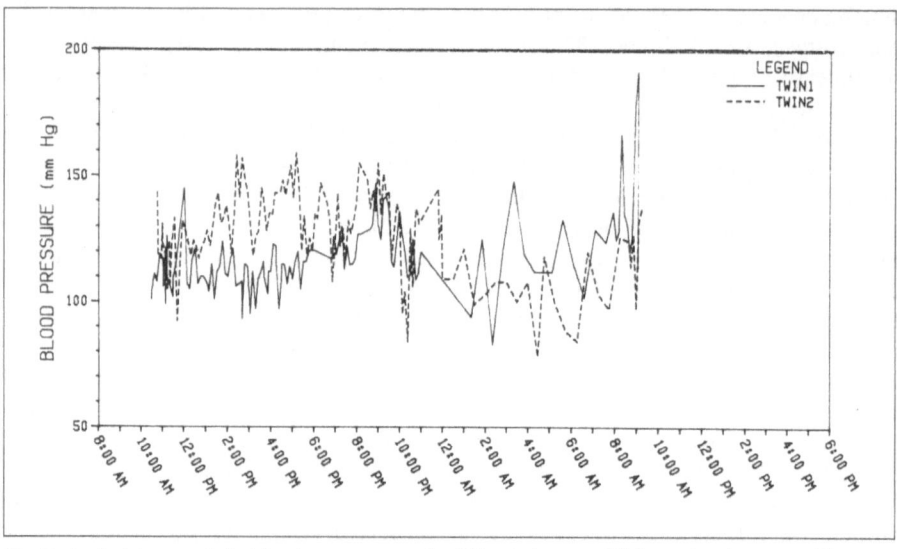

Fig. 3. Ambulatory systolic blood pressures, male, DZ cotwins, age 28, hypertensive parent(s)

genetic variance in the lability, as well as level, of the SBP data. Figures 1–3 suggest that parallel analyses of the ambulatory profiles will yield further evidence of genetic influence on lability of SBPs. Finally, individuals at elevated risk for EH by virtue of a con-

Table 1: Lability and level of systolic blood pressure are stable characteristics of individuals.

	Level of SBP	Lability of SBP
Stability Over Time[1] N = 136	0.81 (p < 0.01)	0.49 (p < 0.01)
Stability Over Measurement[2] N = 27	0.73 (p < 0.01)	0.36 (p < 0.05)

[1] Correlations of level (means) and lability (standard deviations) of morning with afternoon pressures self measured for 21–30 days.

[2] Spearman Rank Correlations of level and lability of SBPs from ≥ 20 days at-home monitoring with those from 15–24 hour ambulatory recording.

firmed history of the disease in one or both parents tend to exhibit more lability in the month of at-home data and in the 24-hour ambulatory profiles.

To sum up, although our initial use of ambulatory monitoring has been as a validity check on self-measurement of blood pressure, it is apparent that ambulatory records from normotensive twins have value in and of themselves. We are evaluating profiles of ambulatory pressure as predictive of stress-reactivity to standardized laboratory stress. We expect that profile analyses of the records, using distance functions and curve-fitting techniques, will reveal genetic influences on the patterning of pressure over 24-hour periods. And finally, we expect that the level and lability of ambulatory blood pressure will be associated with familial history of risk for hypertensive disease.

Acknowledgements

The skilled assistance of Cheryl K. Tanner and Meloni Muir Ditto and the compliance and cooperation of participating families in the Indiana University Twin Panel is gratefully acknowledged. This research was supported by HL-20034 and HL-26761.

References

1. Rose RJ, Miller JZ, Grim CE, Christian JC: Aggregation of blood pressure in the families of identical twins. Amer J Epidemiol 109: 503–511 (1979).
2. Rose RJ, Fulker DW, Miller JZ, Grim, CE, Christian, JC: Heritability of systolic blood pressure: Analysis of variance in MZ twin parents and their children. Acta Genet Med Gemellol 29: 143–149 (1980).
3. Rose RJ, Miller JZ, Grim CE: Familial factors in blood pressure response to laboratory stress: A twin study. Psychophysiol 19: 583 (1982).
4. Grim CE, Miller JZ, Rose RJ: Inherited influence on blood pressure response to psychophysiological testing: Studies in twins and singletons. Circulation 66: II-105 (1982) (abst.).
5. Falkner B, Onesti G, Angelakos ET, Fernandes M, Langman C: Cardiovascular response to mental stress in normal adolescents with hypertensive parents. Hypertension 1: 23–30 (1979).

6. Pickering TG, Harshfield GA, Kleinert HD, Blank S, Laragh JH: Blood pressure activities, sleep, and exercise. JAMA 247: 992–996 (1982).
7. Rose RJ, Tanner CK, Christian JC: Familial influences on lability of blood pressure: Data from normotensive twins. Circulation 68: II-344 (1983) (abst.).

Address for correspondence:
Richard J. Rose, Ph.D.
Indiana University
Dept. of Psychology, Room 150
10th Street
Bloomington, Indiana 47 405

The role of ambulatory blood pressure monitoring in the evaluation of adolescent hypertension induced by exercise

Bruce N. Garrett, Jose R. Salcedo, Anne M. Thompson

Summary: We performed 24-hour ambulatory blood pressure monitoring in a group of adolescents with hypertension induced by dynamic exercise. Ten patients with a mean age of 15.1 years (12–18) developed systolic blood pressure greater than 240 mmHg after 15 minutes of graded exercise (initial load 400 KPM; increased every 3 minutes to 1000 KPM, then 1 minute at 1800 KPM) on a stationary bicycle. Ambulatory blood pressure monitoring was performed using a Del Mar Avionics PIII recorder with recordings taken every 7½ minutes for 24 hours. Data was expressed as the mean systolic and diastolic blood pressure for each hour of recording, for the total 24 hour recording period, for the period from 8 a.m. to 8 p.m. (daytime), and for the period from 8 p.m. to 8 a.m. (night-time). Variability was defined as one standard deviation of the mean systolic and diastolic blood pressure obtained in each recording period. There was little inter-individual variation in mean hourly blood pressure and the difference between mean hourly readings was not significant. Mean 24-hour ambulatory blood pressure was 130.2/80.7 mmHg. Mean 24-hour systolic variability was 18.3 mmHg and diastolic variability was 12.9 mmHg. There was no significant change in blood pressure between daytime and night-time recording periods. There was no significant difference in variability between day and night. The normal fall in blood pressure seen during the early morning hours in adults and normotensive adolescents and the lack of reduction in variability seen in the night-time in the same groups suggested abnormal circadian variation. In adolescents with systolic hypertension induced by dynamic exercise, ambulatory blood pressure monitoring may be used as a predictive marker of early adult essential hypertension.

Introduction

Exercise-induced hypertension in adolescents may be a predictive marker of early adult essential hypertension. The normal response to dynamic exercise is a marked rise in systolic blood pressure and heart rate with either no change or a slight fall in diastolic blood pressure. In contrast, isometric exercise produces only a moderate increase in heart rate and a rise in both systolic and diastolic blood pressure. The rise in systolic is less than that seen with dynamic exercise (1). The response to isometric and dynamic exercise has been studied in both normotensive and hypertensive adolescents. In 1978, Strong et al. studied 170 normotensive black children aged 7–14 years. Their systolic blood pressure rose from 104 mmHg at rest to 122 mmHg with isometric exercise and 157 mmHg with dynamic exercise (2). The following year, Fixler et al. compared normotensive to hypertensive adolescents age 14–17. The normotensives rose from a systolic of 108 mmHg at

Division of Renal Diseases, George Washington University Medical Center and
Children's Hospital National Medical Center, Washington, D.C.

rest to 126 mmHg with isometric exercise and 162 mmHg with dynamic exercise. Hypertensives rose from 134 mmHg at rest to 157 mmHg with isometric exercise and 187 mmHg with dynamic exercise (3). A systolic blood pressure greater than 220 mmHg during dynamic exercise was considered a hypertensive response. By contrast, in a comparison of normotensive to hypertensive young adults (18–34), the normotensive adults had a rise in systolic blood pressure from 120–173 mmHg, while the hypertensives rose from 173–234 mmHg (4, 5). Thus, an elevation in systolic blood pressure greater than 220 mmHg with dynamic exercise in an adolescent would be similar to that seen in a hypertensive young adult and suggests early adult essential hypertension.

We evaluated a group of adolescents with resting blood pressure in the 95th percentile, since this group is at the highest risk for developing adult essential hypertension. In addition to dynamic exercise, we attempted to further define this population by employing 24-hour ambulatory blood pressure monitoring. We wanted to see whether "active" but not "exercise" situations could evoke a similar response and whether the pattern of 24-hour blood pressure was "unique" in this population. "Uniqueness" was interpreted as an increase or decrease in variability, the presence or absence of circadian variation, the mean 24-hour blood pressure pattern and the change in blood pressure between hourly intervals. A study by Brenner et al. has compared normotensive adolescents from either hypertensive or normotensive parents. By utilizing ambulatory blood pressure monitoring, they showed that children of a hypertensive parent have a greater daytime systolic blood pressure than children of a normotensive parent. However, most of these groups have similar blood pressures during a sleep period (6). No other information on long term blood pressure recording in adolescents is available at present.

It was the purpose of this study to determine: (1) whether ambulatory blood pressure monitoring could define in greater detail a unique subpopulation of adolescents with exercise-induced hypertension; (2) whether ambulatory blood pressure monitoring could demonstrate any characteristics in this group that were different from those of age-matched normotensives; (3) whether ambulatory blood pressure monitoring had any prognostic significance in terms of future development of essential hypertension.

Patients and methods

Patients

Sixty patients with either systolic and/or diastolic blood pressure in the 95th percentile when adjusted for age, race and sex, were identified from clinic records. The patients performed a standard bicycle ergometer exercise as outlined below. Ten patients, all black males, met three out of four criteria required for referral to ambulatory monitoring. The mean age was 15.1 years (12–18). The mean (resting) blood pressure in this group was 138.4/87.4 mmHg. None of the participants were on anti-hypertensive medication and no patient was on dietary sodium restriction. All patients had normal renal function and no patient had a history of congenital heart disease, diabetes, asthma or secondary cause of hypertension. All patients gave voluntary informed consent to participate in this study and the study was approved by the institutional review boards of both medical centers.

Methods

After an initial resting period, all patients were placed on a standard bicycle ergometer with an initial work load of 400 KPM. Exercise was begun at this work load and continued for three minutes, then the work load was increased by 200 KPM every three minutes up to 1000 KPM. The work load was then increased to 1800 KPM for one additional minute. Blood pressure and pulse were taken at rest and at one minute intervals during each work load. Blood pressure and pulse were then taken after three minutes of maximum work load. Blood pressure was obtained using a standard mercury sphygmomanometer and a standard size cuff. The 5th Korotkoff sound served as the diastolic blood pressure. In order to qualify for ambulatory monitoring, patients had to meet three of the four criteria listed below: (1) a rapid increase in systolic blood pressure at the first work load; (2) systolic blood pressure greater than 240 mmHg at any time; (3) diastolic blood pressure that increased greater than 10 mmHg during the course of exercise; (4) a lack of blood pressure recovery after three minutes of rest.

Twenty-four hour ambulatory blood pressure monitoring was performed with the Del Mar Avionics PIII recorder with recordings taken every 7½ minutes. The reliability of this device has been previously described (7). All recordings were begun at 9 a.m. and all were done on school days. Data was assessed as the mean systolic and diastolic blood pressure for each hour, for the total 24 hours, for the period from 8 a.m. to 8 p.m. (M) and for the period from 8 p.m. to 8 a.m. (E). Variability was defined as one standard deviation of the mean systolic and diastolic blood pressure obtained in each recording period. Statistical analysis was performed by Student's t-test and one way analysis of variance taking into account repeated measures.

Results

Dynamic exercise

Mean resting blood pressure was 147/89 mmHg. Systolic blood pressure then rose significantly to 175 mmHg at 400 KPM, 189 mmHg at 600 KPM, 215 mmHg at 800 KPM and 248 mmHg at 1000 KPM (P < 0.0001 when compared to baseline for all work-loads). Systolic blood pressure rose to 260 mmHg after one minute of exercise at 1800 KPM (P < 0.0001 vs baseline). After three minutes of rest, blood pressure fell back to 172/78 mmHg (P < 0.005 vs baseline). Diastolic blood pressure did not change significantly from baseline in any time period. The pulse was 79 beats/min at rest. This rose significantly to 99 beats/min at 400 KPM, 125 beats/min at 600 KPM, 147 beats/min at 800 KPM, and 162 beats/min at 1000 KPM. Pulse continued to rise to 183 beats/min at 1800 KPM (P < 0.0001 for all work-loads vs baseline). Pulse fell to 105 beats/min after 3 min of exercise (P < 0.005 vs baseline) (Fig. 1).

Blood pressure

Mean 24-hour ambulatory blood pressure was 130.2/82.7 mmHg. Mean blood pressure from 8 a.m. to 8 p.m. was 132.3/84.2 mmHg. Mean blood pressure from 8 p.m. to 8 a.m.

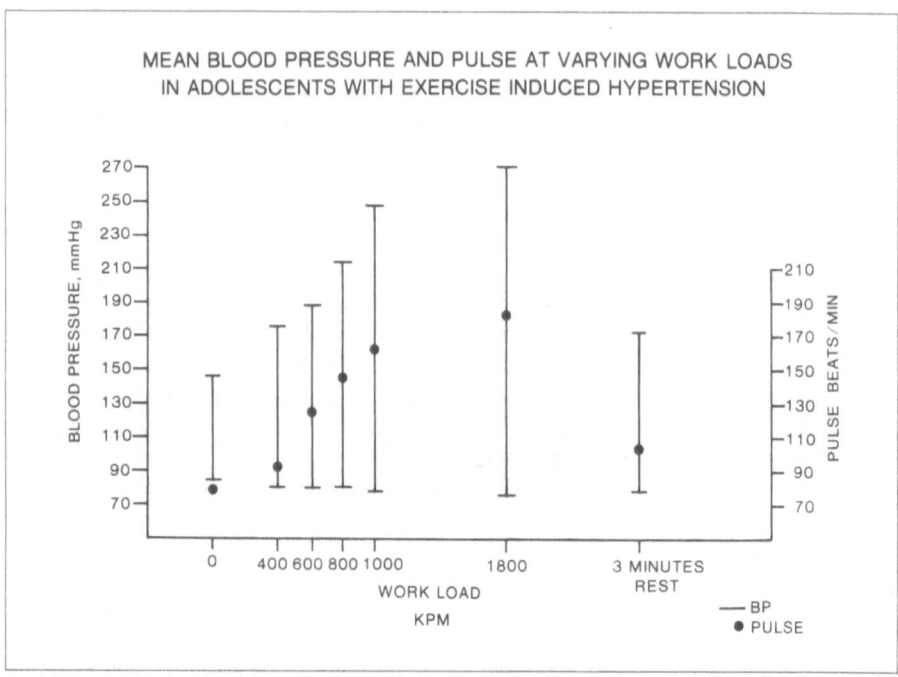

Fig. 1. Mean blood pressure and pulse at rest and at increasing work loads in patients exercised on a standard bicycle ergometer. Work load measured in kilo-pond meters (KPM). For all work-loads versus baseline p < 0.0001 systolic; p = ns diastolic; p < 0.0001 pulse. Three minutes after maximal exercise p < 0.005 systolic; p = ns diastolic; p < 0.005 pulse when compared to baseline.

was 126.5/81.2 mmHg. There was no significant difference in either systolic or diastolic blood pressure when comparing morning to evening time periods. Mean hourly blood pressure did not demonstrate significantly elevated readings at any particular time period. There was no significant difference in mean hourly blood pressure between any two hourly intervals, and there was minimal inter-individual variation in blood pressure. The normal circadian pattern of blood pressure was not seen and the blood pressure patterns remained "linear" throughout the 24-hour recording period (Fig. 2).

Variability

Mean 24-hour variability was 18.3 mmHg systolic and 12.9 mmHg diastolic. Mean variability from 8 a.m. to 8 p.m. (M) was 16.7 mmHg systolic and 11.1 mmHg diastolic. Mean variability from 8 p.m. to 8 a.m. (E) was 14.3 mmHg systolic and 11.5 mmHg diastolic. There was no significant difference in either systolic or diastolic variability when comparing morning to evening time periods. There was no reduction in variability in the evening (sleep) recording period.

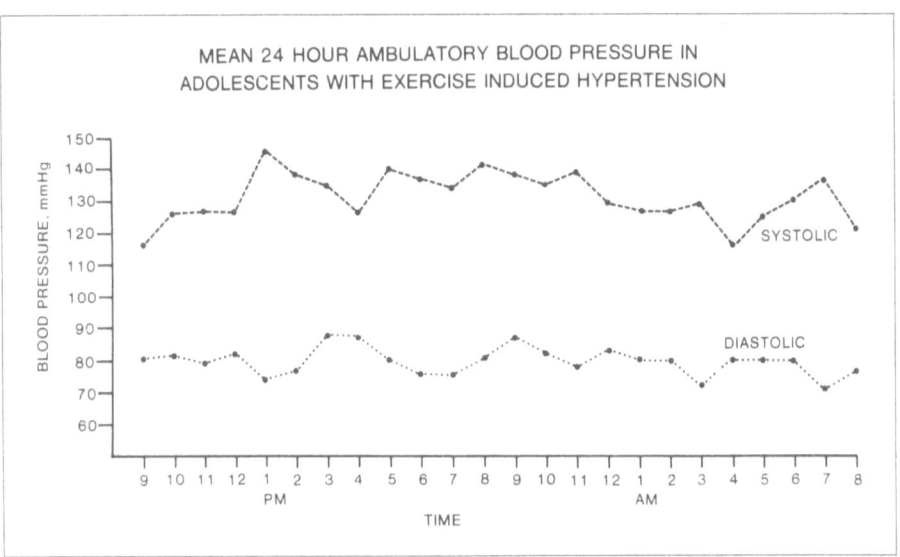

Fig. 2. Mean hourly systolic and diastolic blood pressure when measured over 24-hours with a Del-Mar Avionics P III recorder. All recordings began at 9 a.m. and were recorded on a school day. There is no significant elevation in blood pressure at any specific time and there is no significant difference between any pair of hourly blood pressure measurements.

Discussion

Patients with a resting blood pressure in the 95th percentile are at the greatest risk for developing essential hypertension. Exercise studies in black children have already delineated maximal work-loads and blood pressure for various age groups (8, 9). Dynamic exercise has shown that an adolescent patient with an exercise systolic blood pressure greater than 220 mmHg is similar in magnitude to a young adult with essential hypertension. This suggests that adolescent exercise-induced hypertension is itself a marker of early adult essential hypertension. The rôle of ambulatory blood pressure monitoring in the hypertensive evaluation has been well described (10, 11, 12). Its use as a tool for diagnostic, prognostic and therapeutic applications is apparent (13). Thus it would seem that the combination of dynamic exercise and ambulatory blood pressure monitoring would be additive in its ability to isolate and critically define an "at risk" population.

Exercise-induced hypertension is a distinct physiologic phenomenon. Of sixty patients screened in this study, ten patients developed systolic blood pressure greater than 240 mmHg when subjected to dynamic exercise by bicycle ergometer. Twenty-four hour ambulatory blood pressure monitoring was then performed in an effort to determine whether elevated blood pressures could be obtained in "active" but not "exercise" situations. In addition, monitoring was performed to see if the blood pressure pattern or variation were different from normotensive adolescents and hypertensive and normotensive adults. This study clearly demonstrates that patients with exercise-induced hypertension clearly have an abnormal and unique 24-hour blood pressure monitoring. There was no significant

177

difference in mean blood pressure between morning and evening values. There was no reduction in mean blood pressure during evening hours and no reduction in pulse pressure during evening hours. There was no significant change in variability between morning and evening values. The blood pressure pattern was "linear" and failed to show circadian variation. The variability was not reduced during sleep, as is commonly seen in adults. The abnormal circadian variation may be due to an increased catecholamine secretion during sleep, though this is only theoretical at present.

Normotensive adolescents have a blood pressure pattern which mimics normal circadian variation (14). Normotensive and hypertensive adults have similar blood pressure patterns though of different magnitude (15). Ambulatory blood pressure monitoring demonstrated a failure to reduce variability during sleep plus the absence of circadian variation, thus defining this subpopulation as being unique and different from either normotensive adolescents or hypertensive or normotensive adults. The combination of dynamic exercise plus ambulatory blood pressure monitoring delineates those patients who have distinct physiologic properities. This combination may have prognostic significance as a predictive marker of early adult essential hypertension.

Conclusion

In sixty adolescents with baseline blood pressure in the 95th percentile, bicycle ergometer produced a systolic blood pressure greater than 240 mmHg in ten patients. During bicycle ergometer, these ten patients showed no significant change in diastolic blood pressure from baseline values. Pulse rose in linear fashion with increased work load. There was no significant change in ambulatory systolic or diastolic blood pressure between morning and evening recording periods. There was no significant change in systolic or diastolic variability between morning and evening recording periods. Ambulatory blood pressure monitoring confirmed a lack of circadian variation and a failure to reduce variability during sleep in this population. In patients with exercise-induced hypertension, ambulatory blood pressure monitoring may have prognostic significance as a predictive marker of early adult essential hypertension.

References

1. Nutter DO, Schlant RC, Hurst JW: Isometric exercise and the cardiovascular system. Mod Conc Cardiovasc Dis 41: 11–15 (1972).
2. Strong WB, Miller MD, Striplin M, Salehbhai M: Blood pressure response to isometric and dynamic exercise in healthy black children. Am J Dis Child 132: 587–591 (1978).
3. Fixler DE, Laird WP, Browne R, Fitzgerald V, Wilson S, Vance R: Response of hypertensive adolescents to dynamic and isometric exercise stress. Ped 64: 579–583 (1978).
4. Amery A, Julius S, Whitlock LS, Conway J: Influence of hypertension on the hemodynamic response to exercise. Circulation 36: 231–237 (1967).
5. Julius S, Amery A, Whitlock LS, Conway J: Influence of age on the hemodynamic response to exercise. Circulation 36: 222–230 (1967).
6. Brenner JI, Dischinger PC, Ferencz C, Wilson PD, Berman MA: Twenty four hour blood pressure monitoring in adolescents. Circulation 68: III–396 (1983).
7. Harshfield GA, Pickering TG, Laragh JH: A validation study of the Del-Mar Avionics ambulatory blood pressure system. Ambulat Electrocardiol 4: 7–12 (1979).

8. Nudel DB, Gootman N, Brunson S, Shenker RI, Gauthier BG, Stenzler A: Exercise performance of adolescents with essential hypertension. Pediatr Res 12: 366 (1978).
9. Strong WB, Spencer D, Miller MD: Physical working capacity of healthy black children. Am J Dis Child 132: 244–248 (1978).
10. Watson RD, Stallard TJ, Finn RM, Littler WA: Factors determining direct arterial pressure and its variability in hypertensive man. Hypertension 2: 333–341 (1980).
11. Horan MJ, Padgett NE, Kennedy HL: Ambulatory blood pressure monitoring: recent advances and clinical applications. Am Heart J 101: 843–848 (1981).
12. Pickering TG, Harshfield GA, Kleinert HD, Laragh JH: Ambulatory monitoring in the evaluation of blood pressure in patients with borderline hypertension and the role of the defense reflex. Clin Exp Hypertens 4: 675–693 (1982).
13. Mallion JM, de Gaudemaris R, Debru JL, Doyon B, Perdrix A, Morin B, Cau G: Mesure de la pression arterielle par methode automatique. Arch Mal Coeur 73: 95–101 (1979).
14. Brenner JI, Dischinger PC, Ferencz C, Wilson PD, Berman MA: Twenty four hour blood pressure monitoring in adolescents. Ped Card 3: 346 (1982).
15. Pickering TG, Harshfield GA, Kleinert HD, Blank S, Laragh JH: Blood pressure during normal daily activities, sleep and exercise. Comparison of values in normal and hypertensive subjects. JAMA 247: 992–996 (1982).

Address for correspondence:
Bruce N. Garrett, M.D.
George Washington University Medical Center
2150 Pennsylvania Ave., N.W.
Washington, D.C. 20037

Essential hypertension in the elderly: circadian variation of arterial pressure

Isaac Kobrin, Francis G. Dunn, Wille Oigman, Ajay Kumar,
Hector O. Ventura, Franz H. Messerli, Edward D. Frohlich

Summary: Continuous 24-hour arterial pressure (BP) recordings (Del Mar Avionics Pressurometer II) in elderly essential hypertensive patients revealed that while all patients had daytime ambulatory systolic pressure significantly lower than in the office, two different patterns emerged during the night. In 14 patients both systolic and diastolic pressures continued to fall to significantly lower levels than daytime ambulatory BP. However, in seven other patients, systolic pressures increased to similar levels as the office BP recording, although diastolic pressures remained unchanged. The prevalence of clinical cardiovascular complications was 43% in those with a nocturnal drop in pressure and 100% in those patients with a nocturnal increase in pressure (x^2, 6.46; $p < 0.025$). We conclude that, in elderly patients, outpatient office BP recording may give a misleading impression of the individual's integrated arterial pressure. The presence or absence of a nocturnal fall in pressure may be helpful in predicting a patient's risk of developing future cardiovascular complications.

Arterial hypertension in the elderly is associated with increased cardiovascular morbidity and mortality (1–4) but there are no hard data on the benefits of treatment in this population (5). Furthermore, drug treatment of elderly patients in general may be difficult, exposing these patients to the unwanted effects of drugs (2, 5–8). However, it is believed that the evidence indicting hypertension as a major risk factor for cardiovascular problems in this age group does provide a theoretical basis at least for lowering pressure in some patients (2, 5, 7, 8).

We have been struck by the finding that in many elderly patients office blood pressure (BP) measurements are substantially higher than in other settings. Similar observations were also reported by Mancia et al. in younger patients with essential hypertension (9). Thus, the present study was undertaken to determine whether significant differences exist between office and other pressure measurements and whether different patterns of 24-hour BP measurements in elderly patients with essential hypertension might be related to a different cardiovascular risk.

Patients and methods

Twenty-one elderly patients, all over 65 years of age (mean: 70 ± 1; range: 65–87 years) were included in this study. All had established hypertension with office systolic or dias-

Department of Internal Medicine, Section on Hypertensive Diseases, Ochsner Clinic and the Research Division, Alton Ochsner Medical Foundation, New Orleans, LA.

tolic pressures persistently above 160 and 90 mmHg, respectively. The group was comprised of 14 men and 7 women who either had never received antihypertensive therapy or had discontinued medications at least four weeks previously. Clinical evaluation and definition of established essential hypertension followed established guidelines (10). Target organ involvement was assessed by electrocardiogram (ECG), chest x-ray, biochemical indices of renal function, and funduscopic examination. Thus, it was possible to assess the presence of clinical evidence of cardiovascular diseases (CVD) as follows: (a) cardiac involvement: congestive heart failure, angina pectoris, myocardial infarction, and ECG evidence of left ventricular hypertrophy; (b) cerebrovascular disease: history of transient ischemic attacks and cerebrovascular accident; (c) peripheral arterial disease: femoral arterial bruit, disappearance of pulses below the femoral arteries, history of aortofemoral bypass or intermittent claudication, carotid arterial bruit or a history of carotid arterial surgery; (d) renovascular disease: arteriographic evidence of occlusive atherosclerotic renal arterial disease.

Ambulatory BP measurements were recorded every 7.5 minutes as previously reported (11). Repetitive analyses of the 24-hour BP monitoring were made for each group of patients, and x^2 value was obtained for the incidence of CVD.

Results

During the daytime, ambulatory systolic but not diastolic pressures were significantly lower than in the office in all patients ($p < 0.01$) (Table 1). In 14 patients (Group 1), both the systolic and diastolic arterial pressures continued to fall in the evening and night reaching levels lower than office and daytime ambulatory pressures. In contrast, in seven other patients (Group 2), the systolic pressure increased to levels significantly higher than the daytime ambulatory measurements ($p < 0.05$), indeed even reaching office BP measurements in some patients.

Further analysis between these two groups revealed significant differences with regard to clinical evidence for cardiovascular disease ($x^2 = 6.4615$; $p < 0.025$). In only six men of Group 1 (43%), but in every patient in Group 2, there was clinical evidence of cardiovas-

Table 1. Clinical evidence of CVD in patients with nocturnal fall (Group 1) and patients without nocturnal fall in BP (Group 2).

	Cerebro-vascular disease	Left ventricular hypertrophy	Femoral artery disease	Carotid artery disease	Renovascular disease	Clinical evidence of CVD (total no.)
Group 1 (n = 14)	1	3	2	3	0	6 (43%)*
Group 2 (n = 7)	2	4	3	1	1	7 (100%)

* A two by two contingency table was made giving a Chi square value of 6.4615 with a $p < 0.025$.
CVD = Cardiovascular diseases.

cular disease (Table 2). There were no differences between groups with respect to other risk factors such as: age, smoking history, fasting blood sugar and lipids, uric acid, creatinine, and body weight.

Table 2. Diurnal variation of heart rate (HR), systolic (SAP) and diastolic (DAP) arterial pressures in elderly patients with (Group 1) and without (Group 2) nocturnal fall in blood pressure.

	Office	9.00 a.m. 1.00 p.m.	1.00 p.m. 5.00 p.m.	5.00 p.m. 9.00 p.m.	9.00 p.m. 1.00 a.m.	1.00 a.m. 6.00 a.m.	6.00 a.m. 9.00 a.m.
Group 1 (n = 14)							
SAP (mmHg)	177	157	150	142	131	126	141
	± 3	$\pm 4^{1)}$	$\pm 5^{2)}$	$\pm 4^{2)}$	$\pm 4^{2)4)}$	$\pm 4^{2)4)}$	$\pm 7^{2)}$
DAP(mmHg)	97	93	91	85	77	74	83
	± 2	± 2	± 3	± 3	$\pm 3^{2)4)}$	$\pm 3^{2)4)}$	$\pm 4^{1)}$
HR (beats/min)	76	80	78	78	78	70	76
	± 3	± 3	± 2	± 3	± 3	± 2	± 4
Group 2 (n = 7)							
SAP (mmHg)	175	147	154	168	163	170	167
	± 6	$\pm 4^{2)}$	$\pm 3^{1)}$	$\pm 7^{3)}$	$\pm 8^{3)}$	$\pm 8^{3)}$	± 11
DAP(mmHg)	92	88	88	93	89	89	92
	± 4	± 4	± 4	± 6	± 3	± 4	± 6
HR (beats/min)	86	84	80	79	72	72	79
	± 4	± 4	± 5	± 4	± 3	± 4	± 5

Each number represents the mean ± 1 SE.

[1]) $p < 0.05$; [2]) $p < 0.01$ compared with office measurements; [3]) $p < 0.05$; [4]) $p < 0.01$ compared with daytime measurements (9.00 a.m.–6.00 p.m.).

Discussion

The present study shows that diurnal variations of arterial pressure had two distinct patterns in elderly patients with essential hypertension. While all patients had daytime systolic ambulatory pressures lower than their daytime office measurements, two different patterns emerged during the night. In one group of patients both the systolic and diastolic pressures continued to fall, whereas in the other group the systolic pressure increased to the same levels as in the office.

Since the development of methods for recording BP accurately during normal daily activities (11–13), studies have shown that BP measurements recorded in the outpatient clinic setting tend to be higher than at home. This has been attributed to the "anxiety" associated with a visit to a physician's office (9, 14). Acknowledgment of these facts is of particular importance in the elderly patient when antihypertensive therapy associated with its own particular hazards may be unduly excessive (2, 5–8). All patients in the present study had significantly lower ambulatory systolic daytime pressures as compared with their office measurements. Although systolic hypertension is common in this age group and systolic pressure increases with age (5, 15), many patients may very well have lower or even normal pressures during routine daily activities. Moreover, the reduced distensibility of the larger vessels due to atherosclerosis may contribute to disproportionately higher office systolic pressures (16, 17). Thus, office pressure measurements may be misleading in elderly patients with systolic hypertension for whom the decision whether or not to start treatment is difficult.

Although these findings are preliminary due to the small number of patients in this study, the observation of a significant difference in the prevalence of clinical CVD is most important. Moreover, this finding strengthens the assumption that patients with higher night pressures (Group 2) may suffer from more advanced vascular disease. Therefore, treatment might prove more beneficial in these patients than in the patient with lower nighttime pressures. Moreover, antihypertensive treatment in the patients with the night fall in BP could lower arterial pressure to hypotensive levels which might compromise blood flow to vital organs (15). However, larger groups of patients would be necessary to prove that 24-hour pressure monitoring in elderly patients with essential hypertension may help to predict the likelihood of clinical CVD.

References

1. Forette F, Henry JF, Hervy MP, Fagard R, Lijnen P, Staessen J, Amery A: Hypertension in the eldery. In: Amery A, Fagard R, Lijnen P, Staessen J, (eds). Hypertensive cardiovascular disease: pathophysiology and treatment. Pp. 347–364, Martinus Nijhoff Publishers (The Hague/Boston/London 1982).
2. Kirkendall WM, Hammond JJ: Hypertension in the elderly. Arch Intern Med 40: 1155–1161 (1980)
3. Dyer AR, Stamler J, Shekelle RB, Schoenberger JA, Farinaro E: Hypertension in the elderly. Med Clin North Am 61: 513–529 (1977).
4. Astfeld AM, Shekelle RB, Klawans H, Tuf HM: Epidemiology of stroke in an elderly welfare population. Am J Pub Health 64: 450–458 (1974).
5. Koch-Weser, O'Malley K, O'Brien E: Drug Therapy: Management of hypertension in the elderly. N Engl J Med 302: 1397–1401 (1980).
6. Jackson G, Pierscianoski TA, Mahon W, Condon J: Inappropriate antihypertensive therapy in the elderly. Lancet 2: 1317–1318 (1976).
7. Gifford RW Jr: Isolated systolic hypertension in the elderly. Some controversial issues. JAMA 247: 781–785 (1982).
8. Finnerty FA Jr: Hypertension in the elderly. Special consideration in treatment. Postgrad Med 65: 119–125 (1979).
9. Mancia G, Bertinieri G, Grassi G, Pomidossi G, Parati G, Gregorini L, Ferrari A, Zanchetti A: Hemodynamic alterations triggered by blood pressure assessment by the doctor. Clin Sci 63: 387s–389s (1982).
10. Messerli FH, deCarvalho JGR, Christie B, Frohlich ED: Systemic and regional hemodynamics in low, normal, and high cardiac output borderline hypertension. Circulation 58: 441–448 (1978).
11. Messerli FH, Glade LB, Ventura HO, Dreslinski GR. Suarez DH, MacPhee AA, Aristimuno GG, Cole FE, Frohlich ED: Diurnal variations of cardiac rhythm, arterial pressure, and urinary catecholamines in borderline and established essential hypertension. Am Heart J 104: 109–114 (1982).
12. Pickering TG, Harshfeld GA, Kleinert HD, Blank S, Laragh JH: Blood pressure during normal daily activities, sleep, and exercise. JAMA 247: 992–996 (1982).
13. McCall WC, McCall VR: Diagnostic use of ambulatory blood pressure monitoring in medical practice. J Fam Pract 13: 25–30 (1981).
14. Harshfield GA, Pickering TG, Kleinert HD, Blank S, Laragh JH: Situational variations of blood pressure in hypertensive patients. Psychosom Med 44: 237–245 (1982).

15. Koch-Weser J: The therapeutic challenge of systolic hypertension. N Engl J Med 289: 481–483 (1973).
16. Koch-Weser J. Correlation of pathophysiology and pharmacotherapy in primary hypertension. Am J Cardiol 32: 499–510 (1973).
17. Colandrea MA, Friedman GD, Nichaman MZ, Lynd CN: Systolic hypertension in the elderly. An epidemiologic assessment. Circulation 41: 239–245 (1970).

Address for correspondence:
Dr. Frohlich, Vice President
Education and Research
Alton Ochsner Medical Foundation
1516 Jefferson Highway
New Orleans, LA 70121.

Non-invasive assessment of cardiac anatomy and blood pressure in patients with borderline hypertension

R. Dimitriou, R. De Gaudemaris, J. L. Debru, A. Camaleonte, F. Dubois, A. Perdrix, J. M. Mallion*

Summary: Extensive non-invasive evaluation of cardiac function and blood pressure was performed in 26 subjects with borderline hypertension. The degree of cardiac hypertrophy was assessed in these subjects using echocardiographic techniques. Blood pressure and its variability were measured using a 24-hour ambulatory monitoring technique and blood pressure measurements obtained during exercise testing.

An abnormal blood pressure pattern was found during exercise testing in 57% of patients and during ambulatory monitoring of blood pressure in 38%. The echocardiogram revealed an abnormal interventricular septal thickness in 23% of patients and an abnormal posterior wall thickness in 12 percent of patients with borderline hypertension.

Patients with an abnormal blood pressure pattern during ambulatory monitoring or exercise testing had a greater ventricular wall thickness than those with a normal blood pressure (p < 0.001).

The correlation between the average 24-hour systolic blood pressure and septal thickness, posterior wall thickness and left ventricular mass were highly significant. Discriminatory analysis of the data show that an abnormal ambulatory blood pressure pattern is more predictive of cardiac hypertrophy than blood pressure patterns found during exercise testing. Thus, extensive non-invasive evaluation of patients with borderline hypertension allows better assessment of the relationship between blood pressure and abnormalities in cardiac muscle mass.

Introduction

Borderline hypertension poses diagnostic as well as therapeutic problems. The diagnostic approach is now based on repeated measurements at rest, and other more specialized examinations such as the exercise test blood pressure profile (ETP) and the ambulatory blood pressure load (BPL).

Therapy is justified as a means to avoid early lesions of target organs. The echocardiogram permits the precise detection of morphological anomalies of the myocardium which are related to hemodynamic impairment. It would be interesting to look for a correlation between cardiac reactivity, quantified by ETP and BPL, and cardiac strain measured by echocardiography.

* Centre de consultations et d'explorations d'hypertension artérielle Médecine Interne et Cardiologie C.H.U. Grenoble, France.

Population studied

The group studied was composed of 26 patients (19 males and 7 females) with borderline essential hypertension according to the W.H.O. criteria (resting systolic blood pressure (SBP): 140–160 mmHg; resting diastolic blood pressure (DBP): 90–95 mmHg, both measurements occurring at several readings). The average age was 29 ± 8 years for males and 34 ± 10 years for females.

None of the patients had been treated previously and none had congenital or acquired cardiac disease. All subjects had a sinus rhythm (EKG) without conduction anomalies. None of the patients participated in competitive sports.

Methods

The 26 patients underwent successively an echocardiogram, a stress test and a 24-hour ambulatory blood pressure recording. The maximum interval between each test was 10 days.

Echocardiographic study

This was performed using a wide-angle Sectorscan apparatus* with systematic recording of the parasternal incidence (long and short axis for cardiac cavities incidence).

The dimensions of the left ventricle were determined on the TM curve and recorded at the extremity of the mitral valve which was located with bi-dimensional echography in order to avoid errors due to angulation of the ultrasonic beam. All recordings and interpretations of the curves were carried out by the same observer.

The following parameters were studied: diastolic and systolic interventricular septum thickness (IVS); diastolic and systolic posterior wall thickness (PWT); internal diastolic (IDD) and internal systolic (ISD) left ventricle dimensions. The left ventricular mass (LVM) was calculated according to the Reicheck-Devereux method (1).

Stress test (EST)

This was performed on an ergometric bicycle using a previously reported method (2). The blood pressure curve was interpreted with respect to a normal curve established as a function of age and sex.

Ambulatory blood pressure load (BPL)

The BPL was recorded with a full automatic and ambulatory device**. Patients followed their normal working activities. Data are expressed:

---

* Robert et Carriere RC 2000.
** Del Mar Avionics Pressurometer.

– in reference to normal curves established during previous studies (3) and
– as average values of SBP/DBP during the active period (8 a.m. to 8 p.m.) and over a
  24-hour period.
The BPL is considered high in all patients who present more than 50% of their values at
levels higher than the 90th percentile of normal subjects.

Statistical analysis

Tests of means are done by variance analysis, and correlation coefficients are found.

Global results

1) Study during exercise
Fifteen patients (57%) had a pathologic exercise test BP profile for the SBP and/or the
DBP.

2) Study during ambulatory activity
Ten patients (39%) had a high BPL.

3) Echocardiographic study
The IVS was greater than 11 mm in 6 patients (23%). The PWT was greater than 11 mm
in 3 patients (11.5%). The relationship between the two (IVS/PWT) was greater than 1.3
in 2 patients and the IDD and the ISD of the left ventricle were normal in all cases.

Comparative results

1) Relationship between ETP/BPL and IVS/PWT

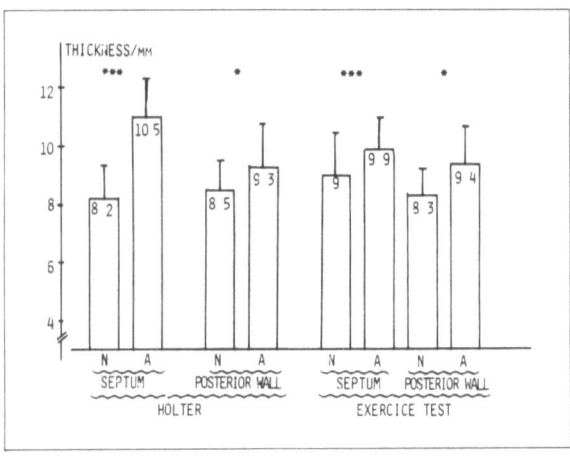

Fig. 1. Average values of the septal and posterior wall thickness of the L.V. for the exercise test (E.T.) and the measurement of the ambulatory BP (holter) * P < 0.05, ** P < 0.01, *** P < 0.001.

The subjects whose ETP and/or BPL was pathologic had average values of IVS and PWT significantly higher (P < 0.001) than the normal subjects (Fig. 1).

2) Correlation coefficient between the average values of the ambulatory BP (during activity and 24 hours) and the different echocardiographic parameters (Table 1)

Table 1: Correlations between the average values of SBP and DBP (during activity or 24 hours) and echocardiographic measurements (septal and posterior wall thickness, left ventricular mass).

	Septum	Posterior wall	left ventricular mass
SBP – 24 h	r = 0.63***	r = 0.52***	r = 0.44*
SBP – activity	r = 0.61***	r = 0.53***	r = 0.34^{ns}
DBP – 24 h	r = 0.37*	r = 0.26^{ns}	
DBP – activity	r = 0.30^{ns}	r = 0.20^{ns}	

Blood pressure load and echocardiographic linear correlations.
  * P < 0.05
 ** P < 0.01
*** P < 0.001.

Interventricular septum: a significant correlation was found for values of SBP during activity (r = 0.61, P < 0.001) and over 24 hours (r = 0.63, P < 0.001).
A correlation was found with the DBP over a 24-hour period (r = 0.37, P < 0.05) but was not found for DBP during activity (r = 0.30, P = NS).
Posterior wall: there was a good correlation for the SBP during activity (r = 0.53, P < 0.001) and over 24 hours (r = 0.52, P < 0.001). A correlation was observed with the DBP over 24 hours (r = 0.68, P < 0.005) but not found with DBP during activity.
Left ventricular mass: a correlation was seen with SBP over 24 hours (r = 0.44, P < 0.05) but no significant correlation was found for SBP during activity or for DBP.

3) Other parameters
There were no differences observed between the groups and no significant correlation seen for IDD, ISD and left ventricular septal and parietal systolic thicknesses. The double product (HR × BP) was not correlated with any of these measurements.

Discussion

The results of this study confirm the presence of the effect of borderline hypertension (left ventricular hypertrophy, appraised by echocardiography) in a certain number of patients (4).
Some authors, including ourselves, have suggested than the development of myocardial hypertrophy is better related to ambulatory BP measurements of patients subjected to their day-to-day physical and psychosensorial pressures than to BP measurement at rest (5, 6).

Previous studies all concerning true hypertension have confirmed a much better correlation between ambulatory BP values and left ventricular hypertrophy than with resting values (7). Until now, no study had been done with borderline hypertensive patients.

BP variation is dependent on various factors. While the ETP allows a more specific approach to the variations due to physical effort and cardiovascular reactivity, the ambulatory BPL is related to physical and psychosensorial pressures.

The echocardiogram enables the detection of ventricular myocardial alterations which negatively affect cardiac performance and coronary circulation (8).

It is for these reasons that we looked for a correlation between echocardiographic alteration of the left ventricle and the data of these other two examinations.

More particularly, measurement of the BPL has suggested that imposed daily constraints must be taken into account.

These morphological changes in the myocardium seem to be related to both mechanical and neurohormonal factors (8, 9) which occur simultaneously.

The demonstration of correlations between ETP, BPL and echocardiographic data justifies the practice of these investigations in the borderline hypertensive patient as a prognostic and therapeutic guide.

Few subjects having discordances between ETP, BPL and echocardiographic measurements let us suggest that these 3 tests should be performed on each patient. When all 3 tests are in agreement, treatment would seem logical. If only one of the examinations is pathologic, the dicision becomes more difficult, and in this case an annual checkup would be appropriate.

Conclusions

Our data confirm the necessity of rigorous management of borderline hypertensive patients in order to detect early stages of ventricular hypertrophy.

The cardiac modifications are closely related to daily occupational constraints; measurements at rest is important for epidemiologic studies but is of much less value at the individual level.

These findings justify the use and repetition of these different types of investigations in the diagnosis, therapy and prognosis of borderline hypertension.

References

1. Devereux RB and Reichek N: Echocardiographic determination of left ventricular mass in man: anatomic validation of the method. Circulation 55: 613–618 (1977).
2. Mallion JM, Bonhoure JP, Broustet JP, Cahen JP, Lesbre JP, Letac B, Serradimigni A, Wagniart P: Guide pour les épreuves d'effort par le groupe de travail "Epreuve d'Effort et réadaptation" de la Société Française de Cardiologie. Arch Mal Coeur 72, N° spécial: 1–30 (1979).
3. Mallion JM, De Gaudemaris R, Debru JL, Villemain P, Daver H, Perdrix A, Cau G: Mesure de la pression artérielle en ambulatoire. Ann Cardiol Angéiol 31: 503–509 (1982).
4. Culpepper WS, Sodt PC, Messerli FH, Ruschhaupt DG, Arcilla PA: Cardiac status in juvenile borderline hypertension. Ann Int Med 98: 1–7 (1983).
5. Mallion JM, Debru JL, De Gaudemaris R, Perdrix A, Cau G: Mesure tensionelle de repos, charge tensionnelle d'activité. Nouv Presse Méd 10: 2877–2879 (1981).

6. Rowlands DB, Glover DR, Ireland MA, McLeay RAB, Stallard TJ, Watson RDS, Littler WA: Assessment of left ventricular mass and its response to antihypertensive treatment. Lancet (I): 467–470 (1982).
7. Devereux RB, Pickering TG, Harshfield GA, Kleinert HD, Denby L, Clark L, Pregibon D, Jason M, Kleiner B, Borer J, Laragh JH: Left ventricular hypertrophy in patients with hypertension: importance of blood pressure response to regularly recurring stress. Circulation, 1983, 68, 470–476.
8. Tarazi RC, Levy MN: Cardiac responses to increased after-load. Hypertension 4 (Suppl. II): 11–18 (1982).
9. Safar ME, Lehener JM, Vincent MI, Plainfosse MI, Simon AC: Echocardiographic dimensions in borderline and substained hypertension. Am J Cardiol 44: 930–935 (1979).

Address for correspondence:
Dr. R. de Gaudemaris
Service Medecine Interne et Cardiologie
Centre Hospitalier Regional
Et Universitaire De Grenoble
BP 217 X
38043 Grenoble Cedex, France

Ambulatory monitoring of blood pressure: the importance of blood pressure during work

Thomas G. Pickering, Gregory A. Harshfield, Richard B. Devereux

Summary: Studies of 24-hour blood pressure (BP) patterns in patients with mild untreated hypertension have shown that BP is highest while at work, intermediate while at home, and lowest during sleep. Since the majority of these patients had sedentary jobs, the higher pressures during work are attributed to psychosocial factors rather than to physical activity.
Three lines of evidence support the view that work blood pressure could have a disproportionate effect on target organ damage. Firstly, left ventricular hypertrophy correlates closely with 24-hour ambulatory BP on a working but not on a non-working day; secondly, patients showing higher work BP are more likely to have left ventricular dysfunction; and thirdly, patients with higher work systolic BP are more likely to have ventricular premature contractions.

One of the most consistent findings with ambulatory blood pressure (BP) monitoring has been the enormous variations of BP which occur over 24 hours. In the majority of people, BP is highest during the day, lower during the evening, and lowest of all during the night. Although it has been suggested that there is an intrinsic circadian rhythm of blood pressure which accounts for these changes, it is our belief that the normal pattern of BP variation is determined largely by environmental factors. The highest pressures during the day normally coincide with the hours of work, and fall during the evening hours of relaxation and watching television, with the lowest levels always occurring during sleep (Figure 1). The importance of environmental influences is shown in Figure 2, which represents the BP changes occurring in a night shift worker: in this case the lowest pressures occurred when the subject went to sleep in the afternoon, and remained high during the night when he was at work.

In a study of untreated hypertensive patients (1) we found that the average pressure was 147/101 mmHg during work, 138/95 at home, and 121/85 during sleep. The pressures recorded in the clinic were generally similar to those at work, but not very closely correlated with them. We do not believe that the higher work pressures are due to differences in physical activity, since most of our subjects had sedentary jobs, and we are generally unable to make ambulatory BP measurements during physical activity of any intensity. It seems most probable that these differences are due to the psychosocial aspects of the work environment. For people who did not go to work on the day of their BP recording we have established a hierarchy of blood pressures associated with different activities.

Cardiovascular Center, Cornell University Medical Center, New York Hospital, New York, NY 10021

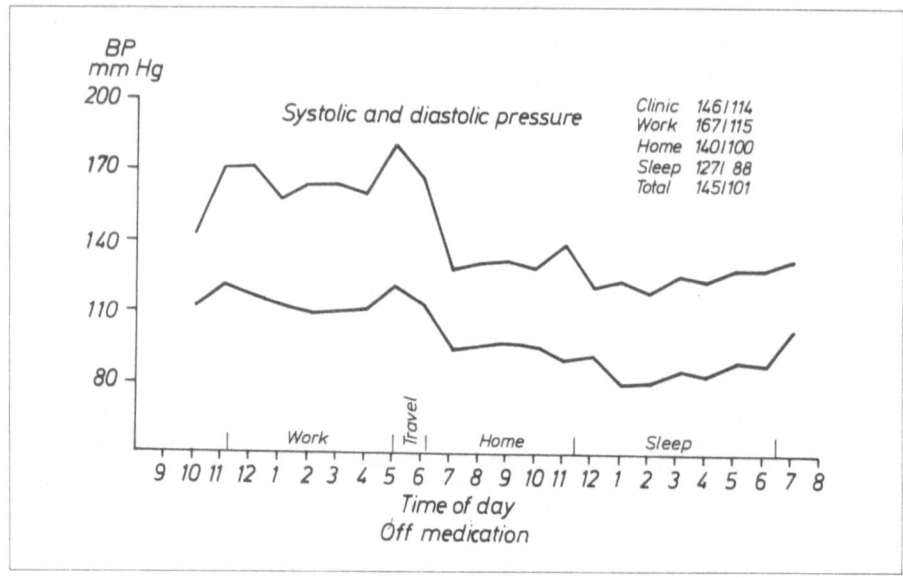

Fig. 1. 24-hour BP recording in an untreated hypertensive patient.

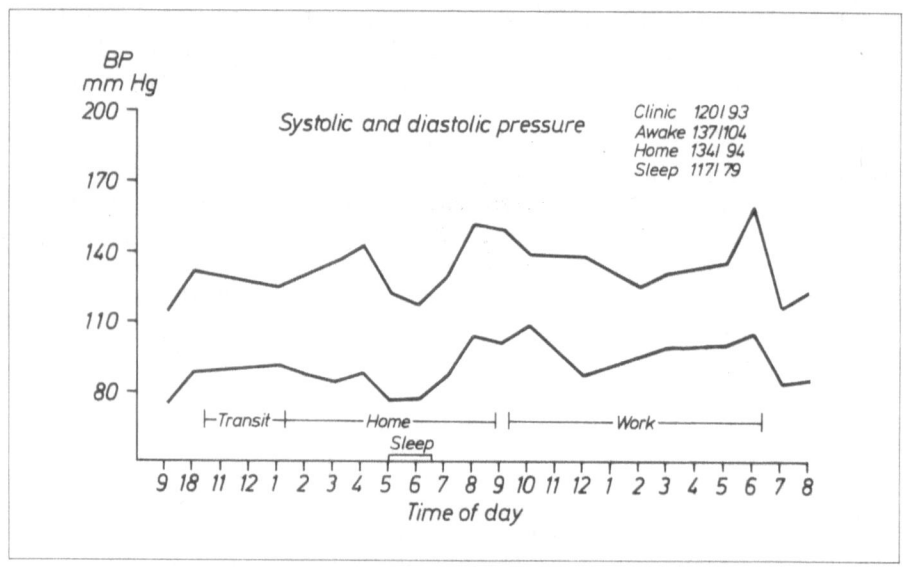

Fig. 2. 24-hour BP recording in a patient who worked at night. Contrast with Fig. 1.

The highest pressures were seen during activities such as eating, walking, talking (especially on the telephone), or being in the doctor's office, and the lowest while reading, relaxing, watching TV, or sleeping. It is clear that both psychological and physiological sti-

194

muli can influence blood pressure, but of particular interest was the finding that work conducted at home did not appear to raise BP.

We next sought to see if it was possible to demonstrate whether the higher pressures at work have any significance for the development of target organ damage and morbid events. So far we have been able to look at three measures of cardiac function which could be related to development of morbidity.

In the first study we correlated various indices of blood pressure with left ventricular hypertrophy (LVH). Since LVH is thought to be a consequence of the level of blood pressure to which the circulation has been exposed over long periods of time, these correlations could indicate which index of blood pressure has the most pathogenic significance. In a study of 100 subjects with either normal or mildly raised blood pressure we found that 24-hour blood pressures correlated much more closely with LVH (r = 0.50) than the physician's office blood pressures (r = 0.24) (2). Closer examination of the 24-hour pressures, however, revealed that the correlation was only significant if the recording was performed on a working day. In patients who stayed at home there was no correlation between 24-hour pressure and LVH. And work blood pressure correlated most closely with relative wall thickness (r = 0.59). These findings suggested to us the possibility that the transient increases of pressure associated with work might be particularly important in causing LVH, in the same way that LVH develops in athletes who only exercise for a small part of the day. Other studies have also reported greater correlations for 24-hour blood pressures with LVH than for clinic blood pressures (3, 4), but ours is the first to raise the possibility that it may not simply be the average level of pressure that determines the degree of LVH.

In a second study (5) we evaluated ventricular function by radionuclide cineangiography (RNCA), which is one of the best non-invasive methods of diagnosing coronary artery disease. The characteristic finding is a failure to increase or an actual decrease of left ventricular ejection fraction (EF) during exercise. We classified 21 hypertensive patients into two groups – those who showed the normal increase of EF with exercise, and those who showed a subnormal change. EF was normal in all these patients at rest, and none had overt coronary artery disease. Although there were no differences in the clinic blood

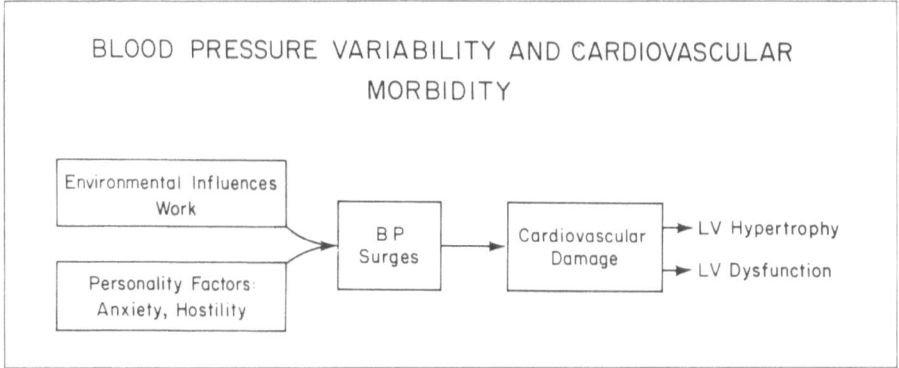

Fig. 3. Hypothetical schema for interaction of psychosocial factors on blood pressure and cardiovascular damage.

195

pressures between the two groups, the patients with the subnormal increase of EF during exercise showed significantly bigger increases (16 mmHg) of blood pressure from home to work than the patients with normal hearts (5 mmHg).

Another index of cardiac function that may be related to the development of morbid events is ventricular premature contractions (VPCs). Using an ambulatory monitor which records ECG (continuously) as well as blood pressure (intermittently) we found that there was no correlation between the frequency of VPCs and clinic or average 24-hour pressures, but there was a correlation with work systolic pressure (6), such that systolic pressure was higher at work (153 mmHg) in patients with complex VPCs than in those with simple VPCs (140 mmHg) or no VPCs (128 mmHg).

These findings, using three independent measures of cardiac dysfunction, are all consistent with the hypothesis that the increased pressure at work has a disproportionate role in causing target organ damage. They do not, however, prove a cause and effect relationship. Thus, it is conceivable that patients who have hypertrophied ventricles also have hypertrophied arterial walls, and consequently show an increased pressor response to stressful stimuli.

In another related study the cause and effect relationship appears more clear cut: women who showed the biggest increases of pressure at work (as compared to their home pressures) scored highest on psychometric tests of certain personality variables including anxiety and obsessiveness (7). Many studies have previously tried to relate personality and hypertension but with little success. Our own view is that it is an interactive relationship rather than a direct one, and our current hypothetical model of this interaction is shown in Figure 3.

Support for such an interaction between personality and environmental factors on blood pressure is provided by a study by Chesney et al (8), who correlated Type A Behaviour Pattern (perhaps not really a measure of personality) and occupational stress with blood pressure in a group of 384 Lockheed employees. Although neither variable was correlated with blood pressure on its own, there were significant interaction effects such that blood pressure was highest in Type A subjects who were in settings where peer cohesion was low, whereas Type B subjects showed higher blood pressures when peer cohesion was high.

There is a growing body of literature which suggests that occupational stress may increase the risk of developing coronary heart disease. A 10 year prospective survey of men working in two Belgian banks, one of which was a private bank and the other a semi-public savings bank, demonstrated higher blood pressures and also a higher incidence of major coronary events in men in the private bank. Traditional coronary risk factors could not completely account for the increased morbidity, but a job stress score was higher in the private bankers than the public bankers (9). Another prospective survey of Swedish working men found a higher incidence of coronary heart disease in men with "high strain" jobs characterized by high psychological demand and low decision latitude (10).

It is not yet known whether the pathophysiological connection between occupational stress and coronary heart disease is mediated through high blood pressure, but our findings of a relationship between blood pressure at work and cardiac dysfunction would certainly be consistent with this. There is at the present time very little information about the relationship between work stress and blood pressure, but if it can be established that there is a correlation, it would provide important evidence supporting a role for behavioral factors in the development of human hypertension, which has for many years been

196

the subject of considerable controversy. A recent study from Sweden suggest that the type of work may be an important factor in this relationship (11). Men who were normotensive showed relatively small differences between work and home blood pressures, but in hypertensive men the differences were more marked, particularly in those who had "high strain" jobs. Another study of normotensive men did not report higher pressures during work (12), which differs from our findings, but would be consistent with the view that the work pressure may vary considerably depending on the level of occupational strain.

Another question on which ambulatory monitoring might throw some light is whether the damage done by hypertension is solely a function of the average level of pressure over time, or whether the peaks of pressure have any special significance. While the literature from animal experiments is inconsistent on this point, our own work would suggest that the latter possibility should at least be considered. The answer to this question is of particular relevance to those interested in the behavioral aspects of hypertension, because it is likely that the majority of behavioral influences on blood pressure are transient.

References

1. Pickering TG, Harshfield GA, Kleinert HD, Blank S, and Laragh JH: Blood pressure during normal daily activities, sleep, and exercise. JAMA 247: 992–996 (1982).
2. Devereux RB, Pickering TG, Harshfield GA, Kleinert HD, Denby L, Clark L, Pregibon D, Jason M, Kleiner B, Borer JS, and Laragh JH: Left ventricular hypertrophy in patients with hypertension: importance of blood pressure response to regularly recurring stress. Circulation 68: 470–476 (1983).
3. Rowlands DB, Glover DR, Ireland MA, McLeay RAB, Stallard TJ, Watson RDS, and Littler WA: Assessment of left-ventricular mass and its response to antihypertensive treatment. Lancet 1: 467 (1982).
4. Drayer JIM, Weber MA, and DeYoung JL: BP as a determinant of cardiac left ventricular muscle mass. Arch Int Med 143: 90 (1983).
5. Jason M, Devereux RB, Borer JS, Pickering TG, Fisher J, Harshfield GA, Berkowitz A, and Laragh JH: 24-Hour arterial pressure measurement: improved iprediction of left ventricular dysfunction in essential hypertension. J Am Coll Cardiol 1: 599 (1983).
6. Kornienko WA, Kligfield P, Devereux RB, Pickering TG, Harshfield GA, and Laragh JH: Ventricular arrhythmias in mild essential hypertension: Association with workplace systolic blood pressure and left ventricular mass. J Am Coll Cardiol (in press).
7. Thailer SA, Friedman R, Harshfield GA, and Pickering TG: Relevance of situational changes in blood pressure to personality factors in female hypertensives. Circulation 68: III-286 (1983).
8. Chesney MA, Sevelius G, Black GW, Ward MM, Swan GE, and Rosenman RH: Work environment, type A behavior, and coronary heart disease risk factors. J Occupat Med 23: 551 (1981).
9. Kittel F, Kornitzer M, and Dramaix M: Coronary heart disease and job stress in two cohorts of bank clerks. Psychother Psychosom 34: 110 (1980).
10. Alfredsson L, Karasek R, and Theorell T: Myocardial infarction risk and psychosocial work environment: an analysis of the male Swedish working force. Soc Sci Med 16: 463 (1982).
11. Theorell T, Knox S, Svenson J, and Waller D: Blood pressure variations during a working day at age 30 – effects of different types of work and blood pressure level at age 18. Submitted.
12. Kennedy HL, Horan MJ, Sprague MK, Padgett NE, and Shriver KK: Ambulatory blood pressure in healthy normotensive males. Am Heart J 106: 717–722 (1983).

Address for correspondence:
Thomas G. Pickering, M.D., D.Phil.
Cardiovascular Center
The New York Hospital-Cornell Medical Center
1300 York Avenue
New York, N.Y. 10021

Usefulness of several devices for intermittent blood pressure monitoring in the assessment of the efficacy of antihypertensive therapy

Adesh Jain, F. Gilbert McMahon, Jerome R. Ryan

Summary: Clinic blood pressure measurements using the mercury sphygmomanometer, twice-daily home blood pressures (Lumitronic III instrument), and hourly daytime blood pressures (Physiometrics) were obtained in each of 34 patients before and during antihypertensive therapy with alpha-methyldopa and hydrochlorothiazide. The untreated blood pressure was lower when measured at home than when obtained in the clinic. Moreover, the treatment response derived from the home blood pressures was less than that found using the clinic blood pressures. Blood pressure variability was measured before and during treatment with atenolol in 12 patients using data obtained with the Physiometric device. Atenolol significantly lowered blood pressure and heart rate, but the diurnal variability in blood pressure was not attenuated during atenolol therapy. In another study, the variability of blood pressure was measured in hospitalized patients using multiple blood pressures obtained with the mercury sphygmomanometer, the Physiometrics device, and the Pressurometer III (Del Mar Avionics). The within-subject variability in circadian blood pressure in these ambulatory hypertensive patients was $9/5 \pm 3/2$ with the mercury sphygmomanometer and $12/7 \pm 2/2$ with the Physiometric device, both being significantly lower than that with the Del Mar Avionics system (PIII) $18/13 \pm 7/6$ mmHg. The PIII systolic blood pressure measurements correlated well ($r = 0.74$) but diastolic correlated poorly ($r = 0.38$) with measurements with a mercury sphygmomanometer during 48 hours of intermittent ambulatory monitoring. Malfunctioning of PIII and frequent artifacts resulted in substantial data loss. Within the limitations of the study designs presented here, we found mercury measurements to be consistently more dependable and reproducible than measurements by other devices evaluated.

Introduction

Human arterial blood pressure is a variable biological phenomenon. This variability is due partly to true variation in the subject's arterial pressure and partly to differing measurement errors (1). The mercury sphygmomanometer remains the standard device for measuring blood pressures in clinical practice and in clinical or epidimiological research. Modified versions such as the Hawksley random zero and London School of Hygiene sphygmomanometers have reduced the problem of observer bias but, inaccuracy resulting from differences between observers remains (1, 2). To eliminate this, many portable, semi-automated or fully automated indirect blood pressure recording devices have been introduced (3–6). However, their use has been criticized on the grounds that they are inaccurate or not dependable or perhaps not cost effective.

Clinical Research Center, Inc. New Orleans, LA 70112

199

This paper briefly summarizes our experience with several semi-automated (Lumintronic III, Infrasonde® Model 3010, Physiometrics®) and one fully automated device (Del Mar Avionics Pressurometer III) used by us to monitor home, clinic, or 24-hour ambulatory blood pressure in patients admitted to our research unit as part of several study protocols, and compares the performance of these devices with that of a standard cuff mercury sphygmomanometer under similar clinic or hospitalization conditions.

Methods and results

Study 1

In a double-blind study designed to compare the efficacy of a combination of alpha-methyldopa 500 mg and hydrochlorothiazide 50 mg (Aldoril-D-50), given once daily (qd) with that of half the combination dose (Aldoril-25) given twice daily (bid), we used three different devices to monitor home or clinic blood pressures. The details of this study are reported elsewhere (7). The morning clinic blood pressures were recorded approximately 24 hours following the previous day's a.m. dose by a trained nurse (as far as possible, the same observer for a given patient) using an appropriate sized arm cuff, a mercury sphygmomanometer and recommended techniques (8), phase 1 for systolic and phase 5 of the Korotkoff sounds for diastolic readings. An average of three sets of readings, each following 10 minutes in recumbent position and 2 minutes in erect position, represented the respective supine and erect blood pressures for that visit. Home blood

Table 1. Mean changes in clinic and home morning blood pressures during treatment with a methyldopa-hydrochlorothiazide combination (Aldoril D-50) given once or (Aldoril-25) twice daily.

	Clinic BP (supine)mmHg[1]		Home BP (sitting)mmHg[2]	
	Aldoril D-50	Aldoril-25	Aldoril D-50	Aldoril-25
n =	34	34	34	29
	Sys/Dias	Sys/Dias	Sys/Dias	Sys/Dias
Placebo BP	165/103	164/103	157/99	151/95
Change from placebo:				
Week 2	18/11	22/11	12/6	16/7
Week 4	18/7	26/13	16/8	19/7
Week 6	24/12	26/15	19/10	19/10
Week 8	22/11	28/16[3]	19/10	14/11
Week 10	26/11	29/14	21/11	22/11
Week 12	24/14	27/15	20/13	20/10
Mean	22/11	26/14	18/10	18/9

[1]) Clinic blood pressures were recorded by conventional mercury sphygmomanometer.
[2]) Home blood pressures were recorded by Lumi-Tronic III.
[3]) P < 0.05 (Aldoril D-50 vs. Aldoril-25)

200

pressures were recorded twice daily (on arising in the morning and then 12 hours later) throughout the study by Lumitronic III(R) (a portable, BP instrument) by the patients who were instructed in the proper use of the device. In addition, at the end of 6 weeks of single blind placebo and 12 weeks of double blind treatment, 10 hour clinic blood pressures were monitored by an automated recorder (Physiometrics) at -2, -1 and 0 hours prior to dosing at 10 a.m. and then hourly for 8 hours (6 p.m.). The pressures by this device were recorded on discs which were interpreted by the same individual.

The mean baseline morning home blood pressures were noted to be lower than those in the clinic (Table 1). The corresponding evening baseline blood pressures were 155/96 (qd) and 149/94 (bid). Both regimens of active treatment produced a significant ($p < 0.01$) reduction in home and clinic blood pressures; however, a somewhat smaller home blood pressure response was noted. Furthermore, significant differences noted at week eight between the two active regimens based on clinic blood pressures were not observed from home blood pressure data.

The mean 10-hour clinic diastolic blood pressures as recorded by the Physiometrics device in the same study are shown in Figure 1. No significant differences were noted in the efficacy of the two active regimens based on 10-hour clinic diastolic blood pressures which were noted to be fairly stable. Systolic reponses were similar (7). The 6 p.m clinic blood pressures were reduced by 35/23 on qd regimen and 33/17 on bid regimen. Respective evening home blood pressure improvements were 20/10 and 17/10 mmHg.

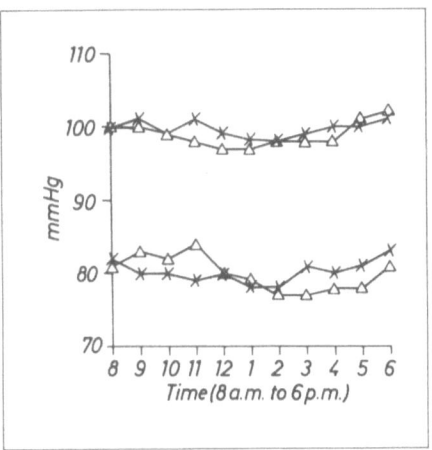

Fig. 1. Mean supine diastolic blood pressures following dosing at 10 a.m., after 6 weeks placebo (upper lines) and 12 weeks alpha-methyldopa/hydrochlorothiazide (lower lines), once daily $\triangle - \triangle$ (QD) and twice daily X– –X (BID) treatments (n = 36 QD, n = 32 BID).

Study 2

The Physiometrics device was also used for recording 24-hour blood pressures in another study designed to evaluate 24-hour efficacy of a 100 mg, once-daily dose of atenolol. Twelve patients who had previously responded to atenolol during a four-week prescreening period were admitted during the last three days of the three-week treatment period, each with placebo or atenolol. Blood pressures were recorded hourly from 8 a.m to 10 p.m and then at midnight, 2 a.m. and 6 a.m. for three consecutive days. An average of three readings at each observation was recorded.

Diurnal trends in blood pressure readings were observed after both placebo and atenolol, blood pressure during night (sleep) being low (Fig. 2). The mean 24-hour supine diastolic blood pressure was reduced from a range of 105–107 mmHg on placebo to 88–91 mmHg on atenolol, significant reductions in systolic blood pressures and heart rate were also observed (9).

Fig. 2. Mean supine diastolic blood pressure during 76 hours of monitoring. 0 hour correlates with once daily dose of placebo △. . ..△ or atenolol O—O (n = 12).

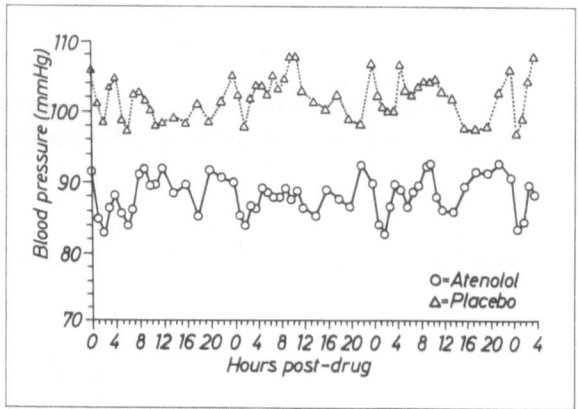

Study 3

In another study we compared the performance of the Del Mar Avionics (Irvine, Calif.) Pressurometer III device with that of the mercury sphygmomanometer. This double-blind crossover study consisted of two 14-day periods of treatment with either a once-daily or twice-daily dose of a combination of clonidine-chlorthalidone (Combipres (R)) separated and preceded by a two-week placebo period. The patients were hospitalized on the thirteenth and fourteenth day of each treatment period for monitoring of 48-hour blood pressures. Our original protocol called for a total of 96 pressure measurements daily at 15 minute intervals, to be recorded by the automated equipment, but 15 standard mercurial measurements at periodic intervals per day were also required, which was fortunate because the automated equipment simply failed to work properly despite numerous emergency repairs.

Eleven out of 24 patients completing the study had blood pressures recorded by both devices at least during the initial placebo phase. A 1979 Pressurometer Charter (Del Mar Avionics) was used to print the data monitored by the automated device. After deleting markedly inconsistent changes in systolic and diastolic readings or artifactual readings, or readings with very low pulse pressure, we lost more than 30% of the data in 6 of the 11 patients analyzed. Data loss was also partly due to the periodically malfunctioning device.

202

For the purpose of this presentation, we have only compared blood pressures recorded simultaneously or within +/– 5 minutes by the two devices, and we have excluded artifactual readings. A poor correlation was noted for the diastolic readings (r = 0.38) obtained by the two devices (Fig. 3), but correlation for systolic blood pressures was much better (r = 0.734), (Fig. 4).

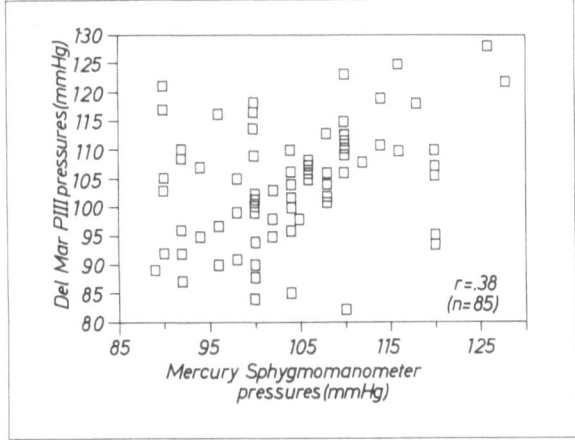

Fig. 3. Correlation between diastolic blood pressure values obtained using Del Mar Avionics PIII and mercury sphygmomanometer, during 48 hours of simultaneous, intermittent monitoring (r = 0.38).

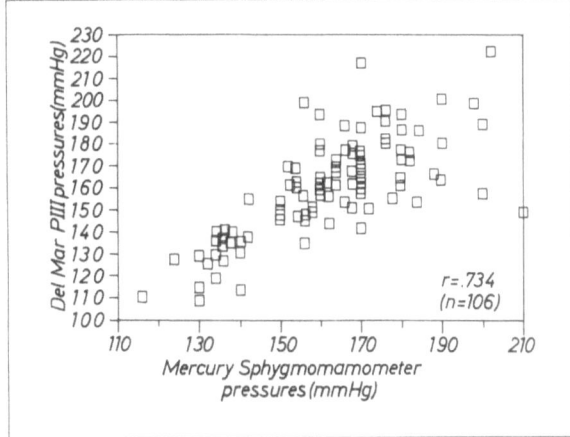

Fig. 4. Correlation between systolic blood pressure values obtained using Del Mar Avionics PIII and mercury sphygmomanometer, during 48 hours of simultaneous, intermittent monitoring (r = 0.734).

Table 2 shows within-subject variability in the recorded 24-hour blood pressure in hypertensive patients of similar demographic backgrounds admitted to our research unit for various study protocols. Only data obtained during the initial placebo phase were compared. Blood pressure was generally taken hourly from 8 a.m. to 10 p.m. and then every two to four hours until 8 a.m. for two or more consecutive days. In general, variability of systolic BP was greater than that of diastolic BP. The within-subject variability of the

Table 2. Variability of BP measurements by different devices

BP Device	Mean ± S.D. Age (yrs)	Sex	Percent overweight	Mean Sys/Dias (mmHg)	Between subject variance	Within subject variance*)	Readings in 24 hrs
Mercury (n = 24)	52 ± 11†	17F, 7M	23 ± 19†	150/100	21/7	9/5 ± 3/2†	18
Del Mar Avionics PIII (n = 10)	51 ± 4	8F, 2M	22 ± 12	160/105	26/8	18/13 ± 7/6	50–80
Physio-metrics (n = 12)	54 ± 5	11F, 1M	12 ± 9	146/105	15/6	12/7 ± 2/2	18

*) Variance is defined as the standard deviation of all readings obtained during 24 hours.
F = female, M = male, Sys = systolic, Dias = diastolic, † mean ± S.D.

24-hour blood pressure by the Avionics device was significantly higher than that of the Physiometrics or mercurial manometer.

Comments

In the first two studies, as an alternative to 24-hour continuous blood pressure monitoring, we were able to obtain meaningful data by intermittent blood pressure recordings at home, or in the clinic, or in ambulant in-patients, using conventional manometry or the Physiometrics device. Our observation that home blood pressures were lower than those in the clinic is in accordance with several similar reports (3–5). The observation of somewhat smaller improvement in treated blood pressures at home as opposed to in the clinic may be due to a lower baseline, relatively more activity at home or measurement errors. Lumitronic III was simple to operate and its overall performance in the hands of our patients, who were mainly of low socio-economic status, was judged to be fair. Malfunctioning units resulted in the loss of study data on few occasions. Although periodic rechecking of the units resulted in good correlation with the mercury sphygmomanometer, the accuracy and precision of this simple unit were felt to be far from desirable.

The Physiometrics device appears to be a good alternative to conventional manometry, although no substantial advantage seemed to be gained considering its cost, bulkiness, need for frequent calibration and possible observer error in interpreting systolic and diastolic readings from the discs. Furthermore its reproducibility was noted to be no better than that of the mercury sphygmomanometer using more than one observer (unpublished data).

To minimize observer error, our unit has also used the Infrasonde (R) Model 3010 (cost $1000), a lightweight, portable, electronic sphygmomanometer (quite precise and accurate but perhaps not cost effective) and the Hawksley random zero sphygmomanometer. Since multiple readings with the Hawksley tend to be more painful and time-consuming than conventional mercurial measurements, we have reserved the use of the Hawksley device for training purpose and at times to evaluate intra- or inter-observer differences, and have heavily relied on conventional mercury sphygmomanometer for most study data. Proper training of the observer in the use of the mercury manometer (8) and a good study design (7, 9, 10) are key to the successful outcome of a study.

Although several investigators have reported meaningful ambulatory blood pressure data in normals and hypertensive subjects with the Del Mar Avionics PIII using 1979 charter (4–6), our experience with the device has been rather disappointing. Malfunctioning units and frequent inconsistent changes in systolic and diastolic readings or artifactual readings resulted in substantial loss of study data in the only study in which we had hoped to obtain true ambulatory data. Our published results of this study comparing efficacy of two regimens of a combination of chlorthalidone-clonidine were solely based on mercurial measurements (10). The mean percent. overweight of the study population was 22 +/– 12%. No consistent pattern was seen between the frequency of artifactual readings and total bodyweight. Factors like circumference and shape of the arm (in a predominantly female population) may make this device unsuitable for certain patients. We lack experience with direct intra-arterial continuous monitoring which, though precise add ref., appears to have marked practical limitations because of being invasive with its inherent morbidity. Thus within the limitations of the study designs presented and devices evaluated, we found mercurial measurements to be consistently more dependable and reproducible in the efficacy assessment of antihypertensive agents.

References

1. Rose GA, Holland WW, Crowley EA: A sphygmomanometer for epidemiologists. Lancet i: 296–300 (1964).
2. Hunyor SN, Flynn JM, Cochineas C: Comparison of performance of various sphygmamometers with intra-arterial blood pressure readings. Br Med J 2: 159–162 (1978).
3. Horan MJ, Padgett NE, Kennedy HL: Ambulatory blood pressure monitoring, recent advances and clinical applications. Am Heart J 101: 843–848 (1981).
4. Harshfield GA, Pickering T, Laragh J: A validation study of the Del Mar Avionics blood pressure system. Ambulatory Electrocardiography 4: 7–12 (1979).
5. Pickering TG, Harshfield GA, Kleinest HD, Blanks S, Laragh JH: Blood pressure during normal activities, sleep, exercise comparison of values in normal and hypertensive subjects. JAMA 247: 992–996 (1982).
6. Drayer J, Weber MA, DeYoung JL, Wyle FA: Circadian Blood Pressure Patterns in Ambulatory Hypertensive Patients. Am J Med 73: 493–499 (1982).
7. Noveck RJ, McMahon FG, Jain AK: Treatment of elevated blood pressure with a simplified methyldopa-hydrochlorothiazide treatment regimen. Curr Ther Res 32(6): 822–833 (1982).
8. Recommendations for Human Blood Pressure Determination by Sphygmomanometer. American Heart Association Dallas (1980).
9. Ryan JR, LaCorte W, Jain AK, McMahon FG, Rosenberg A: Atenolol in the Treatment of Hypertension. Curr Ther Res 32(6): 834 (1982).
10. McMahon FG, Ryan JR, LaCorte W, Mather FJ: Once Daily vs Twice Daily Clonidine-chlorthalidone: A controlled clinical trial. Curr Ther Res 33(6): 1041 (1983).
11. Goldberg AD, Raftery EB, Cashman PM, Stott FD: Study of untreated hypertensive subjects by means of continuous intraarterial blood pressure monitoring. Br Heart J 40: 656 (1978).

Address for correspondence:
Adesh Jain, M.D.
Clinical Research Center, Inc.
134 La Salle
New Orleans, LA 70112

Blood pressure variability in hypertensive patients during and immediately following treatment with propranolol and clonidine

Andre-Jacques Neusy, John M. Steele Jr.*, Jerome Lowenstein

Summary: The effects of placebo, propranolol and clonidine on blood pressure and blood pressure variability were examined in 9 patients with moderate essential hypertension. Hydrochlorothiazide was given throughout sequential 4–8 week periods of placebo, propranolol and clonidine treatment. During each treatment period, subjects were admitted twice to the clinical research unit for 24-hour blood pressure monitoring. Blood pressure was recorded at 15 minute intervals using an automated non-invasive recorder (Arteriosonde). Blood pressure monitoring was performed during administration of placebo, propranolol and clonidine and repeated 1–2 weeks later during the first 24 hours following the abrupt cessation of placebo or drug administration.
Systolic and diastolic blood pressure readings were averaged and the standard deviation taken as a measure of long term variability (LTV). Systolic and diastolic blood pressures in sequential overlapping blocks of 7 readings were averaged and the standard deviation calculated. Short term variability (STV) was estimated as the average of the standard deviations of the running means.
During placebo administration and withdrawal systolic blood pressure, diastolic blood pressure, LTV and STV were unchanged.
Systolic and diastolic blood pressure did not differ during propranolol administration and propranolol withdrawal. LTV and STV were not different from placebo during clonidine administration or withdrawal but both systolic and diastolic blood pressure increased to values significantly greater than placebo during the final 8-hour monitoring period following discontinuation of clonidine. Rebound hypertension after withdrawal of clonidine was not characterized by increased blood pressure variability.

Regulatory mechanisms maintaining blood pressure within a narrow range have been studied extensively in experimental animals. New blood pressure monitoring devices such as non-invasive automated intermittent blood pressure recorders and intra-arterial blood pressure recorders with computer programs which allow beat-to-beat analysis of blood pressure provide a means for examining the regulation of arterial pressure in man (1, 2). A close relationship between systolic and diastolic blood pressure and blood pressure variability has been demonstrated in essential hypertension (1, 2). Little is known, however, of the effects of antihypertensive therapy on blood pressure variability. Lability of the blood pressure is a distinctive feature of neurogenic hypertension in experimental animals (3, 4). Changes in sympathetic activity induced by sympatholytic drugs are associated

---

Renal and Hypertensive Disease Section Department of Medicine, New York University Medical Center
* deceased

with a reduction of mean arterial pressure but little is known of their effects on blood pressure variability. Clonidine, a central α_2 adrenergic agonist, is believed to exert its hypotensive effect via a reduction of sympathetic outflow from the brain (5). Similarly, propranolol has been reported to exert its blood pressure lowering effect through changes in sympathetic nerve function via central actions of the drug (6, 7) and possibly via inhibition of presynaptic beta adrenoceptors which modulate per pulse norepinephrine release (8).

In the present study we have compared blood pressure variability in patients receiving placebo with blood pressure variability during administration of propranolol and clonidine. Further, we examined the changes in blood pressure and blood pressure variability during the 24-hour period following abrupt cessation of drug administration (withdrawal).

Design of study

After obtaining informed consent, 14 patients with mild to moderate essential hypertension were enrolled in the study (Fig. 1). Patients were treated with hydrochlorothiazide (50 mg daily) for 4 weeks. Those whose blood pressure remained elevated ($>140/90$ mmHg) entered into the first placebo control period and were given a placebo tablet to be taken twice daily for a period of 4–6 weeks and were seen in clinic biweekly. Hydrochlorothiazide was given throughout the remainder of the study. The subjects were then randomized to propranolol or clonidine treatment. Propranolol was given initially at a dose of 40 mg twice daily and titrated to a maximum dose of 160 mg twice daily; clonidine was given initially at a dose of 0.1 mg twice daily and increased to 0.2 mg twice daily if needed to attain a blood pressure at or below 140/90 mmHg. A second 4 week placebo control period intervened between the administration of the two active drugs. Twice during each treatment period the patient was admitted to the Clinical Research Unit (C.R.U.) for 24-hour blood pressure monitoring. The initial study examined the effect of continued administration of the placebo or active drug. Several weeks later, while still receiving the placebo or the active drug, the patient was readmitted to the C.R.U. for study of the effects of drug withdrawal. The 8 a.m. dose was omitted and BP was monitored during the subsequent drug-free 24 hours. The blood pressure was recorded every 15 minutes beginning at 8.00 a.m., using a non-invasive automated intermittent recorder (Arteriosonde). Heart rate was not monitored. The times of sleeping, waking and restricted ambulation in the room were recorded by a nurse assigned to the project. Nine of the 14 subjects completed all 8 phases of the study; in the remaining 5 complete data were available for the first placebo and both drug periods. The detailed data to be presented will include only the nine patients who underwent all eight monitoring periods.

Data analysis

Blood pressure variability over the whole 24-hour period or during eight hour time blocks (8 a.m. to 4 p.m., 4 p.m. to midnight, midnight to 8 a.m.) was assessed by averaging all the systolic and diastolic pressures during the 24 or 8 hour period and calculating the standard deviation of the mean pressure ("long term variability"). In order to assess

208

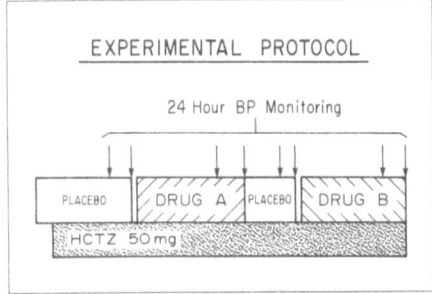

Fig. 1. Experimental protocol. Patients were assigned to receive propranolol or clonidine as the initial drug in random sequence. Arrows indicate the 24-hour blood pressure monitoring periods.

blood pressure variability over shorter time intervals, since the number of BP values recorded in each patient over a 24 hour period was relatively small, we chose a method of analysis which would minimize the contribution to variability of single widely divergent blood pressure readings. To this end, we measured a moving average and moving standard deviation in sequential overlapping blocks of 7 pressure recordings. For each block of 7 pressure recordings, a mean and standard deviation were calculated for systolic and diastolic pressure (Fig. 2). "Short term variability" was estimated by averaging the standard deviations of the running means of overlapping blocks of seven blood pressure recordings. Artefactual misreadings of the BP recorder accounted for less than 2% of all the measurements and were excluded from analysis.

In order to examine the effects of drug withdrawal on BP and BP variability, we compared the data obtained during the first 8 hours of monitoring with those obtained during the last 8 hours of monitoring on days during which drug (or placebo) administration was continued as contrasted with days during which drug (or placebo) administration was abruptly discontinued.

Statistical analysis was performed by analysis of variance.

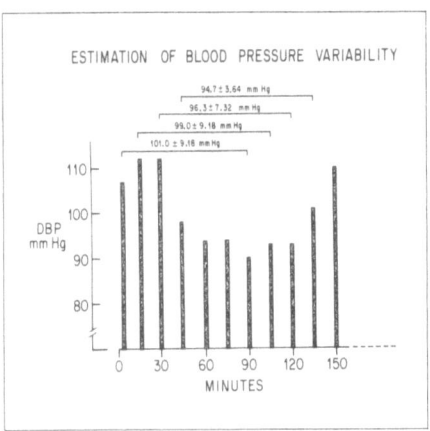

Fig. 2. Estimation of blood pressure variability (example). To assess short term variability, a running mean of systolic and diastolic pressures averaged over sequential overlapping blocks of 7 pressure recordings was calculated. The standard deviation of each block was averaged to yield STV (short term variability).

Results

Clonidine (average dose 0.23 mg/day) and propranolol (average dose 108.5 mg/day) exerted significant and comparable antihypertensive effects as judged by the blood pressures recorded in the outpatient clinic at the visit immediately preceeding the 24-hour blood pressure monitoring (Table 1).

The measured 24-hour mean systolic and diastolic blood pressures were consistently lower than the blood pressure recorded in the outpatient clinic whether the patient was receiving placebo, propranolol or clonidine. This difference was relatively large during placebo administration and clonidine administration. A comparable difference between outpatient clinic blood pressure and mean 24-hour blood pressure averaging 18/10 mmHg was noted by Watson et al. (2). Twenty-four hour mean blood pressure, was, however, only minimally lower than the blood pressure recorded in the outpatient clinic in patients receiving propranolol.

During administration of placebo we observed a small, but significant decrease in systolic and mean arterial pressure over the course of the 24-hour monitoring period. A similar

Table 1: Blood pressure and blood pressure variability during treatment with placebo, propranolol and clonidine and following abrupt cessation of drugs.

	Blood pressure (Outpatient)		Inpatient Blood pressure Monitoring					
			24 hours		Initial 8 hours		final 8 hours	
	Systolic	Di-astolic	Sys-tolic	Di-astolic	Sys-tolic	Di-astolic	Sys-tolic	Di-astolic
Placebo	Mean 151.7	100	Mean 130.7	90.1	135.1	91.9	125.2	88.5
	Sem 7.2	2.5	LTV 13.7	9.6	10.9	8.4	12.4	9.4
			STV 10.4	7.8	9.4	7.5	11.0	8.2
Placebo Withdrawal	–		Mean 130.8	89.2	132.3	87.9	126.5	89.7
			LTV 11.5	7.8	11.1	6.9	11.1	7.4
			STV 9.7	6.6	9.7	6.4	10.4	6.9
Propranolol	Mean 136.9	89.6	Mean 131.1	87.3	130.8	87.1	126.8	84.3
	Sem 8.4	14.5	LTV 13.7	9.9	10.3	8.2	15.2	10.6
			STV 10.3	7.9	8.8	7.4	13.3	9.2
Propranolol Withdrawal	–		Mean 131.8	87.4	133.4	87.1	129.7	87.2
			LTV 12.6	9.5	10.3	8.3	11.9	10.2
			STV 10.2	7.9	9.0	7.3	10.2	8.7
Clonidine	Mean 138.4	90.2	Mean 117.8	80.1	119.9	80.1	114.1	79.1
	Sem 4.8	2.7	LTV 13.0	9.8	11.6	9.2	12.9	9.9
			STV 10.2	7.8	9.8	7.5	10.4	8.4
Clonidine Withdrawal	–		Mean 138.0	91.5	131.4	86.8	141.5	94.3
			LTV 14.0	10.1	12.0	9.1	12.2	9.0
			STV 10.3	7.7	9.7	7.8	10.7	7.8

Sem = Standard error of the mean
LTV = (long term variability) = standard deviation of mean systolic or diastolic pressure
STV = (short term variability) = the mean of the standard deviations of the running mean systolic or diastolic pressures.

trend was found when we compared the initial and final eight hour periods of observation in patients receiving either propranolol or clonidine. This finding, seen with placebo and active drug treatment, might reflect an effect of acclimatization to the hospital environment and/or the monitoring procedure, or the fall in BP seen during periods of sleep (9).

Blood pressure and its variability during placebo administration and placebo withdrawal

Systolic and diastolic pressure did not differ during placebo administration, as compared with the period of placebo withdrawal, considering the 24 hours as a whole. During both the placebo administration and placebo withdrawal days systolic pressure was significantly lower during the last 8-hour period as compared with the initial 8-hour period. The standard deviation of systolic, diastolic and mean arterial pressure was similar indicating that long term variability of blood pressure was not different during placebo administration and placebo withdrawal. Short term variability was generally somewhat less than long term variability and also did not differ significantly during placebo administration and placebo withdrawal.

Blood pressure and its variability during propranolol administration and propranolol withdrawal

Considering the entire 24-hour period, systolic and diastolic pressure did not differ during propranolol administration as compared with the period of propranolol withdrawal indicating that there was no rebound hypertension during the 24 hours following propranolol withdrawal. Comparing the initial and final 8-hour periods there was a small but significant decrease in systolic pressure on both the propranolol administration and propranolol withdrawal days. Neither long term variability nor short term variability was different during propranolol administration or withdrawal from that observed during placebo administration or withdrawal.

Blood pressure and its variability during clonidine administration and withdrawal

Systolic and diastolic blood pressures were significantly lower throughout the 24-hour period of clonidine administration as compared with the periods of placebo or propranolol administration. Systolic and diastolic pressure were greater during the 24-hour period of clonidine withdrawal than during the 24-hour period of clonidine administration. Comparison of the first 8 hour of clonidine withdrawal with the last 8 hours revealed a significant increase in systolic and diastolic pressure during the last 8 hours, a pattern not seen during continued clonidine administration or propranolol or placebo administration or withdrawal. While no instances of alarming rebound hypertension were observed in this study, this finding confirms the occurrence of rebound increase of BP during the first 24 hours of clonidine withdrawal (10, 11). Neither the long term variability nor the short term variability of systolic or diastolic blood pressure differed between clonidine administration and clonidine withdrawal studies.

Discussion

This study examined the effects of administration and abrupt withdrawal of clonidine and propranolol on the level of arterial pressure and blood pressure variability in patients with essential hypertension.

We did not observe a significant difference in blood pressure during the 24-hour period of propranolol withdrawal as compared with the 24-hour period of propranolol administration, nor did either systolic or diastolic blood pressure tend to increase during the course of the 24-hour period of propranolol withdrawal. The absence of blood pressure "rebound" following abrupt cessation of propranolol therapy is in agreement with the findings of others (12). Heart rate was not monitored; we cannot exclude the possibility that rebound tachycardia occurred.

Neither long term nor short term blood pressure variability was different during propranolol administration from that during placebo administration. This finding appears to be in conflict with the report of Watson et al. who described decreased blood pressure variability measured as the standard deviation of systolic and diastolic pressure, during propranolol treatment (13). It should be noted however that reduced blood pressure variability in Watson's study was associated with, and closely paralleled, reduced mean systolic and diastolic blood pressure. While it is not firmly established that blood pressure variability is always proportional to the absolute level of blood pressure such a relationship was suggested in the comparison of mild, moderate and severe hypertensives reported by Mancia et al. (1).

Administration of clonidine resulted in a significant decrease of systolic and diastolic pressure when compared with placebo administration. Abrupt cessation of clonidine administration was associated with an increase of the systolic and diastolic pressures throughout the 24-hour monitoring period. This "rebound" effect was already evident during the first 8 hours of monitoring off clonidine, in that systolic and diastolic pressures were higher than the corresponding pressures recorded during the first 8 hours of monitoring during clonidine administration. Systolic and diastolic blood pressures recorded during the last 8 hours of the 24-hour period following discontinuation of clonidine were significantly higher than those recorded during the corresponding period during clonidine administration and exceeded pressures recorded during the corresponding time periods of placebo administration or withdrawal.

We observed that blood pressure variability during clonidine administration did not differ from that during placebo administration, indicating that this central α_2 adrenergic agonist does not influence blood pressure variability despite its hypotensive effect. During clonidine withdrawal, blood pressure variability remained unchanged despite the clear cut blood pressure rebound to pretreatment level, indicating that clonidine withdrawal does not affect blood pressure variability during the first 24 hours following cessation of the drug.

Acknowledgement

The authors thank Margaret Lyman, M.D. and Howard Spivak Ph.D. for their valuable assistance.

This work was supported by a grant from Boehringer Ingelheim.

References

1. Mancia G, Ferrari A, Gregorini L, Parati G, Pomidosei G, Bertinieri G, Grossi G, diRienzo M, Pedotti A, Zanchetti A: Blood pressure and heart rate variabilities in normotensive and hypertensive human beings. Circ Res 53: 16–104 (1983).
2. Watson RDS, Stallard TJ, Flinn RM, Littler WA: Factors determining direct arterial pressure and its variability in hypertensive man. Hypertension 2: 333–341 (1980).
3. Reis DJ: The brain and arterial hypertension: Evidence for a neural imbalance hypothesis. In: Abboud FM, Fozzard HA, Gilmore JP, Reis Dj (Ed): Disturbances in neurogenic control of the circulation. pp 87–104, Williams and Wilkins (Baltimore, Md. 1981).
4 Carey RM, Dacey RG, Jane JA, Winn HR, Ayers CR, Tyson GW: Production of sustained hypertension by lesions of the nucleus tractus solitarii of the American foxhound. Hypertension 1: 246–254 (1979).
5. Kobinger W and Walland A: Investigations into the mechanisms of the hypertensive effect of 2-(2,6-dichlorophenylamino)-2-imidazoline hydrochloride. Europ J Pharmacol 2: 155–162 (1967).
6. Doward PK and Korner PK: Effect of d, 1-Propranolol on renal sympathetic baroreflex properties and aortic baroreceptor activity. Europ J Pharmacol 52: 61–71 (1978).
7. Lewis PJ, Haeusler G: Reduction of sympathetic nervous activity as a mechanism for the hypotensive effect of propranolol. Nature 256: 440 (1975).
8. Rand MJ, Majewski H, Medgett IC, McCulloch MW, Story DF: Prejunctional receptors modulating autonomic neuroeffector transmission. Circ Res 46: Suppl I 1–70 – I–76 (1980).
9. Littler WA: Sleep and blood pressure: Further observations. Am Heart J 97: 35–37 (1979).
10. Goldberg AD, Raftery EB, Wilkinsen P: Blood pressure and heart rate withdrawal of antihypertensive drugs. Brit Med J 1: 1243–1246 (1977).
11. Reid JL, Wing LMH, Dargie JH, Hamilton CA, Davies DS and Dollery CT: Clonidine withdrawal in hypertension. Lancet 1: 1171–1174 (1977).
12. Nattel S, Rangno RE and Van Loon G: Mechanism of propranolol withdrawal phenomenon, Circ 59: 1158–1164 (1979).
13. Watson RDS, Stallard TJ, Littler WA: Influence of once-daily administration of β-adrenoceptor antagonists on arterial pressure and its variability. Lancet 1: 1210–1213 (1979).

Adress for correspondence:
Jerome Lowenstein, M.D.
New York University Medical Center
560 First Avenue
New York, N.Y. 10016

Evaluation of the posology of pindolol therapy of hypertension with automatic indirect ambulatory blood pressure monitoring

Sheldon G. Sheps, Alexander Schirger, Peter C. O'Brien, Ralph E. Spiekerman, Thomas R. Harman

Summary: Pindolol, a nonselective β-adrenergic blocking drug, lowered systolic and diastolic blood pressure equally well during once daily and twice daily dosage. Absence of supine bradycardia likely was attributable to the intrinsic sympathomimetic activity of pindolol. Automatic ambulatory blood pressure monitoring reliably confirmed office blood pressure recordings and indicated good control throughout the day and night.

The effect on blood pressure of the β-adrenergic blocking drugs is not well correlated with blood levels of the drugs. The dosage must be evaluated clinically in man. The technique of automatic indirect ambulatory blood pressure monitoring, which provides up to 200 blood pressure readings in 24 hours, was used to compare the effectiveness of once a day and twice daily doses of pindolol, a nonselective β-adrenergic drug with high intrinsic sympathomimetic activity, in the control of blood pressure.

Materials and methods

Twenty patients receiving long term therapy with pindolol administered twice daily were entered into a single blind study to evaluate the effect of administration of the same total dose of pindolol as a single dose in the morning for twelve weeks (one patient discontinued the study after four weeks). The patients all had mild to moderate hypertension. The total dose of pindolol was 10 mg per day in one patient, 20 mg in three patients, 30 mg in four patients, and 40 mg in twelve patients. Sixteen patients were receiving additional therapy (hydrochlorothiazide, hydralazine) and this dose remained unchanged throughout the study.

Blood pressure and heart rate were recorded in the Clinic every two weeks for six visits on each regimen; two readings each with the patient in the supine and standing positions. The observations were obtained before the morning medication was taken. In 11 patients, ambulatory indirect blood pressure recordings were made with the Del Mar Avionics equipment (P_2 and P_3) for approximately 24 hours on two occasions at least two weeks apart on each regimen after the patient had been on the regimen for at least one month. Blood pressures were obtained at 7.5 minute intervals throughout the 24 hours

Mayo Clinic and Mayo Foundation Rochester, MN 55905

during daily activities and sleep. The records were edited by a blinded observer and the number of observations averaged 147.35 ± 25.9 (SD-standard deviation) per 24 hours. All patients had at least two ambulatory recordings on one regimen and one on the other regimen.

Results

We had evaluated the Avionics equipment in a previous study (1). Figure 1 illustrates the comparison of the device in the test mode with the technician's observations simultaneously in the same arm. Only 11% of systolic blood pressure and 5% of diastolic blood pressure readings differed by more than 10 mmHg. The median difference was approximately 4 mmHg for both systolic and diastolic averages. Note that 10% of the differences were 0. In the current study the reliability of the device was examined by a comparison of the 24-hour mean systolic pressures on 12 pairs of repeat observations in patients on the same regimen. The absolute difference between days ranged between 0.097 mmHg to 17.298 mmHg, and the median difference was 8.112 mmHg.

The blood pressure and heart rate responses in patients on the once daily and twice daily regimens were compared with each other and with control values. The control values had been obtained before the beginning of therapy at the end of three week washout period with no active drug administered. The control observations had consisted of three readings in each of two circumstances: in the supine position and after two minutes of

Fig. 1. Cumulative distribution of difference (406 observations) without regard to sign, (Δ), between pressure recorded by Avionics device in test mode and technician's recording made simultaneously in same arm. Note that 10% of differences were zero. SBP = systolic blood pressure; DBP = diastolic blood pressure.

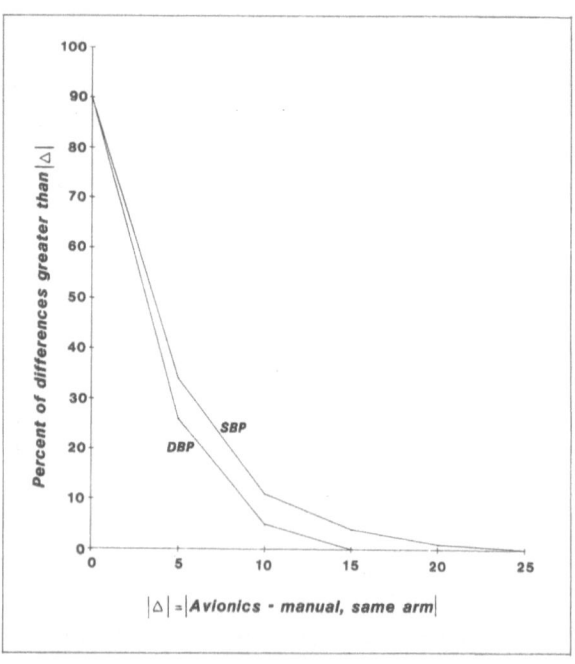

quiet standing; all were averaged for each position. Table I compares the blood pressures obtained in the supine and standing position during the control and on the two pindolol regimens. In all positions the systolic and diastolic blood pressures were significantly reduced from control values on both regimens of pindolol and there was no difference between regimens. In the supine or standing position, the heart rate was not significantly different from the control value. Although the heart rate was not significantly reduced by pindolol, the usual increase in heart rate with standing is blunted as it is with all β-blocking drugs. The morning heart rate was slightly higher on once a day therapy.

Ambulatory blood pressure results are also given in Table I. The blood pressure followed the usual pattern of being lower during sleep and was similar for both regimens when compared for states of being awake and asleep. Figure 2 illustrates the ambulatory blood pressures in patients receiving pindolol administered once daily. Shown are hourly means ± one standard deviation. The waking and sleeping periods are indicated by a break in the graph. The blood pressure is lower at night. As observed with intra-arterial devices, an early morning increase in blood pressure usually occurred, beginning before awakening and affecting patients on both regimens (2). Except for the small and short lived increase at 10 p.m. noted in patients on the once a day regimen, the hourly observations were similar in both treatment groups.

Variability of blood pressure was examined by calculating the mean difference of hourly averages of systolic and diastolic pressure in patients on the two regimens (with 95% confidence limits). There was considerable variability during both waking and sleeping with no significant difference between regimens. Figure 3 illustrates this mean difference (once daily regimen of pindolol minus twice daily regimen) with 95% confidence limits of

Table 1: Blood pressures and heart rates in patient receiving twice daily doses of pindolol compared with those patients receiving once a day doses obtained in the office and by the automatic indirect ambulatory blood pressure monitor.

	Office	Control	Pindolol	
			BID	QD
Supine	S ± SD	158 ± 12.78	140 ± 11.15*	141 ± 10.30*
	D ± SD	103 ± 4.09	86 ± 5.82*	87 ± 5.53*
	HR ± SD	74 ± 10.90	71 ± 9.25	74 ± 9.28
Stand	S ± SD	160 ± 14.37	135 ± 10.91*	137 ± 12.44*
	D ± SD	108 ± 4.38	91 ± 6.34*	90 ± 7.30*
	HR ± SD	80 ± 12.18	74 ± 10.29	76 ± 9.86
Ambulatory	*Awake*			
	S ± SD		128 ± 9.4	129 ± 8.5
	D ± SD		85 ± 2.7	85 ± 3.3
	Asleep			
	S ± SD		118 ± 16.3	118 ± 11.2
	D ± SD		75 ± 8.4	74 ± 8.2

* = $p < 0.01$ When pindolol is compared with control by use of a two-sided paired t-test.

217

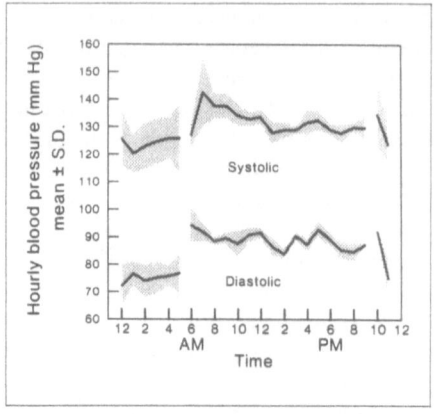

Fig. 2. Ambulatory blood pressures in patients receiving pindolol administered once daily. Shown are hourly means ± one standard deviation. Waking and sleeping periods are indicated by break in graph.

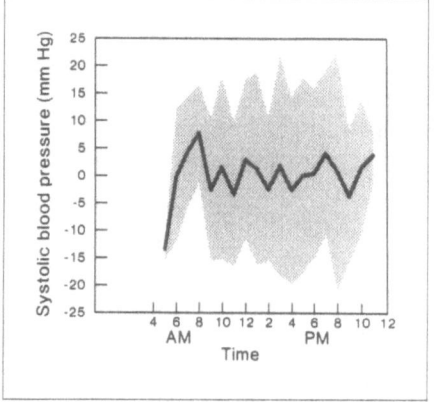

Fig. 3. Mean difference (once daily regimen of pindolol minus twice daily regimen), with 95% confidence limits, of hourly average ambulatory systolic blood pressures while patients were awake.

hourly average ambulatory systolic blood pressures while patients were awake. Figure 4 illustrates cumulative distributions of mean blood pressure differences (day 2 minus day 1) in patients on the two regimens combined. Daily differences of greater than 30 mmHg were quite infrequent but differences of greater than or equal to 10 mmHg occurred approximately 40% of the time.

Discussion

Pindolol is an effective β-adrenergic blocking drug in the lowering of blood pressure (3). It is distinguished from other β-adrenergic blocking drugs by its high intrinsic sympathomimetic activity. The minimal reduction in heart rate after pindolol is of potential value in patients with sinus node dysfunction (4). Gonasun (5) showed that although a dose re-

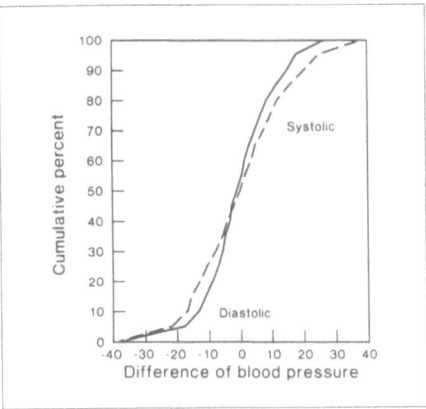

Fig. 4. Cumulative distribution of mean differences (day 2 minus day 1) of ambulatory systolic and diastolic blood pressures. Regimens are combined.

sponse relationship existed between blood pressure decrement and dose of pindolol, no such relationship existed for the change in heart rate. These findings substantiated the observations that the intrinsic sympathomimetic activity of pindolol does not interfere with its antihypertensive effects. Garrett (6) also studied patients receiving hydrochlorothiazide or pindolol or both with the Del Mar Avionics ambulatory monitoring equipment and demonstrated that no change in pulse rate occurred with pindolol and that pindolol provided better 24-hour blood pressure control.

Raftery (2) used various doses of pindolol in crossover experiments in 12 patients, six of whom completed both phases. As determined by the intraarterial blood pressure device, once daily doses of pindolol were as effective as twice daily doses and neither had much effect during the latter part of the night and early morning. Blood pressure was well controlled in our patients by pindolol alone or combined with hydrochlorothiazide or hydralazine or both. Control was manifest in the supine and standing positions at the office and throughout 24 hours as determined by the ambulatory indirect autromtic blood pressure device. Variability of blood pressure was similar on both regimens. Results were not significantly different between administration of pindolol once daily and the administration of the same dose in two equal portions each day. A once daily regimen that is effective can be expected to increase adherence to a drug program, particularly one of long duration as in hypertension.

The effectiveness of the Del Mar Avionics indirect blood pressure recorder has been validated (1). In contrast to the intra-arterial method which records continuously, this technique allows sampling only as often as every 7.5 minutes to provide 150–200 valid blood pressures per 24 hours; thus, diurnal observations could be considered less reliable. However, DiRienzo et al (7) analyzed data obtained by the intra-arterial method by a single beat sampling at 5, 10, 15 and 30 minute intervals and compared the observation to 24-hour averages of all beats. The results for these intervals corresponded closely to 24-hour averages and thus confirmed the applicability of the indirect technique for ambulatory studies of hypertensive patients. Indeed, the median differences between pairs of 24-hour observations of systolic blood pressure was only 8 mmHg in our study. The Del Mar Avionics automatic ambulatory blood pressure monitor reliably confirmed the office and home blood pressure recordings and indicated good control through the waking and sleeping periods of the day. The monitor contributed additional valuable information to standard methods of assessing dosage of antihypertensive medications.

Conclusions

Pindolol lowered systolic and diastolic blood pressure equally well during once a day and twice daily dosage with few side effects. Supine bradycardia was absent, likely attributed to its intrinsic sympathomimetic activity. Blood pressure variability was similar on both regimens. The Del Mar Avionics automatic ambulatory blood pressure monitor reliably confirmed office blood pressure recordings and indicated good control through the waking and sleeping periods of the day. The monitor contributed additional valuable information to standard methods of assessing dosage of antihypertensive medications.

References

1. Sheps SG, Elveback LR, Close EL, Kleven MK, Bissen C: Evaluation of the Del Mar Avionics blood pressure recording device. Mayo Clin Proc 56: 740–743 (1981).
2. Raftery EB, Mann S, BalaSubramanian V, Millar Craig MW: Once daily pindolol in hypertension: An ambulatory assessment. Am Heart J 104: 417–420 (1982).
3. Fanchamps A: Therapeutic trials of pindolol in hypertension: Comparison and combination with other drugs. Am Heart J 104: 388–406 (1982).
4. Dwyer EM Jr, Pepe AJ, Pindernell BH: Effects of beta adrenergic blockade with pindolol versus placebo in coronary patients with stable angina pectoris. Am Heart J 103: 830–833 (1982).
5. Gonasun LM: Antihypertensive effects of pindolol. Am Heart J 104: 374–387 (1982).
6. Garrett BN: Pindolol and hydrochlorothiazide in essential hypertension: A three-way, double-blind, parallel study with 24 hour ambulatory blood pressure measurement (abstract). Clin Pharmacol. Ther 31: 229 (1982).
7. DeRienzo M, Grassi G, Pedotti A, Mancia G: Continuous vs intermittent blood pressure measurements in estimating 24 hour average blood pressure. Hypertension 5: 264–269 (1983).

Address for correspondence:
Sheldon G. Sheps, M.D.
Mayo Clinic
Rochester, MN 55905

A comparison of once daily and twice daily antihypertensive therapy with enalapril using non-invasive ambulatory BP monitoring

Alan H. Gradman, Cathy L. O'Keefe

Summary: Enalapril (MK-421) is a new angiotensin converting enzyme inhibitor with a prolonged duration of action. In order to determine the feasibility of once-a-day dosing with this agent alone and in combination with hydrochlorothiazide, non-invasive ambulatory blood pressure monitoring was used to compare the antihypertensive effectiveness of b.i.d. and q.d. dosing. Patients were first monitored on the b.i.d. regimen, converted to the same total medication dose q.d., and remonitored. Mean blood pressure for the group was $128 \pm 10.4/87 \pm 3.3$. on b.i.d. and $130 \pm 11.1/85 \pm 7.3$ on q.d. (pNS). Analysis of individual patient data showed that b.i.d. dosing appeared to produce superior blood pressure control in two patients, while in ten equal or lower mean 24-hour blood pressures were noted with q.d. dosing. Circadian blood pressure curves revealed that systolic blood pressure was statistically higher during sleep in patients treated q.d. These data indicate that once daily administration of enalapril is an effective treatment strategy for most patients. The clinical significance of the differing patterns of blood pressure variability over 24 hours seen with the two dosing schedules is, however, unknown. The importance of defining the relationship between patterns of blood pressure variability and long-term hypertensive complications is discussed.

Enalapril (MK-421) is a new angiotensin converting enzyme inhibitor which has been shown to be effective in the treatment of hypertension (1, 2) and congestive heart failure (3). A potential advantage of this agent is its relatively prolonged duration of action and previous studies have documented that partial suppression of angiotensin converting enzyme activity persists for more than 24 hours after single oral dose administration (4). In clinical antihypertensive trials to date, the drug has generally been administered on a twice daily basis, though a recent report has demonstrated significant blood pressure reduction with once daily drug dosing (5).

In this study, non-invasive ambulatory blood pressure monitoring was used to critically compare the antihypertensive effects of once daily and twice daily enalapril and enalapril/hydrochlorothiazide administration in a group of patients whose blood pressures were apparently well controlled on a b.i.d. dosing regimen. Our results indicate that mean 24-hour blood pressure is comparable on the two dosing schedules while nocturnal systolic blood pressures tend to be significantly higher and day-time diastolic pressure lower with once daily drug dosing. These data raise important questions as to what exactly constitutes blood pressure "control" and how the technique of ambulatory blood pressure monitoring can best be used to guide antihypertensive drug therapy.

Cardiology Section, West Haven VA Medical Center and Yale University New Haven, Connecticut

Methods

Patient population

The study population consisted of twelve hypertensive men, mean age 55 years, who were patients in the Hypertension Clinic at the West Haven VA Medical Center. All patients were participants in a multicenter trial evaluating the antihypertensive effects of enalapril alone and in combination with hydrochlorothiazide. At the time of entry into the study, nine were receiving 10 mg of enalapril plus 25 mg of hydrochlorothiazide b.i.d. and three were receiving 10 mg of enalapril alone b.i.d. All patients were considered to be well controlled on their medication and had supine diastolic blood pressures in the clinic $\leqslant 90$ mmHg.

Statistical methods

Data are expressed as mean values $\pm$ the standard deviation. Comparisons of clinic blood pressures before and after therapy, mean 24-hour blood pressures on the two dosing regimens, and q2 hourly mean blood pressure for the group were performed using a paired (two-tailed) t-test. Mean 24-hour blood pressure in individual patients on the two regimens was compared using a t-test for unpaired data.

Protocol

Twenty-four hour non-invasive ambulatory blood pressure monitoring (Avionics Pressureometer III) was first performed on the b.i.d. dosing schedule. Patients were then instructed to take the same total daily medication as a single morning dose. Ambulatory blood pressure monitoring was repeated on the q.d. regimen.

To eliminate spurious values resulting from patient movement or environmental noise and vibration, ambulatory blood pressure data were edited using a modification of previously published criteria (6, 7). Blood pressure readings with the following characteristics were deemed artifactual: (1) diastolic blood pressure $\leqslant 40$ or $\geqslant 140$ mmHg; (2) systolic blood pressure $\leqslant 50$ or $\geqslant 255$ mmHg; (3) pulse pressure $< (0.14 \times$ diastolic blood pressure$) - 17$ mmHg. Using these criteria approximately 10% of the 70–200 readings obtained in each monitoring day were excluded from analysis.

Results

Initial blood pressure response to enalapril and enalapril/HCTZ

The effect of enalapril and enalapril/HCTZ on mean supine systolic and diastolic blood pressure in the clinic is shown in Figure 1. Mean systolic pressure decreased from 156 ± 16 mmHg on placebo to 124 ± 9.7 mmHg (p < 0.001), while mean diastolic blood pressures decreased from 104 ± 3.8 to 84 ± 3.4 mmHg (p < 0.001) on twice daily dosing. As stated above, all patients achieved a supine clinic diastolic blood pressure $\leqslant 90$ mmHg.

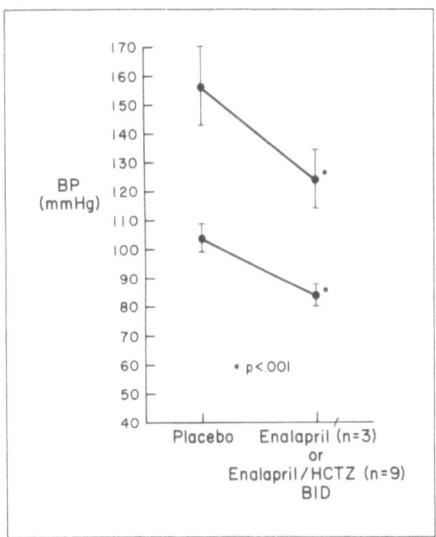

Fig. 1. Effect of enalapril, alone and in combination with hydrochlorothiazide on clinic blood pressures (n = 12).

Comparison of b.i.d. and q.d. drug dosing

A comparison of the mean 24-hour systolic and diastolic blood pressures on the two dosing schedules is given in Figure 2. Mean blood pressure for the group was $128 \pm 10.4/87 \pm 3.3$ on b.i.d. dosing and $130 \pm 11.1/85 \pm 7.3$ during q.d. dosing. No significant difference was noted for either systolic or diastolic pressure. In Figure 3 are shown the mean systolic and diastolic blood pressures for each individual subject on the two dosing regimens. There was no significant difference in either systolic or diastolic pressure in five subjects. In one patient, both systolic and diastolic pressures were statistically higher on the q.d. regimen; in another, a statistically higher systolic but not diastolic pressure was observed with once daily therapy. One subject demonstrated statistically

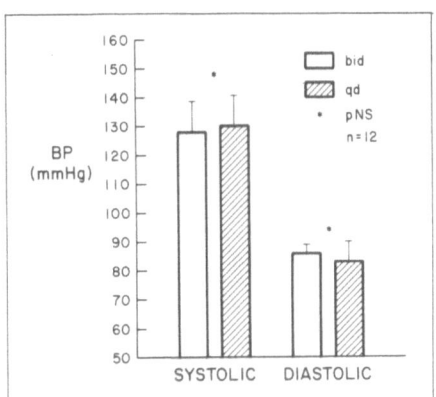

Fig. 2. Comparison of mean 24-hour blood pressure in patients treated b.i.d. and q.d. with enalapril and enalapril/HCTZ (n = 12).

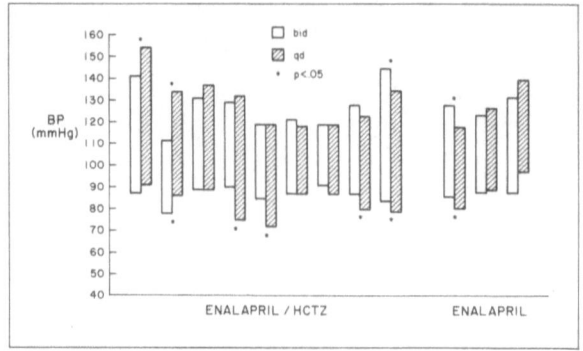

Fig. 3. Comparison of mean 24-hour blood pressure in individual patients treated b.i.d. and q.d. with enalapril and enalapril/HCTZ (n = 12).

lower systolic and diastolic pressures on the q.d. regimen and in four the diastolic but not the systolic pressure was lower with once-a-day dosing. Thus, two subjects appeared to show an advantage of b.i.d. dosing while in ten mean blood pressures were equal or lower during q.d. therapy.

In order to determine the effectiveness of a single a.m. dose in controlling blood pressure over 24 hours, circadian blood pressure curves were constructed for the two dosing regimens (Figure 4). Only patients in whom complete or near complete night-time blood pressures were recorded are included in this analysis (n = 6). The data indicate that systolic blood pressure was statistically higher during the 6 hour period from midnight to 6 a.m. on q.d. therapy. Thus, patients exhibited mean systolic pressures in the 130 mmHg range during sleep on b.i.d. compared to approximately 120 mmHg during q.d. dosing. Diastolic blood pressures were not significantly different during this same time period. In addition, diastolic blood pressure between noon and 2 p.m. (approximately 4–6 hours after a.m. drug ingestion) was statistically lower when patients were given their total medication dose in morning. No other differences in either systolic or diastolic pressures were noted throughout the 24-hour period.

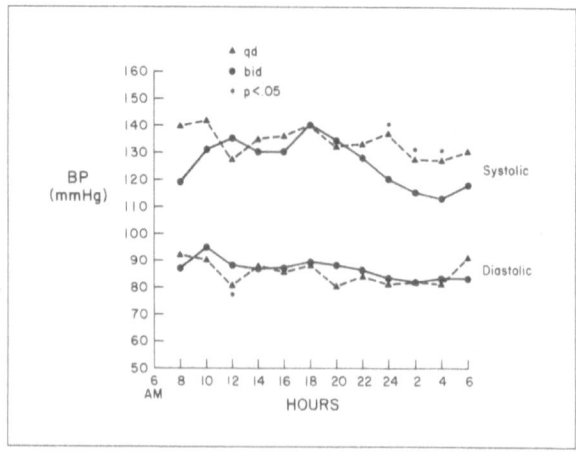

Fig. 4. Mean blood pressure over 24 hours in patients treated b.i.d. and q.d. with enalapril and enalapril/HCTZ (n = 6).

Discussion

The recent upsurge in interest in ambulatory blood pressure monitoring stems from the observation that single or even multiple blood pressure determinations performed in the artificial setting of the physician's office are frequently unrepresentative of a patient's "true" blood pressure status (8). Nevertheless, physicians have long relied upon these imperfect data to guide antihypertensive drug therapy and much of our thinking about what constitutes effective blood pressure "control" is based upon single blood pressure readings. Ambulatory blood pressure monitoring, by sampling blood pressure repeatedly over 24 hours, allows a much more accurate calculation of mean arterial pressure. Previous studies suggest that this 24-hour mean is superior to random clinic pressures in predicting long-term hypertensive vascular complications (9). Presumably, it is also a better guide to the adequacy of drug therapy.

In this study, we sought to use ambulatory blood pressure monitoring to answer seemingly simple clinical questions – must enalapril and enalapril/hydrochlorothiazide be given twice daily to achieve a satisfactory antihypertensive response, or is once daily dosing sufficient? Our results indicate that for the study group, mean arterial pressure is virtually identical on the two treatment schedules. Furthermore, analysis of individual patient data suggests that blood pressure control achieved with q.d. dosing was equal or superior to b.i.d. dosing in 10/12 (83%) patients studied. Based upon these observations, we believe that enalapril is a suitable once-a-day drug and, in fact, have converted many of our patients to this treatment schedule.

It is important to recognize, however, that the above conclusion is based entirely upon a consideration of *mean* 24-hour blood pressure. In addition to allowing more precise calculation of this mean, ambulatory monitoring furnishes additional information concerning blood pressure variability. In this study, analysis of circadian blood pressure patterns on the two dosing schedules reveals that systolic pressure during sleep is significantly higher and day-time diastolic pressure somewhat lower when patients receive their total daily medication as a single morning dose. It is apparent that the two treatment schedules produce comparable mean arterial pressures but differing patterns of blood pressure variability over the course of the diurnal cycle. Whether patterns of blood pressure over time are important determinants of long-term complication rate in hypertensive individuals is presently unknown. In view of this ignorance, it is difficult to conclude definitively that the two dosing schedules are, in fact, equally beneficial.

It becomes apparent that a more sophisticated definition of what constitutes blood pressure "control" is needed. It is easy in the clinic setting to set a goal blood pressure and define control as a pressure equal to or lower than that value. When viewed over 24 hours, however, it is appreciated that blood pressure often varies dramatically. Normotensive individuals frequently exhibit pressures in the hypertensive range and hypertensives frequently display normal or even low pressures for many hours of the day and especially at night. The relative importance of mean blood pressure over time, of blood pressure peaks and of "resting" the vasculature during normotensive sleep on long-term prognosis is currently unclear and may, in fact, be different for different hypertensive complications. Thus, most studies have shown that while conventional antihypertensive drug therapy is successful in reducing the risk of cerebrovascular events, it is not effective in reducing morbidity and mortality from coronary artery disease (10). A better understanding of the pathophysiology of hypertensive complications and the relationship of blood pressure variability patterns to their occurrence are needed if more useful definitions of blood pressure control are to be developed.

There are many reasons to speculate, for example, that peaks in blood pressure may be important determinants of vascular complications. In patients with coronary artery disease, myocardial oxygen consumption is largely determined by the systemic arterial pressure (afterload). If a patient develops a very high blood pressure for even a short period of time, this could precipitate angina pectoris or an acute myocardial infarction. Similarly, in patients with chronic congestive heart failure due to left ventricular dysfunction, acute increases in afterload may well produce pulmonary edema.

The prognostic importance of nocturnal blood pressure reduction in preventing hypertensive vascular damage is also unknown. Investigators have noted that both normotensive and hypertensive individuals usually show significant blood pressure reduction during sleep (11). Established criteria concerning what constitutes normal blood pressure, however, are based entirely upon epidemiologic observations relating to the prognostic implications of day-time blood pressures. While pressures up to 140/90 are generally considered normal in the awake patient, no definition of normal blood pressure during sleep is presently available, and the independent prognostic impact of night-time blood pressure has not been explored. This question is particularly relevant to the current study, as patients receiving enalapril once daily demonstrated systolic pressures that were statistically higher during sleep, though still within what is usually considered to be the normal range. It is impossible to determine based upon current knowledge whether the relatively lower nocturnal systolic pressures achievable with twice daily enalapril dosing constitutes a real advantage or are clinically irrelevant.

An additional problem in the use of ambulatory blood pressure monitoring concerns the interpretation of individual patient, as opposed to grouped, blood pressure responses. Thus, several patients in this study demonstrated statistically different systolic and/or diastolic blood pressures on the two monitoring days. It would be premature to conclude, however, that these differences are due solely to differences in the enalapril dosing schedule. While considerable attention has been paid to hour-by-hour blood pressure variability, little is known about blood pressure variability from day to day. It is well recognized that other clinical variables such as premature ventricular contraction frequency vary greatly from day to day (12). Reproducability studies have shown that statistically different PVC frequencies often occur between monitoring days without intervening change in treatment status. Further studies are needed to determine if this is also the case with ambulatory blood pressure data.

This question is of particular importance in the conduct of antihypertensive drug therapy and in interpreting the results of the present study. It is well known that patients may display significant differences in the absorption, metabolism, and excretion of pharmacologic agents and it is quite possible that some subjects require b.i.d. enalapril dosing while others can be equally well-controlled with once-a-day therapy. Ideally, ambulatory blood pressure data should be used to individualize therapy by directly observing the duration of treatment effects. Until further data are available, however, considerable caution must be exercised before assuming that a single day of monitoring is sufficient to characterize blood pressure status.

In summary, the results of the present study suggests that once daily administration of enalapril alone and in combination with hydrochlorothiazide is an effective treatment strategy for most patients. The study raises many questions, however, as to the long-term implications of diurnal blood pressure variations and the interpretation of individual patient data. It is important to remember that effective blood pressure "control" must be defined as the achievement of a long-term blood pressure profile *not* associated with increased risk of cardiovascular, cerebrovascular or renal complications. As discussed earlier, the determinants of such a "safe" blood pressure profile are largely unknown. By helping to provide answers to these questions, ambulatory blood pressure monitoring may be able to make an extremely important contribution to understanding the pathophysiology and improving the treatment of arterial hypertensive states.

Acknowledgement

The authors wish to express their sincere appreciation to Mrs. Gail Beer for expert assistance in preparation of this manuscript.

References

1. Gavras H, Waeber B, Gavras I, Biollaz J, Brunner HR, Davies RO: Antihypertensive effect of the new oral angiotensin converting enzyme inhibitor "MK-421." Lancet 543–546 (Sept. 1981).
2. Chrysant SG, Brown RD, Kem DC, Brown JL: Antihypertensive and metabolic effects of a new converting enzyme inhibitor, enalapril. Clin Pharmacol Ther. 33: 741–746 (1983).
3. Cody RJ, Covit AB, Schaer GL, Laragh JH: Evaluation of a long-acting converting enzyme inhibitor (enalapril) for the treatment of chronic congestive heart failure. J Am Coll Cardiol 1 (4): 1154–9 (1983).
4. Millar JA, Derkx FHM, McLean K, et al: Pharmacodynamics of converting enzyme inhibitions: The cardiovascular, endocrine and autonomic effects of MK-421 (enalapril) and MK-521. Br J Clin Pharmac 14: 347–355 (1982).
5. Bergstrand R, Johansson, Vedin A, Wilhelmsson C: Comparison of once-a-day and twice-a-day dosage regimens of enalapril (MK-421) in patients with mild hypertension. Br J Pharmacol 14(1): 136P–137P (1982).
6. Pickering TG, Harshfield GA, Kleinert HD, Blank S, Laragh JH: Blood pressure during normal daily activities, sleep, and exercise. JAMA 247: 992–1003 (1982).
7. Kennedy HL, Padgett NE, Horan MJ: Performance reliability of the Del Mar Avionics non-invasive ambulatory blood pressure instrument in clinical use. Ambulatory Electrocardiology 1(4): 13–16 (1979).
8. Perloff D, Sokolow M, Cowan R: Clinical relevance of ambulatory blood pressure measurements. Biotelemetry Patient Monitg 8: 67–80 (1981).
9. Perloff D, Sokolow M, Cowan R: The prognostic value of ambulatory blood pressures: JAMA 249: 2792–2798 (1983).
10. Kaplan NM: Systemic Hypertension: Therapy. In: Braunwald E, Heart disease: A textbook of cardiovascular medicine. pp. 922–951, W.B. Saunders Company (Philadelphia, London and Toronto 1980).
11. Richardson DW, Honour AJ, Fenton GW, Stott FH, Pickering GW: Variation in arterial pressure throughout the day and night. Cli Sci 26: 445–460 (1964).
12. Morganroth J, Michelson EL, Horowitz LN, Josephson ME, Pearlman AS, Dunkman WB: Limitations of routine long-term electrocardiographic monitoring to assess ventricular ectopic frequency. Circulation 58: 408–414 (1978).

Address for correspondence:
Alan H. Gradman, M.D.
Chief, Cardiology Section/111B
West Haven VA Medical Center
West Spring Street, West Haven
Connecticut 06516

Continuous blood pressure monitoring in the evaluation of the effectiveness of antihypertensive drugs

Marianne Frisk-Holmberg

Summary: The evaluation of the duration of action of antihypertensive agents requires devices that can measure blood pressure repetitively during a prolonged period of observations. In order to be of value in the clinical setting, these devices must be safe, comfortable, and accurate. In this study, the conventional mercury sphygmomanometer has been used to test the accuracy of two automated blood pressure-measuring systems: the Dinamap and the Avionics Pressurometer III. The Dinamap is a non-portable device that is capable of automatically measuring and recording blood pressure at pre-set intervals during a period of several hours. The blood pressure is measured through a conventional cuff, but is dependent upon oscillometric signals rather than the auscultation of the Korotkoff sounds. When blood pressures measured with the Dinamap equipment during the evaluation of antihypertensive therapy were compared with blood pressures measured by a mercury sphygmomanometer, there were strong correlations (in the supine posture) for both systolic ($r = 0.84$) and for mean ($r = 0.82$) blood pressures, although the correlation between the diastolic blood pressures appeared weaker ($r = 0.66$). In the standing position, the correlations for both the diastolic and mean blood pressures were less powerful than they had been in the supine posture; moreover, the regression line did not pass through the origin. The Avionics Pressurometer III is a portable device that repetitively measures blood pressure while the patient is able to go about his daily routine. It utilizes an auscultatory method (via a small microphone under the cuff) for determining the blood pressure. The correlations between Pressurometer and conventional sphygmomanometer blood pressures did not appear to change with posture; for systolic blood pressure the correlations were $r = 0.82$ and $r = 0.80$ in the supine and standing positions, and for diastolic blood pressures the correlations were $r = 0.66$ and $r = 0.60$. Although the accuracy of these automated non-invasive methods for repetitively measuring blood pressures appears to be quite reasonable in this early experience, problems of reproducibility and artifacts remain to be dealt with, and it is also clear that a high degre of patient cooperation and education is required to allow these methodologies to be effective. Thus, more testing may be required before these automated devices can be used confidently in the evaluation of the effectiveness of antihypertensive therapy.

Introduction

When epidemiological studies and clinical drug trials are performed, the following requirements should be fulfilled for repetitive long-term accurate blood pressure measurements. First of all the arterial blood pressure should be recorded by a reliable, comfortable device, and secondly the hazards should be low. Regarding reliability, intra-arterial measurements of pressure seem incomparable, but have strong drawbacks due to hazards and lack of comfort. In the context of comfort, the need for surveillance of the patient and for sterility are major concerns. Non-invasive pressure recorders are therefore those most commonly used.

Clinical Pharmacology, Uppsala University Hospital

Since Riva Rocci introduced the mercury sphygmomanometer most blood pressure re-cordings have been performed with this device (1). However, it is connected with some potential sources for inaccuracy: the manometer; the width of the cuff; the circumference of the patient's arm; and his peripheral circulation (2). For many years several automatic and semi-automatic devices have been used in clinical trial methodoloy and in intensive care units. High expectations have been connected with these devices. Initially, it was thought that they would provide advantages compared to the conventional device, espe-cially concerning time-saving and comfort. The possibility of a simultaneous data com-putation was a further advantage. The initial expectations that these automatic devices could be used for continuous recordings in research, intensive care and as simple home blood pressure devices have, however, not been fulfilled. They have to be used by a skilled observer and a co-operative patient, as will be demonstrated in this presentation.

Methods

The following results are drawn from an investigation in which, during the clinical trial of antihypertensive drugs, the conventional mercury sphygmomanometer, using a ran-dom zero device, has been compared with the Dinamap 845 and the Avionics Pressuro-meter III Model 1978. A mercury sphygmomanometer can be connected to both of these non-invasive automatic devices so as to check their accuracy. The Dinamap works with an oscillometric technique. Its cuff inflates automatically (1–16 minutes interval). Sys-tolic and diastolic, MAP and heart rate are displayed digitally. The device is suitable for continuous measurements, the accurate upper pressure limit being $\leqslant 220$ mmHg. The Avionics is a portable device for continuous recordings, weighs about 1 kg and should be used when the patient pursues his daily activities. The transducer has an accuracy of 1 mmHg in the operating range of 50–220 mmHg. Pressures up to 245 can be recorded. Through a datorized device, time-correlated digital print-outs or graphic plots are made. Time selection for measurements is from 7.5 to 30 minutes (3).
In both trials blood pressures were measured after 10 minutes supine rest or one minute standing, manually on the same arm, either one minute before or one minute after the automatic registration. Four blood pressure measurements in the supine and standing po-sitions were selected randomly from each patient. Comparison of data was made by the paired t-test. Systolic and diastolic blood pressures (phase V) were registered.

Results

In one group of essential hypertensive patients (n = 8) undergoing an effect duration trial of alfuzosine 5 mg b.i.d. (L.E.R.S., an alpha – adrenoceptor blocker in phase II develop-ment) the Dinamap was compared with the conventional method.
The supine systolic blood pressure showed a higher correlation (r = 0.84) than the MAP (r = 0.82) (Fig. 1) and the diastolic blood pressure (r = 0.66). In the standing position the correlations, especially for the MAP and the diastolic pressures, became less (Fig. 2). Moreover, the regression-line did not pass through the origin. The Dinamap in all mea-surements undervalued the sphygmomanometer value. To investigate if the deviations were due to factors in the device or in the patient the blood-pressure was registered twice

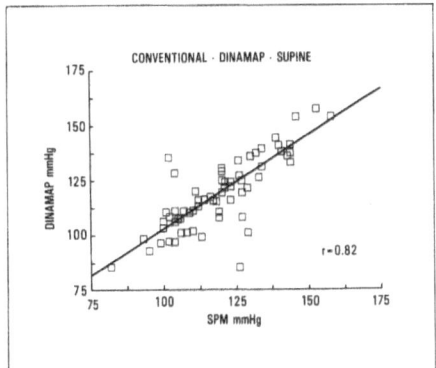

Fig. 1. The relationship betweent the supine MAP (mean arterial blood pressure) when measured by Dinamap (y-axis) and the mercury sphygmomanometer (x-axis): r = 0.82.

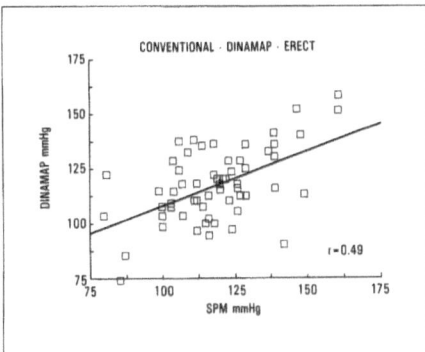

Fig. 2. The relationship between the erect MAP when measured by Dinamap (y-axis) and the mercury sphygmomanometer (x-axis): r = 0.49.

with the Dinamap at two minutes intervals. The correlation coefficient, however, remained the same, indicating that factors in the device were responsible for the low correlation. The measurements were, however, relatively unsensitive to how the cuff was placed. If the device was applied on the same patient at a distance of up to 180 ° from its original position over the brachial artery, the blood pressure recorded change relatively little compared to the original measurements.

The Avionics device was evaluated in another trial (in six hypertensive patients) of the effectiveness and duration of action of the alpha-agonist, guanfacine (Sandoz). The correlation between the systolic blood-pressure (r = 0.82) was higher than for the diastolic (r = 0.66). When the body position was changed from supine to erect, the correlations changed to r = 0.80 and r = 0.60 respectively. Various mistakes in the print-outs were seen and unless patients were carefully superintended, we had several problems with this device (Fig. 3). The most apparent disadvantage was, however, the weight of the device. Moreover it requires a high patient co-operation and the arm must be absolutely still during inflation and measurement to avoid artificial readings.

The present investigation demonstrates a low agreement between blood pressures when measured with automatic devices and the conventional sphygmomanometer. One explan-

231

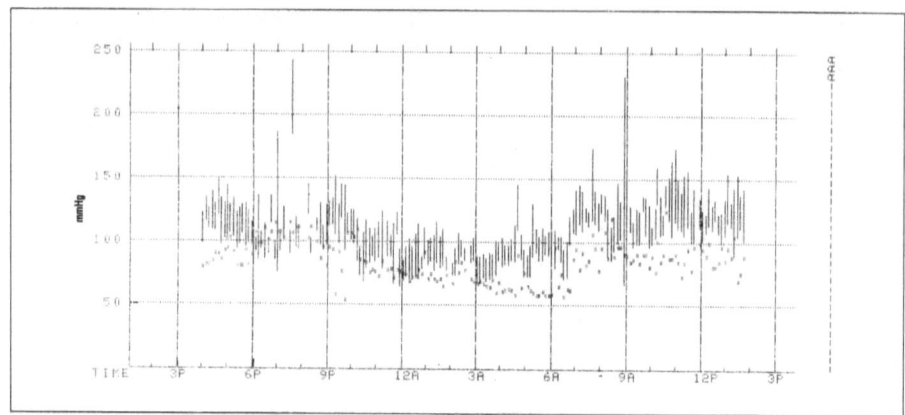

Fig. 3. A real-time data print-out of blood pressure and heart rate when measured by Avionics Pressurometer III.

ation for the disagreement is certainly the fact that different techniques are used; oscillometry, auscultatory microphones, and human auscultation. The advantages of the automatic devices, such as observer and patient freedom, are not counter-balanced by their disadvantages: validity. Another important factor in both clinical surveillance and clinical trials is that the patient/observer contact may be lost. This is usually of the utmost importance for the successful outcome of both the clinical management and clinical trial programme.

References

1. Rushmer RF: Cardiovascular dynamics. pp 176–186, WB Saunder (New York 1976).
2. Krikendall WM, Feinleib M, Freis ED, Mark AL: AHA Committee report recommendations for human blood pressure determination by sphygmomanometers. Circulation 62: 1146 A (1980).
3. Automatic non-invasive blood pressure and heart rate monitoring with tabular and trend write-outs. Del Mar Avionics 1976 (unpublished).

Address for correspondence:
Dr. M. Frisk-Holmberg
Clinical Pharmacology
Uppsala University Hospital
S-75014 Uppsala
Sweden

Intra-arterial ambulatory blood pressure monitoring in the assessment of antihypertensive drugs

R. I. Jones, B. A. Gould, R. S. Hornung, S. Mann, E. B. Raftery

Summary: Direct measurement of blood pressure in ambulatory patients was performed with the intra-arterial "Oxford System" to assess the effectiveness of differing antihypertensive agents. The beta-blocker, metoprolol (200 mg daily), decreased daytimed blood pressure from 174/95 mmHg to 158/85 mmHg; the combination of metoprolol and chlorthalidone (25 mg daily) further decreased the mean daytime pressure to 143/78 mmHg (p < 0.001 systolic, p < 0.005 diastolic). The calcium channel blockers, nifedipine (20–40 mg twice daily) and verapamil (120–160 mg three times daily), each significantly decreased the mean hourly blood pressure during most of the day (23 of 24 hours with nifedipine, 15 of 24 hours of verapamil). Heart rate did not change with nifedipine, but decreased significantly with verapamil. The angiotensin converting enzyme inhibitor, enalopril (20–40 mg daily), significantly decreased blood pressure for 18 of 24 hours, the antihypertensive effect being most pronounced during the daytime period. These experiences indicate that the technique of direct ambulatory blood pressure monitoring is of value in studying both the efficacy and the duration of antihypertensive treatment.

Introduction

Indirect methods of blood pressure measurement for the assessment of antihypertensive drugs allow only a small number of blood pressure readings of limited accuracy to be obtained and the results are susceptible to a placebo effect. The technique of ambulatory recording of direct arterial blood pressure allows a profile of action of such drugs to be obtained throughout 24 hours and the results are not influenced by placebo therapy (1). Using this technique it is also possible to measure blood pressure continuously during various physiological tests and to accurately assess the effect of antihypertensive drugs on the blood pressure responses. We have used this technique to study a number of antihypertensive agents, and in this paper the effects of three differing classes of drugs will be discussed:

1. Beta adrenoceptor blockers
   (a) Metoprolol (200 mg once daily) and placebo (once daily).
   (b) Metoprolol (200 mg) and chlorthalidone (25 mg once daily).

Department of Cardiology & Division of Clinical Sciences, Northwick Park Hospital & Clinical Research Centre, Watford Road, Harrow, Middlesex, HA1 3UJ, UK.

233

2. Calcium ion antagonists
   (a) Nifedipine (20–40 mg twice daily).
   (b) Verapamil (120–160 mg three times daily).

3. Angiotensin converting enzyme inhibitors
   (a) Enalapril (20–40 mg once daily).

Methods

Because of the lack of effect of placebo on directly measured arterial blood pressure, two of these studies were of open design. The third (metoprolol and chlorthalidone) was a double blind randomised crossover study. Patients were included in these studies on the basis of a mean of three clinic blood pressure readings (using a conventional sphygmomanometer) of > 160/100 mmHg after four weeks on no antihypertensive treatment.

The equipment used (the "Oxford System") has previously been described in detail (2). Patients initially underwent a period of 24-hour monitoring on no antihypertensive therapy. During this period they were allowed to be ambulant within their own environment, returning to the hospital at 12-hourly intervals for equipment calibration. Patients then started the active drug, and after a period of dose titration a secod 24-hour period of recording was performed. In the study of metoprolol and chlorthalidone patients were initially randomised to receive either metoprolol and placebo or metoprolol and chlorthalidone. A second intra-arterial recording was then performed after four weeks. Patients were switched to the alternative regime and a third study was performed after a further four weeks.

During each period of ambulatory monitoring patients performed a planned program of physiological testing consisting of:
(1) 20 minutes supine rest
(2) 5 minutes of head-up tilt at 60°
(3) Isometric exercise using a hand grip dynanometer held at 50% maximum voluntary contraction for 2 minutes
(4) Graded cycle ergometry at increasing workloads of 250, 400, 700 and 1000 kpm in three minute stages.

Data analysis

The data from these studies was analysed by means of a hybrid computer (3). Mean hourly data for each patient was pooled for corresponding hours of the day and pre- and post- therapy differences for blood pressure and heart rate were assessed for statistical significance using Student's paired t-test (two-tailed). The supine rest, isometric exercise and dynamic exercise data were computed using a digitising programme on a hybrid computer. During the last five minutes of supine rest a mean pressure over the last 30 beats of each minute was compared. For head-up tilt the mean pressures over consecutive 10 beat periods were computed for the first 200 beats; for isometric exercise the mean systolic and diastolic pressure over 20 beats every 30 s were computed and the peak response extracted; for dynamic exercise the mean pressures over 30 beats at the end of the final minute at each exercise level were digitised for further analysis. For each physiological test heart rate data was derived in the same way as blood pressure data. The pre- and post-therapy differences were for blood pressure and heart rate again assessed for significance using Student's t-test (two tailed) on paired data. When paired data were missing because of different exercise times in the same patient these data were omitted from the analysis.

Results

(a) Metoprolol and chlorthalidone (4)

30 patients took part in this study. The twenty-four hour circadian curves before treatment, and after treatment with metoprolol and placebo and metoprolol and chlorthalidone are shown (Fig. 1). Both treatments appreciably reduced blood pressure and pulse rate; mean daytime intra-arterial blood pressure was reduced from 174/95 to 158/85 by metoprolol plus placebo and to 143/78 by metoprolol plus chlorthalidone. The reduction in blood pressure by the combined treatment was significantly greater than with metoprolol and placebo (p systolic = 0.001, p diastolic = 0.004).

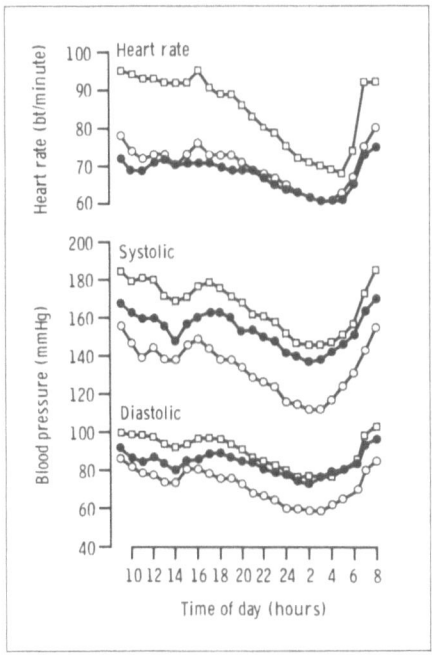

Fig. 1. Circadian curves for systolic and diastolic blood pressure and heart rate (n = 30). □ Pre treatment; ● Metoprolol and placebo; ○ Metoprolol and chlorthalidone.

Side effects

Three patients withdrew with side effects. One because of severe dyspepsia, one because of transient ischaemic attacks and one with depression.

(b) Nifedipine (5)

Seventeen patients completed this study using nifedipine tablets given twice daily. The effects of nifedipine on 24-hour ambulatory blood pressure is shown (Fig. 2). There was a substantial reduction in both systolic and diastolic BP throughout the 24-hour period. A within-patient statistical comparison (paired t test) showed the reduction in both systolic and diastolic BP to be highly significant for 23 of the 24 one hourly periods. The heart rate was not significantly changed by twice daily therapy. Fifteen patients produced suitable data for analysis during physiological testing. At the end of supine rest BP was significantly reduced after therapy with nifedipine (p < 0.001). However, there was no additional orthostatic fall in BP in response to tilting. Peak values for systolic and diastolic BP obtained during isometric exercise were significantly reduced by therapy (p < 0.001) although the rate of rise and magnitude of the response was unaltered (Fig. 3). Similarly during dynamic exercise systolic and diastolic BP were uniformly lower during each minute of exercise although the rate and magnitude of rise were unaffected.

Fig. 2. Circadian curves for systolic and diastolic blood pressure and heart rate before and after treatment with nifedipine.

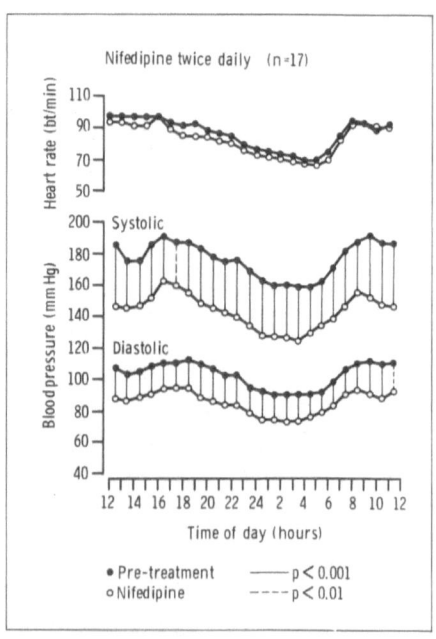

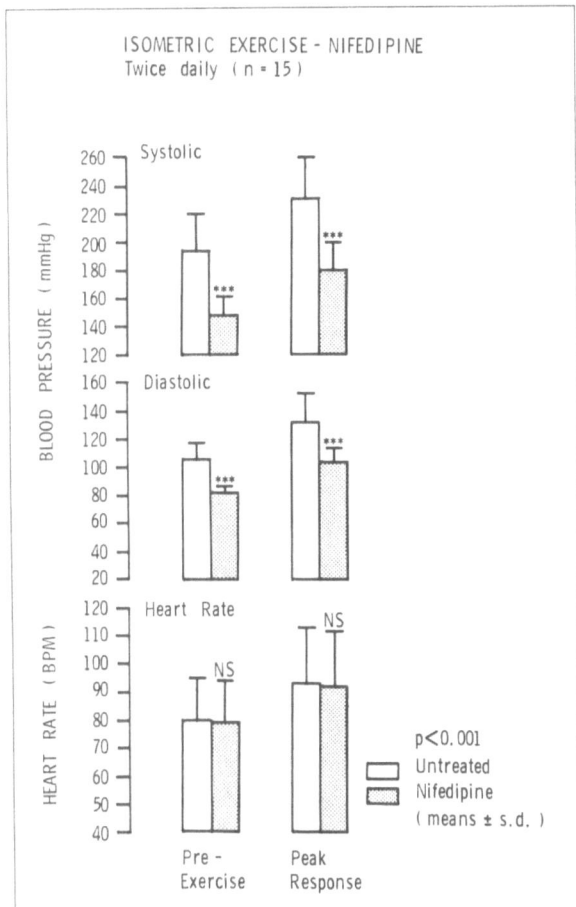

Fig. 3. Systolic and diastolic blood pressure and heart rate at rest and at peak isometric exercise following treatment with nifedipine.

Side effects

No patients developed side effects severe enough to warrant withdrawal of therapy. Three patients developed ankle oedema without change in body weight. One patient developed headache and giddiness and two patients complained of facial flushing within one hour of the dose.

(c) Verapamil (6)

Sixteen patients completed this study. The effect of verapamil on 24-hour ambulatory blood pressure is shown (Fig. 4). There was a statistically significant reduction in systolic and diastolic blood pressure for 15 out of the 24 hours and the hourly mean heart rate was significantly reduced for 19 out of the 24 hours in contrast to nifedipine. There was no evidence of postural hypotension with verapamil and the pressor response to dynamic and isometric exercise was not attenuated.

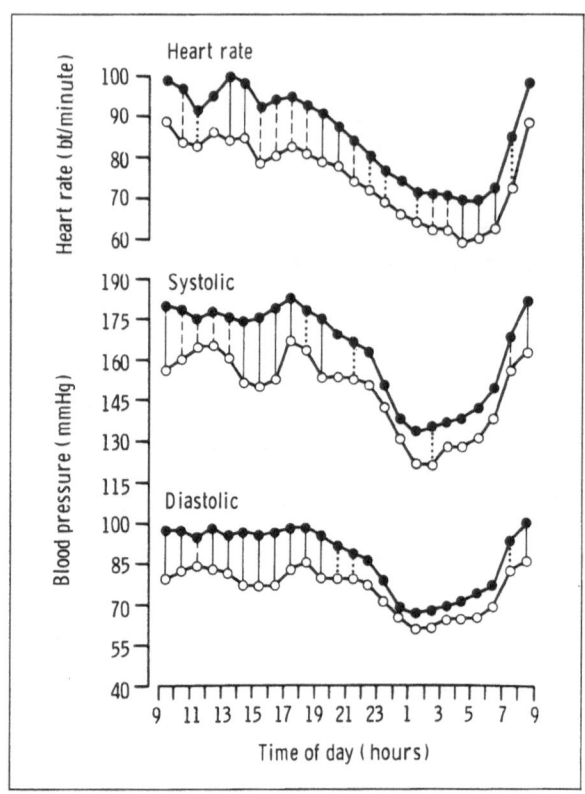

Fig. 4. Circadian curves for systolic and diastolic blood pressure and heart rate before (●) and after (○) treatment with verapamil (n = 16). ····· p < 0.05; --- p < 0.01; ——— p < 0.001.

Side effects

Four patients developed constipation. One patient developed epigastric pain and two patients developed facial pains and burning in the gums.

(d) Enalapril

Fifteen patients completed this study. The effect of enalapril on 24-hour blood pressure is shown (Fig. 5). The mean daytime intra-arterial blood pressure (mmHg) calculated by averaging the mean hourly blood pressure between 12.00 hours and 18.00 hours was reduced from 180 ± 25.3 to 152 ± 26.3 for systolic ($p < 0.01$) and from 109 ± 13.3 to

93 ± 14.9 for diastolic ($p < 0.01$). Both systolic and diastolic blood pressure were significantly reduced for eighteen out of the 24 hours ($p < 0.05$–$p < 0.001$). Three patients increased their blood pressure following therapy with enalapril. For the remaining twelve patients there was a significant correlation between the pretreatment with intra-arterial daytime blood pressure and the reduction in pressure in response to treatment ($r = 0.679$; $p < 0.001$). Following head up tilt there was an additional othostatic fall in blood pressure from $157 \pm 24.5/87 \pm 16.0$ to $138 \pm 25.7/84 \pm 21.6$ ($p < 0.01$ systolic $p = NS$ diastolic) (Fig. 6).

Side effects

One patient complained of mild postural hypotension during this study.

Discussion

The results of these highlight some of the advantages of intra-arterial ambulatory blood pressure monitoring in the study of antihypertensive drugs. The duration of action and ef-

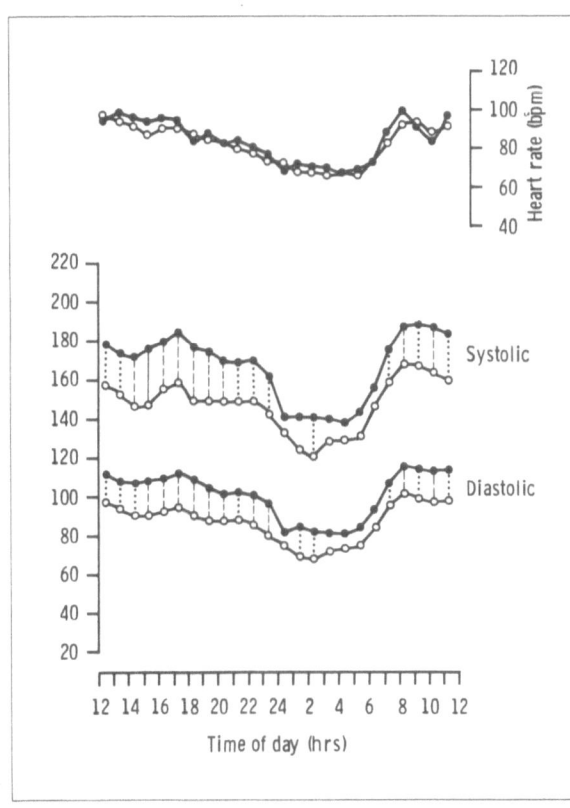

Fig. 5. Circadian curves for systolic and diastolic blood pressure and heart rate before (●) and after (○) 20–40 mg o.d. of enalapril (n = 15). ····· $p < 0.05$; $---$ $p < 0.01$; ———— $p < 0.001$.

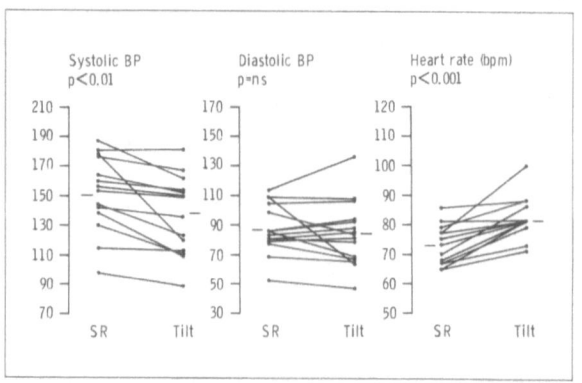

Fig. 6. Individual responses of systolic and diastolic blood pressure and heart rate to 60° head up tilt, following therapy with enalapril (n = 15).

ficacy of antihypertensive drugs can be accurately studies in this way which also provides information on the effect of drugs on the underlying circadian rhythm of blood pressure. Early studies in our department have shown the method to be reproducible and the results not invalidated by short term variations in activity (7, 8). Direct pressure is not affected by placebo therapy which simplifies the way in which such studies can be performed. The results of the metoprolol study demonstrate that this agent alone effectively lowered the daytime blood pressure, but had little effect on blood pressure between 3.00 hours and 8.00 hours. This response is closely similar to that of other beta adrenoceptor blocking drugs that we have reported (9, 10). We have explained this by postulating that the rise of pressure before awakening is due to intense sympathetic activity mediated at the ateriole by an alpha receptor. Thiazide diuretics exert their antihypertensive effect by virtue of direct arteriolar vasodilation and this study demonstrates that the net effect on the circadian curve is an overall lowering of values without any change in the shape of the curve. Therapy with nifedipine produced a smooth reduction in blood pressure throughout 24 hours but the absence of a reflex tachycardia is clearly demonstrated. During both isometric and dynamic exercise there was no alteration of the rate of rise of blood pressure which is consistent with a drug acting directly on smooth muscle without affecting sympathetic reflexes. Verapamil produced a similar reduction in blood pressure to nifedipine. However, the bradycardia following verapamil therapy can be clearly seen, and is in keeping with the drug's known action on the sinus node.

Enalapril is a new long acting angiotensin converting enzyme inhibitor. Twenty-four hour ambulatory monitoring following enalapril therapy suggests that this drug may be effective in a once daily dosage. Separate analyses of the two groups of patients taking 20 mg or 40 mg daily revealed that the fall in blood pressure was greatest in these patients subsequently controlled on 20 mg daily suggesting that increasing the dosage above this level may confer little benefit. Continous monitoring of blood pressure during 60° head up tilt allows the short term effects of drugs on this response to be studied. Following enalapril treatment, the additional othostatic fall in blood pressure occurring during the first fifteen seconds of tilt is clearly demonstrated.

These studies demonstrate that important aspects of antihypertensive therapy can be more closely studied using intra-arterial monitoring. Despite the fact that this technique

240

is invasive we have now performed over 1,500 studies in our department with no major complications and the procedure is well tolerated by patients. Until an entirely accurate method for non-invasively measuring ambulatory blood pressure is developed, this technique must remain one of the most important available for the assessment of antihypertensive drugs.

References

1. Gould BA, Mann S, Davies AB, Altman DG, Raftery EB: Does placebo lower blood pressure? Lancet ii 1377–1381 (1981).
2. Millar Craig MW, Hawes D, Whittington J: A new system for recording ambulatory blood pressure in man. Med Biol Eng & Comput 16: 727–31 (1978).
3. Cashman PMM, Stott FD, Millar Craig MW: Hybrid system for fast data reduction of long term pressure recordings. Med Biol Eng & Comput 17: 629–35 (1979).
4. Kieso HA, Gould BA, Mann S, Hornung RS, Altman DG, Raftery EB: Effect on intra-arterial blood pressure of slow release metoprolol combined with placebo or chlorthalidone. British Med J 287: 717–20 (1983).
5. Hornung RS, Gould BA, Jones RI, Sonecha TN, Raftery EB: Nifedipine tablets for systemic hypertension: A study using continuous ambulatory intra-arterial recording. Am J Cardiol 51: 1323–27 (1983).
6. Gould BA, Mann S, Kieso H, Bala Subramanian V, Raftery EB: The 24-hour ambulatory blood pressure profile with verapamil. Circulation 65: 1 22–27 (1982).
7. Mann S, Millar Craig MW, Melville DI, Bala Subramanian V, Raftery EB: Physical activity and the circadian rhythm of blood pressure. Clin Sci 57: 291s–294s (1979).
8. Mann S, Millar Craig MW, Bala Subramanian V, Cashman PMM, Raftery EB: Ambulant Blood Pressure: Reproducibility and the assessment of interventions. Clin Sci 59: 497–500 (1980).
9. Millar Craig MW and Raftery EB: The effect of conventional and slow release oxprenolol on the 24-hour arterial blood pressure in essential hypertension. British J Clin Practice 32 (Suppl) 33 (1978a).
10. Raftery EB, Mann S, Bala Subramanian V, Millar Craig MW: Once daily pindolol in hypertension, an ambulatory assessment. Am Heart J 1042: 417–20 (1982).

Address for correspondence:
Dr. E. B. Raftery,
Consultant Cardiologist,
Northwick Park Hospital & Clinical Research Centre,
Watford Road, Harrow, Middlesex, HA1 3UJ, UK.

241

Effects of atenolol on 24-hour arterial pressure and heart rate in essential hypertension

Hector O. Ventura[1]), Franz H. Messerli[2]), Francis G. Dunn[3]),
Edward D. Frohlich[4])

Summary: Ambulatory arterial pressure and continuous ECGs were recorded simultaneously (Del Mar Avionics Pressurometer-II) during 24 hours in 7 patients with mild established essential hypertension before (placebo) and four weeks following the administration of atenolol 100 mg once daily. Systolic arterial pressure was reduced by 12% (130 ± 7 mmHg vs 115 ± 6 mmHg), diastolic by 15% (90 ± 5 mmHg vs 77 ± 5 mmHg), heart rate by 17% (65 ± 5 beats/min vs 56 ± 4 beats/min) and the product of heart rate and systolic pressure by 46% (8432 ± 800 mmHg/beats/min vs 6561 ± 685 mmHg/beats/min) throughout the 24 hour period. Despite the fall in arterial pressure, diurnal variation of pressure and heart rate remained unchanged. Variability of arterial pressure and heart rate was less with atenolol although the variation coefficients were not significantly different. It is concluded that atenolol once a day provides a smooth control of arterial pressure during 24 hours. The pronounced effect on the product of heart rate and systolic pressure indicates a significantly reduced cardiac workload and oxygen consumption, and could, therefore, be responsible for the cardioprotective properties of atenolol.

Introduction

Atenolol is a cardioselective, beta-adrenergic blocking agent without intrinsic sympathomimetic activity and membrane stabilizing properties. It has been shown to be effective, when administered once a day, for the treatment of hypertension (1–8). Its antihypertensive effect appears to be quantitatively similar to those of other beta-blockers (9, 10), methyldopa (11), and thiazide diuretics (2, 9). Disparate results have been reported about the efficacy of atenolol once daily on 24-hour arterial pressure in the treatment of essential hypertension (12, 13). This study was designed to determine the effectiveness of atenolol once daily on 24-hour arterial pressure and heart rate in patients with mild established essential hypertension.

Methods

Seven patients (6 men and 1 woman) with mild established essential hypertension were included in this study. Each subject provided informed consent to a protocol previously approved by our institution's review committee. All subjects were evaluated to exclude

---
[1]) Hypertension Research Division, Alton Ochsner Medical Foundation, New Orleans.
[2]) Ochsner Clinic and Alton Ochsner Medical Foundation, New Orleans, Clinical Associate Professor of Medicine, Tulane University School of Medicine, New Orleans.
[3]) Stobhill General Hospital Glasgow, Scotland.
[4]) Education and Research, Alton Ochsner Medical Foundation; Department of Internal Medicine, Section on Hypertensive Diseases, Ochsner Clinic; Clinical Professor of Medicine and Adjunct Professor of Pharmacology, Tulane University School of Medicine, New Orleans.

secondary forms of hypertension and other concomitant disorders. Mean age was 44 ± 5 years, body weight 86 ± 4 kg, body surface area 2.01 ± 0.1 square meters. Patients were enrolled if, after discontinuation of all medications for at least four weeks, the diastolic pressure (Phase V of Korotkoff sounds) in the supine and standing positions was at least 90 mmHg and did not exceed 114 mmHg.

Twenty-four hour ambulatory blood pressure and heart rate were determined at the end of a three-week placebo phase and four weeks after the administration of atenolol 100 mg once daily, as previously described (14). In brief, blood pressure was recorded every 7.5 minutes by indirect measurement and simultaneously with a continuously recorded electrocardiogram (Pressurometer II, Del Mar Avionics) during one 24-hour period beginning at 9.00 a.m. before (placebo) and at the conclusion (atenolol) of the study. Systolic and diastolic pressures, heart rates, and the product of systolic pressure and heart rate were averaged for each patient for each four-hour period and during day and night.

Statistical analysis was performed using an analysis of variance with repeated measurements and the subsequent Tukey significant difference test (15).

Results

Systolic and diastolic pressures were reduced by atenolol by 12% (130 ± 7 mmHg vs 115 ± 6 mmHg) and 15% (90 ± 5 mmHg vs 77 ± 5 mmHg) respectively throughout the 24-hour period. Moreover, systolic pressure fell 17 mmHg during the day and 12 mmHg during the night (Table 1).

Twenty-four hour heart rate was decreased by 17% and the product of systolic pressure and heart rate by 46% in all seven patients (Table 1). The reduction in heart rate was more pronounced during the day (19%) than at night (9%) (Table 1). Nevertheless, despite the pressure fall, the diurnal variation of pressure remained unchanged (Fig. 1). The variability of arterial pressure and of heart rate was less during atenolol therapy although the variation coefficients were not significantly different.

Table 1: Blood pressure and heart rate changes before and after the administration of atenolol (100 mg) (mean ± standard error of the mean).

	Day		Night		24 Hours	
	Placebo	Atenolol	Placebo	Atenolol	Placebo	Atenolol
Systolic art. pressure (mmHg)	139 ± 6	122 ± 6*	120 ± 7	108 ± 6*	130 ± 7	115 ± 6*
Diastolic (mmHg)	96 ± 4	81 ± 5**	83 ± 5	73 ± 5**	90 ± 5	77 ± 5**
Heart rate (beats/min)	71 ± 5	58 ± 4**	58 ± 5	53 ± 4**	65 ± 5	56 ± 4**
Systolic pressure & heart rate (mmHg × beats/min)	9873 ± 857	7212 ± 712**	6991 ± 742	5909 ± 659**	8432 ± 800	6561 ± 685**

* p < 0.0002 vs placebo
** p < 0.0001 vs placebo

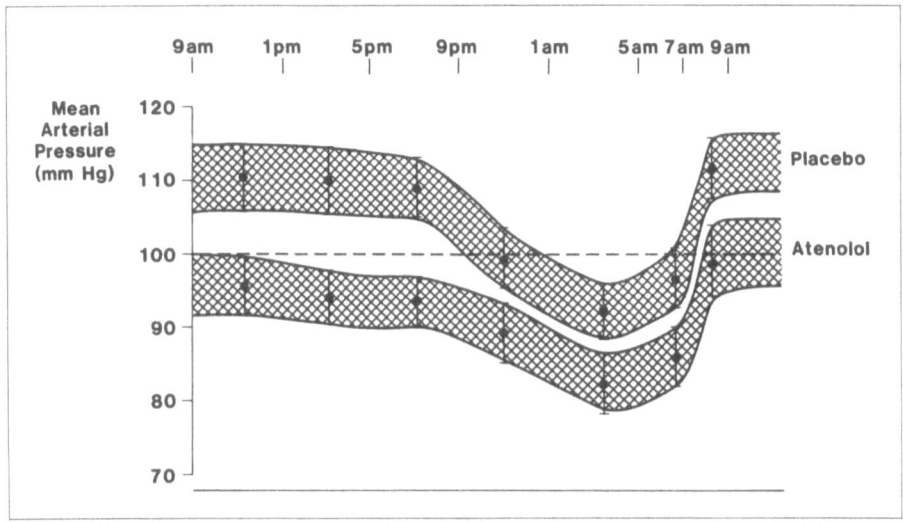

Fig. 1. Diurnal variation of mean arterial pressure before and after atenolol 100 mg once daily.

Discussion

This study demonstrated the 24-hour effectiveness of a single dose of atenolol (100 mg) in patients with early established essential hypertension. Atenolol was well tolerated and no side effects were observed during the four-week period.

Numerous placebo-controlled clinical trials (1–8) have documented the antihypertensive properties of atenolol once a day. Moreover, Floras et al. (12), assessing the control of blood pressure over a 24-hour period, demonstrated that the decreased pressure three hours following the administration of atenolol was similar to the fall observed at 24 hours. Our results confirmed this efficacy of atenolol in controlling blood pressure over a 24-hour period.

Beta-blockers have been shown to be effective in the reduction of cardiovascular mortality (16–18). Atenolol has been reported to decrease heart rate, arterial pressure, and the product of heart rate and systolic pressure in response to treadmill exercise in patients with angina pectoris (19). In addition, atenolol has reduced the incidence of completed myocardial infarction in patients with threatened infarction and reduced infarct size in patients with definite myocardial infarction (20). The decreased heart rate and the fall in the heart-rate pressure product (an indicator of myocardial oxygen consumption) in our patients lend support to this cardioprotective effect.

In conclusion, atenolol once a day provided a smooth control in arterial pressure during 24 hours. The pronounced effect on the double product indicates a significantly reduced cardiac workload and oxygen consumption and could, therefore, be responsible for its cardioprotective property.

References

1. Frishman WH: Beta-adrenoceptor antagonists: New drugs and new indications. N Engl J Med 305: 500–506 (1981).
2. Heel RC, Brogden RN, Splight TM, Avery GS: Atenolol: a review of its pharmacological properties and therapeutic efficacy in angina pectoris and hypertension. Drugs 17: 425–460 (1979).
3. Dreslinski GR, Messerli FH, Dunn FG, Suarez DH, Reisin E, Frohlich ED: Hemodynamic, biochemical, and reflexive changes produced by atenolol in hypertension. Circulation 65: 1365–1368 (1982).
4. Douglas-Jones AP, Cruickshank TM: Once-daily dosing with atenolol in patients with mild or moderate hypertension. Br J Clin Pharmacol 5: 415–419 (1978).
5. Myers MG, Lewis GRJ, Steiner J, Dollery CT: Atenolol in essential hypertension. Clin Pharmacol Ther 19: 502–507 (1976).
6. Jeffers TA, Webster J, Petrie JC, Barker NP: Atenolol once-daily in hypertension. Br J Clin Pharmacol 4: 523–527 (1977).
7. Ibrahim MM, Mossallam R: Clinical evaluation of atenolol in hypertensive patients. Circulation 64: 368–374 (1981).
8. Lund-Johansen P, Ohm OJ: Haemodynamic long-term effects of beta-receptor blocking agents in hypertension: a comparison between alprenolol, atenolol, metoprolol, timolol. Clin Sci Mol Med 48: Suppl 3; 15–35 (1976).
9. Wilcox RG: Randomized study of six beta blockers and a thiazide diuretic in essential hypertension. Br Med J 2: 383–385 (1978).
10. Wall-Manning HJ: Atenolol and three nonselective beta blockers in hypertension. Clin Pharmacol Ther 25: 8–18 (1979).
11. Webster J, Jeffers FA, Galloway DB, Petrie JC, Barker NP: Atenolol, methyldopa and chlorthalidone in moderate hypertension. Br Med J 1: 76–78 (1977).
12. Floras JS, Vann Jones J, Fox P, Hussan MO, Turner KL, Sleight P: Effect of longterm, once-daily administration of atenolol on ambulatory blood pressure of hypertensive patients. J Cardiovasc Pharmacol 3: 958–964 (1981).
13. Miller-Craig MW, Kenny D, Mann S, Balasubramanian V, Raferty FB: Effect of once daily atenolol on ambulatory blood pressure. Br Med J 1: 237–238 (1979).
14. Messerli FH, Glade LB, Ventura HO, Dreslinski GR, Suarez DH, MacPhee AA, Aristimuno GG, Cole FE, Frohlich ED: Diurnal variations of cardiac rhythm, arterial pressure and urinary catecholamines in borderline and established essential hypertension. Am Heart J 104: 109–114 (1982).
15. Snedecor GW, Cochran WG: Statistical Methods. 6th ed. Iowa State University Press (Ames, Iowa 1957).
16. Norwegian Multicenter Study Group. Timolol-induced reduction in mortality and reinfarction in patients surviving acute myocardial infarction. N Engl J Med 304: 801–807 (1981).
17. Hjalmarson A, Elmfeldt D, Herletz J, Holmberg S, Malek I, Nyberg G, Ryden L, Swedberg K, Vedin A, Wasgstein F, Waldestrom A, Waldestrom L: Effect on mortality of metoprolol in acute myocardial infarction. A double blind randomized trial. Lancet 2: 823–827 (1981).
18. Beta blocker Heart Attack Trial Research Group: A randomized trial of propranolol in patients with acute myocardial infarction. I. Mortality Results. JAMA 247: 1707–1714 (1982).
19. Jackson G, Schwartz J, Kates RE, Winchester M, Harrison DC: Atenolol: once-daily cardioselective beta blockade for angina pectoris. Circulation 61: 555–560 (1980).
20. Yusuf S, Ramsdale D, Peto R, Furse L, Bennett D, Bray C, Sleight P: Early intravenous atenolol treatment in suspected acute myocardial infarction: preliminary report of a randomized trial. Lancet 2: 273–276 (1980).

Address for correspondence:
Franz H. Messerli, M.D.
Division of Education and Research
Alton Ochsner Medical Foundation
1516 Jefferson Hwy.
New Orleans, Louisiana 70121 USA

Subject Index

Authors' Index